Oral Premalignancy

1981.

ORAL PREMALIGNANCY

Proceedings of the First Dows Symposium

EDITED BY
IAN C. MACKENZIE
ERIK DABELSTEEN
CHRISTOPHER A. SQUIER

UNIVERSITY OF IOWA PRESS, 1980

Library of Congress Cataloging in Publication Data

Main entry under title:

Oral premalignancy.

1. Oral mucosa—Cancer—Congresses. 2. Mucosa—Cancer—Congresses. I. Mackenzie, Ian C., 1939– II. Dabelsteen, Erik. III. Squier, Christopher Alan. IV. Dows Institute for Dental Research. [DNLM: 1. Precancerous conditions—Congresses. 2. Mouth mucosa—Pathology—Congresses. 3. Mouth neoplasms—Congresses. 4. Neoplasms, Glandular epithelial—Congresses. W3 D0768 1st 1977o / WU280 D752 1977o]

RC280.M6075 616.99'431 80–17988

ISBN 0–87745–103–6

University of Iowa Press, Iowa City 52242

Printed in the United States of America

Contents

Participants

WILLIAM H. BINNIE
Department of Oral Medicine and Pathology
Guy's Hospital
London SE1 9RT
England

ERIK DABELSTEEN
The Royal Dental College
2100 Copenhagen
Denmark

CHRISTOPHER D. FRANKLIN
Department of Oral Pathology
School of Clinical Dentistry
University of Sheffield
Sheffield S10 2TA
England

MURRAY W. HILL
Dows Institute for Dental Research
College of Dentistry
University of Iowa
Iowa City, Iowa 52242
U.S.A.

NEWELL W. JOHNSON
Department of Oral Pathology
London Hospital Medical College
London E1 2AD
England

IVOR R. H. KRAMER
Institute of Dental Surgery
Eastman Dental Hospital
University of London
London WC1 X8LD
England

EDNA B. LAURENCE
Mitosis Research Laboratory
Birkbeck College
University of London
London WC1E 7HX
England

IAN C. MACKENZIE
Dows Institute for Dental Research
College of Dentistry
University of Iowa
Iowa City, Iowa 52242
U.S.A.

ARTHUR MASHBERG
Oral Surgery Section
Veterans Administration Hospital
East Orange, New Jersey 07019
U.S.A.

HENRY C. OUTZEN
The Jackson Laboratory
Bar Harbor, Maine 04609
U.S.A.

JENS J. PINDBORG
The Royal Dental College
2100 Copenhagen
Denmark

WILLIAM G. SHAFER
Department of Oral Pathology
Indiana University School of Dentistry
Indianapolis, Indiana 46202
U.S.A.

HAROLD C. SLAVKIN
Laboratory for Developmental Pathology
Ethel Percy Andrus Gerontology Center
University of Southern California
Los Angeles, California 90007
U.S.A.

COLIN J. SMITH
Department of Oral Pathology
School of Clinical Dentistry
University of Sheffield
Sheffield S10 2TA
England

DENNIS B. SOLT
Department of Pathology
6315 Medical Science Building
University of Toronto
Toronto, Ontario M55 1A8
Canada

CHRISTOPHER A. SQUIER
Dows Institute for Dental Research
College of Dentistry
University of Iowa
Iowa City, Iowa 52242
U.S.A.

EUGENE J. VAN SCOTT
Skin and Cancer Hospital
3322 North Broad Street
Philadelphia, Pennsylvania 19140
U.S.A.

CHARLES A. WALDRON
Department of Oral Pathology
Emory University School of Dentistry
Atlanta, Georgia 30322
U.S.A.

GEORGE D. WILBANKS
Department of Obstetrics and Gynecology
Rush University Medical College
600 South Paulina St.
Chicago, Illinois 60612
U.S.A

Introduction

The idea of a symposium on Oral Premalignancy arose during informal discussion between oral pathologists and research workers with an interest in oral epithelium. It was suggested that although premalignant lesions of the oral mucosa are of clinical importance, their nature is poorly understood and most investigation has focused on the clinical problems or on histopathological diagnosis. Consequently, it seemed worthwhile to bring together in a workshop setting a group of people who would be able to discuss some of the problems to be faced and whose interaction might stimulate a better understanding of the biology of premalignancy.

The general aims of the symposium were (a) to examine the concept of oral premalignancy; (b) to discuss what is known about the nature and behavior of premalignant lesions; (c) to explore which of the many recent advances in the basic sciences may offer hope of improving methods of diagnosis and prognosis, as well as providing direction for new areas of investigation.

The participants at the symposium were both pathologists with a particular interest in premalignancy and basic scientists whose area of research was related to various aspects of the problem. It was hoped that such a group would be able to generate free discussion and an interchange of ideas about concepts of oral premalignancy. The framework of the symposium was a series of presentations covering various facets of the problem so as to provide a general background of information for those participants who were not familiar with the whole field. They were arranged in a sequence expected to provide some order of progression for the discussion which was considered to be a most important feature of the meeting.

The discussion, in its unedited form, amounted to some 350 pages of typed transcript. Participants were encouraged to modify their original manuscripts to cover topics of importance raised during the discussion: many of the points raised during discussion have now been incorporated into the papers themselves. Remaining points of interest from the discussion have been grouped throughout the text in relation to the presentations concerned.

It was the hope of the organizers to extract from the symposium a balanced account of the present state of knowledge about oral premalignancy together with some rational ideas for future work. While the proceedings may go some way toward meeting the former objective, it became clear that such large gaps exist in our knowledge of many aspects of oral premalignancy that a compilation of specific suggestions for future research would be impractical. For example, the meeting indicated that there is, as yet, a lack of a consensus concerning such basic problems as the definition and clinical significance of oral premalignant lesions. Many participants expressed concern about the subjective nature of present methods of histopathological diagnosis and about the uncertain reliability of a prognosis based on such procedures. Too little appears to be known about human premalignant lesions to allow their mechanism of development and progression to be clearly related to basic concepts, such as initiation and promotion in carcinogenesis, which have developed from animal studies. Further, no demonstrably suitable animal model for studying oral premalignancy appears to be available and work is only just reaching the stage where current ideas about control of normal epithelial differentiation and growth can be applied in attempting to understand the changes occurring in oral lesions. Such problems deserve examination and most of them require coordinated clinical and laboratory investigation. We therefore feel that there is still a strong need to further the exchange of ideas by means of meetings such as this one in which the basic scientist becomes aware of the problems of clinical diagnosis and patient management and the pathologist more familiar with progress in the laboratory in fields related to his or her specialty.

The organizers wish to express their gratitude for financial support for the workshop which was provided by grants from the International Union Against Cancer and the American Cancer Society, Iowa Division, and partly from funds made available to the University of Iowa College of Dentistry by gifts from the Sutherland and Frances Dows Trusts.

We have been ably assisted throughout the planning of the symposium, during the meeting itself and in the subsequent work on the manuscript by the secretarial staff of the Dows Institute. Our editorial assistant Nellie Kremenak assisted with every stage of the project and played a major part in producing the final manuscript. Without her help this volume would not have been possible.

PART ONE
CLINICAL AND HISTOPATHOLOGICAL CONCEPTS

1

Lesions of the Oral Mucosa to be Considered Premalignant and Their Epidemiology

J. J. PINDBORG

Department of Oral Pathology, The Royal Dental College and Department of Oral Medicine and Surgery, University Hospital, Copenhagen, Denmark

1. INTRODUCTION

Many attempts have been made to define precancer and its synonym premalignancy. At a World Health Organization (WHO, 1973) "Meeting of Investigators on the Histological Definition of Precancerous Lesions" in Geneva 1972 a *precancerous lesion* was defined as "a morphologically altered tissue in which cancer is more likely to occur than in its apparently normal counterpart." In an additional note it was mentioned that some lesions have a very high probability (20% or more) of developing cancer, others are much lower, while the potential of many is unknown.

Premalignant lesions include leukoplakia and erythroplakia (each of which can be divided into homogeneous and nodular types) and palatal changes associated with reverse smoking (Mehta et al. 1977). These palatal changes should not be confused with leukokeratosis nicotina palati (syn. nicotinic stomatitis).

A *precancerous condition* was defined as "a generalized state associated with a significantly increased risk of cancer." Examples of precancerous conditions are syphilis, sideropenic dysphagia, oral submucous fibrosis, discoid lupus erythematosis, and xeroderma pigmentosum. Apart from these groups are some generalized diseases (for example, lichen planus) which may make the mucosa more susceptible to action of carcinogens and the development of cancerous lesions.

When the above definitions are applied to the oral mucosa a classification emerges, which is shown in Table 1.

2. PREMALIGNANT LESIONS

2:1 LEUKOPLAKIA

In this paper leukoplakia is defined as a white patch which cannot be removed by scraping and cannot be attributed to any other diagnosable disease.

2:1:1 *Epidemiology of oral leukoplakia*

House-to-house studies of oral leukoplakia are rare except in India. Table 2 summarizes the available studies. In India, 176,000 people have

TABLE 1

Classification of Oral Precancerous Lesions and Conditions

Precancerous lesions
- Leukoplakia
  - Homogeneous
  - Nodular (speckled)
- Erythroplakia
  - Homogeneous
  - Nodular (speckled)
- (Palatal changes associated with reverse smoking)

Lichen planus

Precancerous conditions
- Syphilis
- Sideropenic dysphagia
- Submucous fibrosis
- Discoid lupus erythematosus
- Xeroderma pigmentosum

TABLE 2

Prevalence of Oral Leukoplakia in Unselected Populations

Country	*Investigator*	*Size of sample*	*Prevalence*
India			
Villages	Mehta et al. (1969, 1972a)	152,000	0.2-3%
Suburban	Zachariah and Pindborg (unpublished material)	24,000	2%
Sweden	Axéll (1976)	20,000	3.6%
Hungary	Bruszt (1962)	5,000	4%

been surveyed in unselected populations, mostly among villagers, but also including a large suburban sample. The prevalence rates of leukoplakia in India vary between 0.2 and 3%; and are similar to findings in Hungary. The most extensive study in the West is that of Axéll (1976) in Sweden who found a prevalence of 3.6% in adults. It is pertinent to ask whether the same diagnostic criteria have been applied in all these surveys so that a comparison is permissible. It should be noted that the criteria in all the Indian surveys were identical, and that the Swedish investigator calibrated with the author who initiated the Indian surveys.

In India, it has also been possible to make incidence studies in some states, for example in Gujarat and Kerala (Table 3). The incidence (rate) of leukoplakia is much higher in Kerala than in Gujarat, especially among females.

TABLE 3

Annual Incidence of Leukoplakia in a 7-year period.
After Mehta, Pindborg, Bhonsle, and Sinor (1976).

		No. new leukoplakias per 100,000 per year	
	Follow-up rate	*Females*	*Males*
Gujurat	61%	0	190
Kerala	71%	400	330

2:1:2 *Follow-up studies of oral leukoplakia*

The premalignant nature of a given lesion or condition may be demonstrated by the simultaneous occurrence of the lesion (condition) and cancer, or through follow-up studies of presumed premalignant lesions and conditions.

Clinical follow-up studies

The simultaneous occurrence of leukoplakia and oral cancer has been reported by Silverman et al. (1963), who found that this ranged from 11 to 60% in 10 studies. The range reveals more about difference in criteria applied by the investigators than about true differences in the populations examined.

Follow-up studies can be done in two ways: (1) a sample of leukoplakias (with or without matched controls) can be followed over a number of years, (2) a sample selected on the basis of histologic criteria (e.g. epithelial dysplasia) can be followed.

The most frequent approach is to follow a sample of leukoplakias, and this has been carried out in a number of countries. The malignant transformation rate can be expressed as (1) oral cancer development as a percentage of the entire sample, (2) the yearly oral cancer incidence rate, (3) oral cancer development per 100,000 persons, or (4) oral cancer development per 1,000 lesion person years.

Table 4 gives published information as to oral cancer development as a percentage of the entire sample since 1960 and comprises a sample of more than 100 patients. The malignant transformation rate ranges from 0.8 to 9.9%, these very different figures both coming from India. If, however, these two samples are compared it turns out that the police material of Mehta et al. (1972b) is very homogeneous and is comprised of well-fed individuals who lead a much more regular life than the individuals in Gangadharan and Paymaster's sample (1971). When comparing the six groups from Table 4 it should be kept in mind that the various institutions will have different opinions as to when an oral leukoplakia should be kept

TABLE 4

Oral Cancer Development in Percent of Entire Sample.

Years in which material was observed	*Investigator*	*Size of material*	*Observation period*	*Sex distribution*		*Malignant transformation in per cent of entire sample*
				M	*F*	
1959–69	Mehta et al. (1972)	117	10 yrs.	100%	0	0.8
1920–60	Einhorn and Wersäll (1967)	782	11.7 yrs.	522	260	10 yrs.: 2.4
				67%	33%	20 yrs.: 4
1955–64	Pindborg et al. (1968)	248	3.7 yrs.	62%	38%	4.4
1946–76	Bánóczy (1977)	670	9.8 yrs.	76%	24%	6
1955–66	Silverman and Rozen (1968)	117	1-11 yrs.	57%	43%	6
1941–69	Gangadharan and Paymaster (1971)	626	8.9 mos.	82%	18%	9.9

under observation and when it should be treated, either surgically or by removing possible irritants. With these considerations in mind it is remarkable that the figures for malignant transformation are uniform when compared with estimates made some decades ago.

In an analysis of the Copenhagen material from 1974 (Table 5) it was found that the annual incidence (rate) of malignant transformation was 0.75% based upon a follow-up rate of 96.6% (Roed-Petersen and Pindborg, unpublished material).

Oral cancer development from oral leukoplakia given as cancers per 100,000 persons has been determined by Silverman et al. (1976) in material from 6,718 Indian industrial workers with oral leukoplakia. After 2 years 71% of these patients were reexamined and development of oral cancer established in six individuals, which is 0.13% of the entire sample. This equals an annual incidence of 63 oral cancers per 100,000 persons.

Finally, oral cancer development in leukoplakias has been calculated using the person-year method (Mehta et al. 1976a). The investigators found that 6.5 oral cancers developed per 1,000 leukoplakia years. Table 6 from the same study shows the distribution of oral cancers according to type of leukoplakia and other lesions and conditions. The findings confirm previous observations that the nodular (speckled) type of leukoplakia is more prone to malignant transformation than homogeneous leukoplakia. Table 7 also from the same study shows that leukoplakias caused by chewing habits are more likely to become malignant than leukoplakias caused by other habits.

Histological follow-up studies

In 1972, Mincer et al. published the first study of the natural history of oral epithelial dysplasia. Since then four more studies have been reported on the behavior of oral epithelial dysplasia. Table 8 summarizes the results of these investigations. As for the clinical follow-up studies, a direct comparison is difficult, because it is not easy to standardize the criteria for epithelial dysplasia, although an attempt has been made in that direction (Smith and Pindborg 1969). Moreover, patients with epithelial dysplasia in their leukoplakias have been variously treated, sometimes with excisional biopsy. Even with these reservations, it is interesting to note some common trends: e.g., (1) the malignant transformation rate does not exceed 13%, (2) a substantial number of the lesions associated with epithelial dysplasia remain unchanged during the observation period, and (3) there may even be a reduction of the lesions in some patients. It is noteworthy that the

TABLE 5

Results from the 1974 Analysis of the Copenhagen Oral Leukoplakia Material (Roed-Petersen and Pindborg, unpublished material).

Rate of follow-up	96.6 (451/467)
Median observation period	5.5 years
Cancer development	4.1%
Annual cancer incidence	0.75%

TABLE 6

Malignant Transformation of Oral Lesions in 1 to 8 Years Follow-up in Kerala. From Mehta et al. (1976a).

Previous diagnosis	*Number*	*New oral cancers detected*
Leukoplakia		
Homogeneous	321	7
Nodular (speckled)	21	3
Traumatic	59	–
Preleukoplakia	380	2
Other oral lesion		
Submucous fibrosis	44	1
Lichen planus	303	1
Normals	6,686	–

TABLE 7

Rate of Malignant Transformation of Oral Leukoplakia According to Tobacco Habits in 1 to 8 Years Follow-up. From Mehta et al. (1976a).

Tobacco habits	*Leukoplakia person-years*	*New oral cancers detected*	*Rate of malignant transformation per 1,000 leukoplakia years*
Smoking	388	–	–
Chewing	523	6	11.5
Mixed	623	4	6.4
Total	1,534	10	6.5

malignant transformation rate in India is well below the rate in the U.S.A. and Hungary, despite the absence of surgical treatment.

TABLE 8

Behavior of Oral Epithelial Dysplasia and CIS in 5 Studies.

Investigator *Behavior of leukoplakia*	*Mincer et al. (1972)*	*Pindborg and Roed-Petersen (1973, unpublished material)*	*Bánóczy and Csiba (1976)*	*Pindborg et al. (1977)*
	U.S.A.	Denmark	Hungary	India
No. of dysplasia	45	37	68	61
Observation period	1–8 yrs.		6.3 yrs.	7 yrs.
Malignant transformation	11%	3%	13%	7%
Removed by surgery	44%	51%	65%	0
Recurrence	35%*	16%	20%	0
Increased	11%	8%	4%	2%
Unchanged	22%	27%	15%	54%
Decreased	4%	11%	15%	15%

* Mincer et al. (1972) regarded a lesion as a recurrence even if it appeared in a site that was different from that of the primary lesion.

2:2 ERYTHROPLAKIA

Erythroplakia is a well-defined patch with a fiery red, velvety, surface (homogeneous type). Occasionally, white plaques or nodules are observed in or adjacent to the lesion or in other parts of the oral mucosa (speckled or nodular type). The lesion has been discussed thoroughly by Shear (1972) and Shafer and Waldron (1975) and Mashberg (chapter 18, this vol.). There is agreement that erythroplakia is a serious disease, for about 90% show carcinoma, carcinoma in situ, or severe epithelial dysplasia histologically (Shafer and Waldron, 1975; Mashberg, chapter 18).

Erythroplakia is rare and only one epidemiologic survey has looked specifically for it. In that survey, comprising 50,915 villagers in India, erythroplakia was diagnosed in nine patients (Mehta et al. 1971). So far, no follow-up results of these patients are available.

2:3 PALATAL CHANGES ASSOCIATED WITH REVERSE SMOKING

In a study of 10,000 persons in Srikakulam, Andhra Pradesh in India, where reverse smoking is practiced, 22% of those smoking with the glowing end inside the mouth had palatal changes. Within the same sample an annual, age-adjusted incidence rate of 22 palatal cancers per 100,000 individuals has been established (Pindborg et al. 1975). Since epithelial dysplasia was found in 28% of the individuals showing palatal changes, it was decided to study the impact of an intervention trial. In a pilot survey 101 reverse smokers with palatal change were followed for 1 year (Mehta et al. 1977). Of these patients, 24% stopped the habit completely and 27% changed to the conventional type of smoking. Subsequently, palatal keratosis remained very stable, whereas red areas changed into areas less pigmented than normal mucosa.

2:4 LICHEN PLANUS

The prevalence rate of oral lichen planus has been studied in two surveys. In India, Pindborg et al. (1972) found a prevalence of 1.5% among 7,639 villagers in a house-to-house survey, whereas in Sweden Axell (1976) examined 20,333 persons and found 1.9% with oral lichen planus.

As previously mentioned, the precancerous nature of lichen planus has not yet been established beyond doubt. In the author's opinion the only way to do so is through lengthy follow-up studies. In 1958 we began such a survey in Copenhagen which now (1977) comprises about 600 patients with oral lichen planus (see Table 5). In 1973, Fulling published a preliminary report on a clinical follow-up of 225 patients with a mean observation period of 3.6 years in which time only one patient developed an oral carcinoma. In a subsequent but enlarged study including the above 225 patients, Holmstrup et al. (1975) found 5 carcinomas among 470 patients with lichen planus; 3 were present at the first examination, 2 developed during follow-up. In the same population, 2 patients demonstrated epithelial dysplasia at first examination and 3 more were found during follow-up. Table 6, from the Indian study, shows a malignant transformation in one patient out of 303.

3. PRECANCEROUS CONDITIONS

3:1 ORAL SUBMUCOUS FIBROSIS

Submucous fibrosis is an insidious, chronic disease affecting the mucosa of any part of the oral cavity and occasionally extending into pharynx and esophagus. Although sometimes preceded by and/or associated with vesicle formation it is always associated with a subepithelial inflammatory reaction followed by a fibroelastic change in the connective tissue fibers of the lamina propria with epithelial atrophy leading to stiffness of the oral mucosa, and causing trismus and an inability to eat (Pindborg and Sirsat 1966). In recent years, this condition has been associated with an increased tendency for oral cancer development.

The disease occurs almost exclusively among Indians, but sporadic cases have been observed in China, Nepal, Thailand, and South Vietnam. In India, extensive epidemiologic surveys have been carried out comprising 223,000 individuals of which 119,000 were examined in house-to-house surveys (Table 9). A rough calculation reveals that no less than 250,000 cases of submucous fibrosis are present in India.

The etiology of submucous fibrosis is uncertain. It has been suggested that it may be due to hypersensitivity to chili, to betel nut chewing, or to use of tobacco or vitamin deficiencies.

The possible precancerous nature of submucous fibrosis was first mentioned by Paymaster in 1956, who described the development of a slow-growing squamous cell carcinoma in one-third of the cases of submucous fibrosis seen among patients in the Tata Memorial Hospital in Bombay. The precancerous nature of submucous fibrosis has also been emphasised by the present author (Pindborg 1965; Pindborg and Zachariah 1965) and by Dockrat (1967). Table 10 summarizes the available evidence indicating the precancerous nature of submucous fibrosis. However, more studies on the incidence of oral cancer in patients with submucous fibrosis (cf. Table 6) are mandatory before definite conclusions can be drawn.

At present, one can speculate on the possible mechanism whereby a cancer may develop as a consequence of a submucous fibrosis. A probable prerequisite for cancer development is the action of carcinogens; several studies in India have shown that the chewing of tobacco is the major factor responsible for the extremely high frequency of oral cancer in India.

TABLE 9

Epidemiologic Surveys on Oral Submucous Fibrosis.
From Pindborg (1972) where references can be found.

	Location	*Size of sample*	*Prevalence (Percentage)*
	India		
Urban (Dental Colleges)	Bangalore	10,000	0.2
	Lucknow	10,000	0.5
	Bombay	10,000	0.5
	Trivandrum	5,000	1.2
Rural	Bihar (Singhbhum)	10,000	0
	Maharashtra (Poona)	101,000	0.03
	Andhra Pradesh (Srikakulam)	10,000	0.04
	Bihar (Darbhanga)	10,000	0.07
	Kerala (Ernakulam)	5,000	0.1
	Gujurat (Bhavnagar)	10,000	0.2
	Kerala (Trivandrum)	23,000	0.3
	Kerala (Ernakulam)	10,000	0.4
	Uttar Pradesh (Mainpuri)	7,000	0.6
	South Africa		
Urban	Johannesburg	1,000	0.5
	Pretoria		
	Durban	1,200	0.6
Total		223,000	

TABLE 10

Present Evidence Indicating the Precancerous Nature of Submucous Fibrosis (S.F.).
From Pindborg (1972) where references can be found.

1. Clinical observation of higher prevalence of leukoplakia in S.F.
   27% in 101 cases from North India
   15% in 104 cases from Agra
   13% in 63 cases from India
2. Occurrence of epithelial atypia in S.F.
   14% in 104 cases from Agra
   13% in 220 cases from India
3. Occurrence of S.F. in oral cancer patients
   49% with S.F.(?) among 100 cancers in Travancore
   40% with S.F. among 100 cancers in Trivandrum
4. Histologic cancer in S.F.
   6% in 101 cases from North India
   3% in 104 cases from Agra
5. Incidence of oral cancer in patients with S.F.
   Cancer developed in one-third of ? cancers in Bombay

Submucous fibrosis may have to be regarded as a predisposing situation for the action of carcinogens. The following pathogenesis was suggested by the author in 1966 (Pindborg and Sirsat 1966). Submucous fibrosis starts in the connective tissue, an initial inflammatory reaction followed by fibroelastic degeneration causing degenerative changes in the overlying epithelium which becomes atrophic. As a consequence, the epithelium may be more vulnerable to carcinogens, which are so often present in tobacco. The atrophic epithelium shows first an intercellular edema and later epithelial atypia, associated with moderate epithelial hyperplasia; thereafter, carcinoma may develop any time.

This hypothesis may partly explain the extremely high frequency of oral cancer in India. A parallel can be found in the Western world where senile elastosis of the lip has been claimed to be a precancerous condition. This resembles submucous fibrosis in exhibiting epithelial atrophy associated with degenerative changes in the subepithelial connective tissue (see chapter 11).

3:2 SIDEROPENIC DYSPHAGIA

An explanation for the very high percentage of women with oral cancer in the Scandinavian countries is probably to be found in the rather frequent occurrence of *sideropenic dysphagia.* Long term follow-up studies of sideropenic dysphagia with regard to oral cancer development are still lacking, although Jacobsson's study from 1948 strongly indicated the precancerous nature of the condition.

3:3 DISCOID LUPUS ERYTHEMATOSUS AND SYPHILIS

As chronic *discoid lupus erythematosus* is such a rare condition, it will not be discussed in this context.

Years ago it was a well-established fact that patients with a third stage *syphilis* had an increased risk of developing cancer of the tongue. Given the rarity of this stage nowadays, this etiologic factor will not be discussed in this presentation.

CONCLUSION

There is evidence that certain lesions and conditions of the oral mucosa should be considered premalignant. There is, however, little information concerning the rate of transformation of such lesions and long-term follow-up studies are required.

REFERENCES

Axéll, T. 1976. A prevalence study of oral mucosal lesions in an adult Swedish population. *Odont. Din.* **27**, Suppl. 36, 1–103.

Bánóczy, J. 1977. Follow-up studies in oral leukoplakia. *J. Maxillofac. Surg.* **5**, 69–75.

Bánóczy, J. and Csiba, A. 1976. Occurrence of epithelial dysplasia in oral leukoplakia. *Oral Surg.* **42**, 766–774.

Borghelli, R. F., Stirparo, M., Andrade, J., Barros, R., Centofanti, M., and de Estevez, O. T. 1975. Leukoedema in addicts to coca leaves in Humahuaca, Argentina. *Community Dent. Oral Epidemiol.* **3**, 40–43.

Bruszt, von P. 1962. Stomato-onkolgische Reihenuntersuchungen in sieben Gemeinden Südungarns. *Schweiz. Monatsschr. Zahnheilk.* **72**, 758–766.

Dockrat, I. S. 1967. Oral submucous fibrosis as a precancerous condition. *S. Afr. Cancer Bull.* **11**, 103–111.

Einhorn, J., and Wersäll, J. 1967. Incidence of oral carcinoma in patients with leukoplakia of the oral mucosa. *Cancer* **20**, 2189–2193.

Fulling, H. J. 1973. Cancer development in oral lichen planus. A follow-up study of 327 patients. *Arch. Dermatol.* **108**, 667–669.

Gangadharan, P., and Paymaster, J. C. 1971. Leukoplakia: An epidemiologic study of 1504 cases observed at the Tata Memorial Hospital, Bombay, India. *Br. J. Cancer* **25**, 657–668.

Holmstrup, P., Neumann-Jensen, B., and Pindborg, J. J. 1975. Follow-up of 611 patients with oral lichen planus. Abstract. *J. Dent. Res.* **54**, International Assoc. for Dent. Res. 53d General Session. Program and Abstracts, p. L120.

Jacobsson, F. 1948. Carcinoma of the tongue: Clinical study of 227 cases treated at Radiumhemmet, 1931–1942. *Acta Radiol.*, Suppl. **68**, 1–184.

Mehta, F. S., Gupta, P. C., Daftary, D. K., Pindborg, J. J., and Choksi, S. K. 1972a. An epidemiologic study of oral cancer and precancerous conditions among 101,761 villagers in Maharashtra, India. *Int. J. Cancer* **10**, 134–141.

Mehta, F. S., Shroff, B. C., Gupta, P. C., and Daftary, D. K. 1972b. Oral leukoplakia in relation to tobacco habits. A ten-year follow-up study of Bombay policemen. *Oral Surg.* **34**, 426–433.

Mehta, F. S., Hamner, J. E., Pindborg, J. J., and Gupta, P. C. 1976a. The natural history of oral leukoplakia. Paper read at Third International Symposium on Detection and Prevention of Oral Cancer 26 April–1 May, New York.

Mehta, F. S., Pindborg, J. J., Bhonsle, R. B., and Sinor, P. N. 1976b. Incidence of oral leucoplakias among 20,358 Indian Villagers in a 7-year period. *Br. J. Cancer* **33**, 549–554.

Mehta, F. S., Jalnawalla, P. N., Daftary, D. K., Gupta, P. C., and Pindborg, J. J. 1977. Reverse smoking in Andhra Pradesh, India: Variability of clinical and histologic appearances of palatal changes. *Int. J. Oral Surg.* **6**, 75–83.

Mehta, F. S., Pindborg, J. J., Gupta, P. C., and Daftary, D. K. 1969. Epidemiologic and histologic study of oral cancer and leukoplakia among 50,915 villagers in India. *Cancer* **24**, 832–849.

Mincer, H. H., Coleman, S. A., and Hopkins, K. P. 1972. Observations on the clinical characteristics of oral lesions showing histologic epithelial dysplasia. *Oral Surg.* **33**, 389–399.

Paymaster, J. C. 1956. Cancer of buccal mucosa: Clinical study of 650 cases in Indian patients. *Cancer* **9**, 431–435.

Pindborg, J. J. 1965. Frequency of oral submucous fibrosis in North India. *Bull. WHO* **32**, 748–750.

Pindborg, J. J. 1972. Is submucous fibrosis a precancerous condition in the oral cavity? *Int. Dent. J.* **22**, 474–480.

Pindborg, J. J., Daftary, D. K., and Mehta, F. S. 1977. A follow-up study of sixty-one oral dysplastic precancerous lesions in Indian villagers. *Oral Surg.* **43**. 383–390.

Pindborg, J. J. Jølst, O., Renstrup, G., and Roed-Petersen, B. 1968. Studies in oral leukoplakia: A preliminary report on the period prevalence of malignant transformation in leukoplakia based on a follow-up study of 248 patients. *J. Am. Dent. Assoc.* **76**, 767–771.

Pindborg, J. J., Mehta, F. S., and Daftary, D. K. 1975. Incidence of oral cancer among 30,000 villagers in India in a 7-year follow-up study of oral precancerous lesions. *Community Dent. Oral Epidemiol.* **3**, 86–88.

Pindborg, J. J., Mehta, F. S., Daftary, D. K., Gupta, P. C., and Bhonsle, R. B. 1972. Prevalence of oral lichen planus among 7,639 Indian villagers in Kerala, South India. *Acta Derm. Venereol.* **52**, 216–220.

Pindborg, J. J., and Sirsat, S. M. 1966. Oral submucous fibrosis. *Oral Surg.* **22**, 764–779.

Pindborg, J. J., and Zachariah, J. 1965. Frequency of oral submucous fibrosis among 100 South Indians with oral cancer. *Bull, WHO* **32**, 750–753.

Shafer, W. G., and Waldron, C. A. 1975. Erythroplakia of the oral cavity. *Cancer* **36**, 1021–1028.

Shear, M. 1972. Erythroplakia of the mouth. *Int. Dent. J.* **22**, 460–473.

Silverman, S., Jr., Bhargava, K., Mani, N. J., Smith, L. W., and Malaowalla, A. M. 1976. Malignant transformation and natural history of oral leukoplakia in 57,518 industrial workers of Gujarat, India. *Cancer* **38**, 1790–1795.

Silverman, S., Jr., Renstrup, G., and Pindborg, J. J. 1963. Studies in oral leukoplakias. III. Effects of vitamin A comparing clinical, histopathologic, cytologic, and hematologic responses. *Acta Odont. Scand.* **21**, 271–291.

Silverman, S., Jr., and Rozen, R. D. 1968. Observations on the clinical characteristics and natural history of oral leukoplakia. *J. Am. Dent. Assoc.* **76**, 772–777.

Smith, C., and Pindborg, J. J. 1969. *Histological Grading of Oral Epithelial Atypia by the Use of Photographic Standards.* Copenhagen.

Tata Institute of Fundamental Research, Bombay. 1971. *Report on Investigations of Oral Cancer and Precancerous Conditions in Indian Rural Populations, 1966–1969.* Munksgaard, Copenhagen.

World Health Organization. 1973. Report from a meeting of investigators on the histological definition of precancerous lesions. CAN/731. Geneva.

2

Basic Clinical Features of Oral Premalignant Lesions

W. G. SHAFER

Department of Oral Pathology, Indiana University School of Dentistry, Indianapolis, Indiana

1. INTRODUCTION

Leukoplakia and erythroplakia are the chief clinical entities recognized as oral premalignant lesions (see chapter 1). While numerous studies have been reported dealing with the premalignant nature of leukoplakia, such information on erythroplakia is very sparse.

2. BASIC CLINICAL FEATURES OF LEUKOPLAKIA AND ERYTHROPLAKIA

2:1 LEUKOPLAKIA

In the older literature most leukoplakias were said to occur in males. In the first edition of Thoma's *Oral Pathology* (1941) the male to female ratio of leukoplakia was thus described as 95 to 5. However, over the years a change seems to have occurred. In a study by Shafer and Waldron (1961) on 321 patients with leukoplakias, only 68% were males, and in a report on the same population from 1975, which included 3,256 patients with leukoplakia, only 51% were males (Waldron and Shafer 1975). The reason for this increase in the frequency of leukoplakias in women over the past few decades is not known, but may very well relate to the change in smoking habits among young women. A 1975 survey thus showed that teen-age girls and young women smoked nearly as much as their male counterparts, which is in marked contrast to the data for 1930 where 30 times more men than women smoked (Meigs 1977).

It is believed that this is the cause for the increased rates of lung cancer among young women, and for the change in the incidence ratio of male to female lung cancer from 4.7:1 in 1945 to 0.9:1 in 1975. As smoking also seems to be an important etiological factor for leukoplakias, it may also be possible to ascribe the decrease in the male to female ratio for leukoplakias to the altered smoking habits in the population.

With respect to age of occurrence of leukoplakia, the disease has generally been described as one of older people, although there are no large series dealing with this in the earlier literature. However, in the 1961 study (Shafer and Waldron 1961), 50% of the group were in the 5th decade or younger, while in the 1975 study (Waldron and Shafer 1975), only 39% of the group were in the 5th decade or younger. It is of interest that there were no cases of leukoplakia in the first decade of life in the 1961 study and only 6 cases (3 males and 3 females) in the second decade. However, in the 1975 study, there were 4 patients (3 males and 1 female) in the first decade and 31 patients (14 males and 17 females) in the second decade.

With respect to location of lesions, Thoma's 1941 text lists the tongue as the *most* common location, while both the 1961 and 1975 studies reported the tongue to be one of the *least* common sites (Table 1). This formerly high incidence of leukoplakia of the tongue may be related to so-called syphilitic glossitis; in fact in one study cited by Thoma, 27% of the patients with oral leukoplakia had a positive Wassermann reaction.

It had been suspected for quite some time that there might be "high-risk" and "low-risk" sites for leukoplakia occurring in the mouth. In other words, experience seemed to indicate that leukoplakias in certain sites were histologically more serious than in other sites. However, it was not until the study of Waldron and Shafer (1975) that a definite value representing degree of risk could be assigned to each anatomic site. As can be seen in Table 2, the floor of mouth is the highest risk site for leukoplakia with 124 of 289 cases or 43% representing some degree of epithelial dysplasia, carcinoma in situ or invasive carcinoma (see also chapter 14). Following this were lips, with 24%, and tongue, with 24%, being histologically serious or potentially serious. In contrast, only 12% of leukoplakias in the retromolar area were in this category, with 15% each on the mandibular ridge, gingiva, and mucobuccal fold, and 15% with a similar maxillary location, representing serious or potentially serious lesions histologically.

TABLE 1 Leukoplakia—Site

	Male		*Female*		*Total*	
	N	*Per cent*	*N*	*Per cent*	*N*	*Per cent*
Lips	285	15.6	61	4.0	346	10.3
Max. mucosa	163	8.9	196	12.8	359	10.7
Mand. mucosa	388	21.2	457	29.8	845	25.2
Palate	218	11.9	143	9.3	361	10.7
Bucc. mucosa	422	23.1	314	20.5	736	21.9
Tongue	104	5.7	123	8.0	227	6.8
Fl. mouth	110	6.0	179	11.7	289	8.6
Retrom.	138	7.6	59	3.9	197	5.9
Total	1828		1532		3360	

From: Waldron and Shafer (1975).

TABLE 2 Leukoplakia—Site and Relative Risk at Site

		Dysplasia/Cancer	
	Per cent of Cases	*No. of Cases*	*Per cent*
Lips	10	83/346	24
Max. mucosa & sulcus	11	53/359	15
Mand. mucosa & sulcus	25	123/845	15
Palate	11	68/361	19
Buccal mucosa	22	121/736	17
Tongue	7	55/227	24
Floor of mouth	9	124/289	43
Retromolar	6	23/197	12
Total		650/3256	20.0%

From: Waldron and Shafer (1975).

Correlation of the clinical grading of leukoplakia with the histology has been popular for many years (McCarthy 1936). Most workers in the field today disagree with this concept and believe that the clinical appearance of leukoplakia is not a reliable index for predicting the seriousness of the microscopic changes. Lesions considered clinically to be possible squamous cell carcinomas often showed only extensive keratosis on microscopic examination, while conversely, a clinically innocuous leukoplakia occasionally proved to be an early infiltrating squamous cell carcinoma (Waldron and Shafer 1975).

There are several interesting geographical differences in findings in the basic clinical features of leukoplakia (see chapter 1). One of the geographical differences that has been reported was in a study of leukoplakia between patients from the area of Emory University in Atlanta, Georgia, and Indiana University in Indianapolis, Indiana. The sex ratio of the patients in Emory was 50.3 male to 49.7 female, while in Indiana it was 58.3 male to 41.7 female. Furthermore, the incidence of leukoplakia in the biopsy or surgical material was considerably different between the two locations over the same period of time: from Emory, there were 1,626 specimens of leukoplakia in 17,538 cases (9.2% of all specimens received) while Indiana has 1,630 specimens of leukoplakia in 34,607 cases (4.7% of all specimens received) (Waldron and Shafer 1975). In other words, leukoplakia appears to be about twice as common in Georgia as in Indiana. The explanation for this is not known as various possible etiologic factors such as differences in the use of snuff could not be evaluated in this study. Finally, although the number of carcinomas in the leukoplakia material was the same at Emory and Indiana (52 cases in each institution), the incidence of epithelial dysplasia in the Emory material was significantly greater (440 cases in 1,666 specimens or 26.5%) than in the Indiana material (126 cases in 1,944 specimens or 7.4%).

2:2 ERYTHROPLAKIA

Erythroplakia has been widely described on the penis, when it is known as erythroplasia of Queyrat, whereas there are only scattered case reports and up to 1975 only one series of cases in the literature describing its occurrence in the oral cavity (Shear 1972).

From the series of cases of oral erythroplakia reported by Shafer and Waldron (1975), it would appear that there is no significant difference in occurrence between the sexes. Of 58 patients, 31 were males (53%) and 27 females (47%). There does appear to be a marked difference in age of occurrence between erythroplakia and leukoplakia. For, in the above study, only 11 of 58 patients (19%) with erythoplakia were in the 5th decade or younger whereas in the comparable group of leukoplakia patients reported by the same authors (Shafer and Waldron), 39%, or approximately twice as many, were in the 5th decade or younger. By contrast, in a study of 100 patients with penile erythroplakia by Graham and Helwig (1973), 49 (49%) were in the 5th decade or younger.

There were also considerable regional differences in location between oral erythroplakia and leukoplakia (Table 3). The mandibular gingiva, alveolar ridge, and mucobuccal fold was the most common site of erythroplakia in females just as it was the most common site of leukoplakia. However, in males this was the least common site for erythroplakia, only 1 case occurring here. By far the most common site of erythroplakia in males was floor of mouth, an uncommon site for leukoplakia in males (6.0% of all male leukoplakias) and relatively uncommon in females (11.7% of all female leukoplakias). The second most common site for erythroplakia in both males and females (total of 18.8% of all cases) was the retromolar area. Strangely, this was the least common site for leukoplakia (total of 5.9% of all cases). (See also chapter 18.)

In the study of oral erythroplakia reported by Shafer and Waldron (1975), 59 of 65 biopsies from 58 patients (91%) were histologically either invasive carcinoma, carcinoma in situ, or severe epithelial dysplasia. The remaining 6 cases (9%) were either mild or moderate epithelial dysplasia and, for this reason, there can be no consideration of "high-risk" and "low-risk" sites for oral erythroplakia. All sites are at high-risk (Table 4).

The clinical appearance of oral erythroplakia has often been described as having one of three forms: (a) homogenous erythroplakia, (b) erythroplakia intermingled with patches of leukoplakia, and (c) speckled erythroplakia (Shear 1972). Since the study of Shafer and Waldron (1975) dealt only with homogenous erythroplakia, there is no information available for a clinicopathologic correlation of the different types or as to whether one is apt to be more serious than the others.

TABLE 3 Erythroplakia—Site

	Male		*Female*		*Total*	
	N	*Per cent*	*N*	*Per cent*	*N*	*Per cent*
Max. mucosa	2	6.0	3	10.0	5	7.8
Mand. mucosa	1	2.9	7	23.3	8	12.5
Palate	5	14.7	3	10.0	8	12.5
Bucc. mucosa	2	5.9	3	10.0	5	7.8
Tongue	4	11.8	4	13.3	8	12.5
Fl. mouth	13	38.2	5	16.7	18	28.1
Retrom.	7	20.6	5	16.7	12	18.8
Total	34		30		64	

From: Shafer and Waldron (1975).

TABLE 4 Erythroplakia—Site and Relative Risk at Site

		Severe Dysplasia/Cancer	
	Per cent of cases	*No. of cases*	*Per cent*
Max. mucosa & sulcus	8	4/4	100
Mand. mucosa & sulcus	13	8/8	100
Palate	13	6/8	75
Buccal mucosa	8	5/5	100
Tongue	13	6/8	75
Floor of mouth	28	18/19	95
Retromolar	19	12/13	92
Total	65(#)	59/65	91%

From: Shafer and Waldron (1975).

3. CLINICAL FEATURES OF LESIONS SHOWING EPITHELIAL DYSPLASIA AND CARCINOMA IN SITU

We have so far been considering the basic clinical features of definite clinical entities that are generally accepted as premalignant lesions. It would be appropriate also to consider this topic from another point of view, that is in terms of the clinical features of lesions histologically classified as premalignant.

3:1 CARCINOMA IN SITU

As the one histologic lesion which is most likely to be premalignant, we should select carcinoma in situ (CIS) (Shafer 1975). There are few studies that have discussed the problem of the progression or regression of epithelial dysplasia and carcinoma in situ of oral mucosa as has been done for the uterine cervix. The best known are those of Mincer and his associates (1972), of Pindborg and his coworkers (1977), of Bánóczy and Csiba (1976), and Bánóczy (1977). Mincer et al. summarized their conclusions by the following interesting statement: "Follow-up study of forty-five of these patients for periods of 1 to 8 years showed that these lesions may be cured surgically (13 out of 20), may recur after removal (7 out of 20),[1] may increase in size of severity (5 out of 20), may regress or disappear without surgical treatment (3 out of 25), may remain static (10 out of 25), or may undergo malignant transformation (5 out of 25)." Nevertheless, it is probable that the vast majority of cases of oral carcinoma in situ will eventually undergo malignant transformation, and it is therefore important to know the basic clinical features of these lesions. There have only been 2 significant series of cases of this disease reported, one by Shedd et al. (1963) on 10 cases and the other by Shafer (1975) on 82 lesions in 77 patients. The disease has also been discussed in detail by Kramer (1973). The material that is presented here is an extension of the 1975 study which now amounts to a series of 112 patients with 127 lesions of oral carcinoma in situ.

The sex ratio of this CIS group was 60% male and 40% female. The sex ratio of a large group of patients with oral epidermoid carcinoma in our files from the same population group is 69% male and 31% female. Whether this 9% difference in the sexes between the two groups is significant is not known. It is interesting to speculate about the reason for this. One conclusion might be that 9% of the females with CIS never progress to invasive cancer, or at least 9% fewer of the females do not progress to cancer.

With respect to age, there were 2 females with CIS between 26 and 30 and 2 females between 31 and 35 years, but there were no males with CIS under 36 years. The mean age of occurrence of CIS was 61 years in males and 60 years in females. By way of comparison, in our series of oral epidermoid carcinoma, the mean age of occurrence was 62 years in males and 61 years in females. These findings might suggest that the duration of carcinoma in situ as a stage in the development of invasive carcinoma is of very short duration. However, we did have information available in 31 males and 22 females on the duration of the lesion according to the patient. These varied over an extremely wide range from 1 week to 10 years in males and 2 weeks to 8 years in females. The mean duration of a "lesion" at the site of the CIS in males was 52 weeks and in females 56 weeks.

[1] Mincer et al. (1972) regarded a lesion as a recurrence, even if it appeared in a site that was different from that of the primary lesion.

Over two-thirds of all cases of CIS occurred in just 3 sites in the oral cavity: floor of mouth, 28%; tongue, 24%; and lips, 16% (Table 5).

TABLE 5 Carcinomona in situ—Site

	Male		*Female*		*Total*	
	N	*Per cent*	*N*	*Per cent*	*N*	*Per cent*
Lips	18	25	2	4	20	16
Max. mucosa	1	1	1	2	2	2
Mand. mucosa	3	4	8	15	11	9
Palate	8	11	3	5	11	9
Bucc. mucosa	4	6	7	13	11	9
Tongue	12	17	18	33	30	24
Fl. mouth	22	31	14	25	36	28
Retrom.	3	4	2	4	5	4
Fauces	1	1	–	–	1	1
Total	72		55		127	

However, there were some differences between the sexes. As might be expected, males had a higher incidence of CIS of the lips (25%) than females (4%). Females had a higher incidence of CIS of the tongue (33%) than males (17%). Several differences in sites of occurrence become less marked however, if CIS of the lip is discounted in the calculations (see chapter 18).

The descriptions of the clinical appearance of this series of CIS was available from the histories in 79 cases. In 49 of the 79 cases (or 62%), the lesions were described as "leukoplakia," "white patch," "keratotic lesion," or some similar phrase. In 9 cases (12%), the lesion was described as a "red lesion" or as "erythroplakia" and 9 additional cases as an ulcerated lesion. In still another 9 cases, the description was of a combination white and red lesion. In 2 cases (3%), the lesions were described as red and ulcerated and in 1 case as white and ulcerated.

4. SUMMARY AND CONCLUSIONS

There are certain clinical entities which may be considered as oral premalignant lesions by virtue of the fact that carcinomatous transformation occurs in these lesions in a significantly high percentage of cases. The two entities are leukoplakia and erythroplakia.

It is of interest that seemingly significant differences exist in certain basic clinical features of these two diseases. For example, although the predilection of leukoplakia for males appears to be decreasing, there are no remarkable sex differences in the occurrence of erythroplakia. Further, while a small but significant number of patients under the age of 20 years develop leukoplakia, erythroplakia is exceedingly uncommon even as young as the third decade of life.

Finally, there are certain differences in the sites of occurrence between leukoplakia and erythroplakia. For example, while the mandibular gingiva, ridge, and mucobuccal fold is the *most* common site for leukoplakia in both males and females and for erythroplakia in females, it is the *least* common site for erythroplakia in males. Whereas the floor of mouth is the second least common site for leukoplakia in males, it is by far the most common site for erythroplakia in males. In fact, its rate of occurrence here is nearly twice that at any other single oral anatomic site. While the retromolar area is a very uncommon site for leukoplakia in both males and females, it is the second *most* common site for erythroplakia in both males and females.

While no definite information is available, these differences in clinical features between the two diseases might suggest differences in their etiologies even though they both culminate in epidermoid carcinoma.

REFERENCES

Bánóczy, J. 1977. Follow-up studies in oral leukoplakia. *J. Maxillofac. Surg.* **5**, 69–75.

Bánóczy, J., and Csiba, A. 1976. Occurrence of epithelial dysplasia in oral leukoplakia. Analysis and follow-up study of 12 cases. *Oral Surg.* **42**, 766–774.

Graham, J. H., and Helwig, E. B. 1973. Erythroplasia of Queyrat. A clinicopathologic and histochemical study. *Cancer* **32**, 1396–1414.

Kramer, I. R. H. 1973. Carcinoma-in-situ of the oral mucosa. *Int. Dent. J.* **23**, 94–99.

McCarthy, F. P. 1936. Etiology, pathology, and treatment of leukoplakia buccalis with report of 316 cases. *Arch. Dermat. & Syph.* **34**, 612–623.

Meigs, J. W. 1977. Epidemic lung cancer in women. *JAMA* **238**, 1055.

Mincer, H. H., Coleman, S. A., and Hopkins, K. P. 1972. Observations on the clinical characteristics of oral lesions showing histologic epithelial dysplasia. *Oral Surg.* **33**, 389–399.

Pindborg, J. J., Daftary, D. K., and Mehta, F. S. 1977. A follow-up study of sixty-one oral dysplastic precancerous lesions in Indian villagers. *Oral Surg.* **43**, 383–390.

Shafer, W. G. 1975. Oral carcinoma in situ. *Oral Surg.* **39**, 227–238.

Shafer, W. G., and Waldron, C. A. 1961. A clinical and histopathologic study of oral leukoplakia. *Surg. Gynecol. Obstet.* **112**, 411–420.

Shafer, W. G., and Waldron, C. A. 1975. Erythroplakia of the oral cavity. *Cancer* **36**, 1021–1028.

Shear, M. 1972. Erythroplakia of the mouth. *Int. Dent. J.* **22**, 460-473.

Shedd, D. P., Hukill, P. B., Kligerman, M. M., and Gowen, G. F. 1963. A clinicopathologic study of oral carcinoma in situ. *Am. J. Surg.* **106**, 791–796.

Thoma, K. H. 1941. *Oral Pathology: A Histological, Roentgenological, and Clinical Study of the Diseases of the Teeth, Jaws, and Mouth.* 1st ed., p. 1222. C. V. Mosby Co., St. Louis.

Waldron, C. A., and Shafer, W. G. 1975. Leukoplakia revisited. A clinicopathologic study of 3,256 oral leukoplakias. *Cancer* **36**, 1386–1392.

3

Basic Histopathological Features of Oral Premalignant Lesions

I. R. H. KRAMER

Department of Pathology, Institute of Dental Surgery, Eastman Dental Hospital, University of London, London, England

Many malignant neoplasms appear to arise by a two-stage process: initiation, and promotion (see chapter 4). It is well established that the interval between these two stages may be very long, and during this interval, whatever the nature of the subtle chemical changes that have taken place in the cells, these changes are not likely to be recognizable to the light microscopist using routine techniques. To the histopathologist, therefore, altered tissue during the interval between initiation and promotion may not be identifiable as a precancerous lesion. However, there may be a third stage, that MacDonald (1975) has referred to as "predisposition." This stage may precede the others, and consists of a changed state of the tissues that makes them more susceptible to the action of an initiating agent, such as a chemical carcinogen.

What, then, is understood by the term "precancerous lesion"? In clinical terms, it is a lesion in which the risk of malignant change is considerably increased. To the histopathologist a precancerous lesion may belong to two main categories. One category includes those lesions that are regarded as precancerous because of what is known about their behavior, quite irrespective of the tissue changes that may be present in any particular case. For example, recent studies by Kramer et al. (1978) show that with floor of the mouth leukoplakia or sublingual keratosis a frighteningly high proportion will proceed to carcinoma even when initially the tissue changes appear entirely innocent. There is little point in considering the histopathology of precancerous lesions in this category, because it is not necessary to resort to the microscope except to confirm the clinical diagnosis.

The histopathologist's second category of precancerous lesions is that in which the microscopic features are a determining factor, and here the main observation is that of epithelial dysplasia. There is fairly general agreement on the light microscope features of epithelial dysplasia, but real problems arise in any attempt to agree on and quantitate observations, and to decide on the proper interpretation of what is seen. As Davidsohn and Ni wrote in 1970, "It is in the nature of morphologic changes that their interpretation is subject to individual variations. Different observers may see different things in the same object and the difference may be mainly in the eyes of the beholder. The subjective element in morphologic diagnosis is most pronounced in the late stages of metaplasia and in dysplasia. This is the source of many diagnostic differences of opinion just at a time when the correct diagnosis is most important."

Acknowledging these problems, it is now appropriate to illustrate and comment on the generally accepted components of epithelial dysplasia. Some of these will be mentioned only briefly in order to deal more fully with others that may be of special importance.

In a nondysplastic oral epithelium the basal cells may have a definable long axis and perhaps some degree of nuclear polarization. One well-accepted component of epithelial dysplasia is "disturbed polarity" of the basal cells (Fig. 1); in isolation, such a change is not necessarily of great significance.

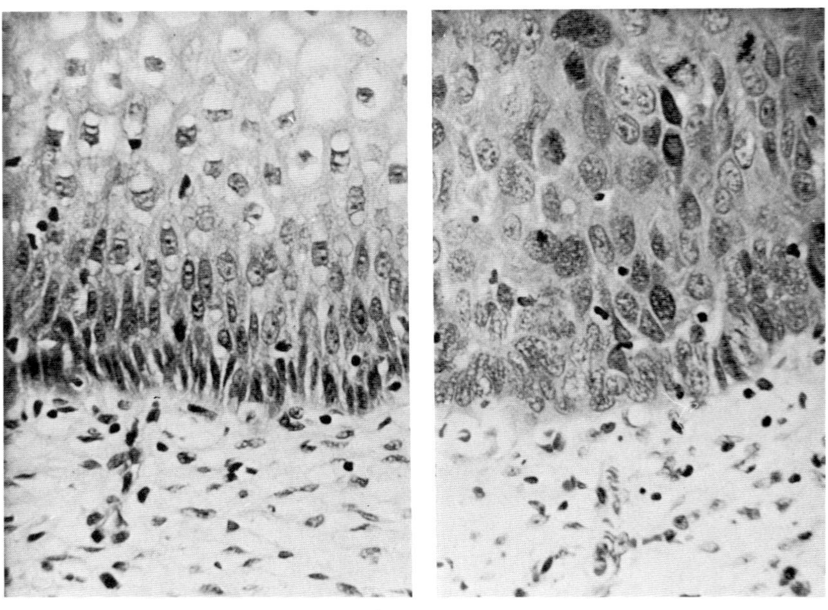

FIGURE 1. a. (or left) Normal well-polarized basal cell layer.
b. (or right) Severe disturbance of polarity.
Hematoxylin and eosin. X 320.

In normal oral epithelium the shape of the rete processes varies considerably from one part of the mucosa to another, but generally they either taper downwards, or they are almost parallel sided with blunt ends.

Rete processes that are wider at their deeper part than they are more superficially are the so-called "drop-shaped" processes. This is an appropriate descriptive term, and such an appearance may represent one of the more ominous features of epithelial dysplasia. It is probably related to a concept that will be discussed later which is the concept of a critical cell number that is a necessary prelude to invasion.

In listing the components of epithelial dysplasia, it is commonplace to refer in some way to variation in cell shape and size, and to variations in nuclear shape and staining. Some writers list pleomorphism and hyperchromatism—usually meaning cellular pleomorphism and nuclear hyperchromatism—whilst others refer to anisocytosis, anisonucleosis, pleomorphism of cells, and pleomorphism of nuclei as four separate entities. This is a degree of refinement that in practice is difficult to achieve. Variation in nuclear size (Fig. 2) tends to fall under another heading, but nuclear hyperchromatism should be identifiable as a separate entity. Gross examples are easily agreed upon, but with less gross changes there may be considerable discrepancy in interpretation. Certainly, what some observers label as hyperchromatic nuclei, others would interpret as probably melanocyte nuclei, or damaged nuclei near the edge of the biopsy, or even nuclei in prophase.

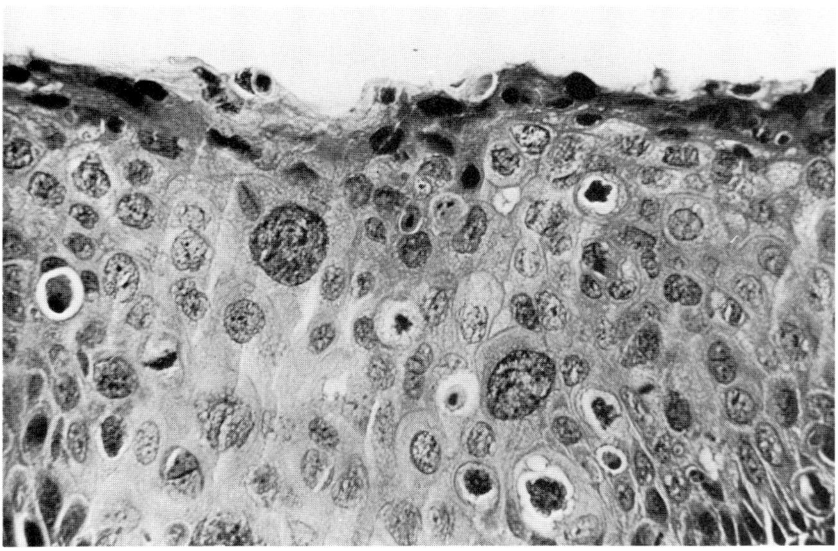

FIGURE 2. Gross variation in nuclear size. Hematoxylin and eosin. X 300.

The next component of epithelial dysplasia, basal cell hyperplasia, is sometimes defined as the development of a basal cell layer that is several cells thick. This is a contradiction in terms, for the basal layer, by definition, is only one cell thick. The presence of several layers of cells that are basaloid in appearance may be genuine, but often it is due to a slightly tangential section through the basal cell layer. Related to the concept of basal cell hyperplasia there is the change often referred to as "irregular epithelial stratification," or disturbed maturational sequence, or some other term conveying the same idea. Such descriptions represent an attempt to put into words that epithelial pattern in which the cells no longer show the proper sequence of morphological and maturational changes as they pass from the basal cell region to the surface (Fig. 3). Perhaps the extreme expression of this change is the sort of pattern sometimes seen in carcinoma in situ, where all the cells, from the basal layer to the surface, look almost exactly alike.

Alteration in the ratio of nuclear to cytoplasmic area or volume is also mentioned in most lists of the components of epithelial dysplasia (Fig. 4). This type of change is readily seen and measured in exfoliative cytology, but it is less readily identified in a section unless one resorts to time-consuming morphometric methods as described by Franklin in chapter 5.

These changes also contribute to another subjective impression—the impression of cell crowding, or an increase in the number of cells per unit area. Basal cell hyperplasia, disturbance of the normal maturational sequence, raised nuclear to cytoplasmic ratio, and "cell crowding" appear to be closely related features, and sometimes they are also related to the formation of drop-shaped rete processes. In a morphometric study of dysplasia and carcinoma of the cervix, Hillemanns et al. (1968a) have related nuclear volume and cytoplasmic-nuclear ratio to the various stages of dysplasia and carcinoma (Fig. 5). They found that there was a steady rise in nuclear volume, and a fall in the cytoplasmic-nuclear ratio, through the stages of dysplasia to carcinoma in situ. Interestingly, when invasion had started, the nuclear volume started to fall again.

In relation to cell crowding, Hillemanns et al. (1968b) have shown that there is also a steady rise in nuclei per unit area up to the stage of carcinoma in situ, and, as with nuclear volume, the value drops when invasion starts (Fig. 6). This observation of cell crowding is related to the concept of Mühlbock (1957) that there is a critical cell number per unit area that must be achieved before invasion can occur. Another interesting expression of cell crowding is to be found from an examination of various levels in the epithelium (Fig. 7), and the following observations are derived

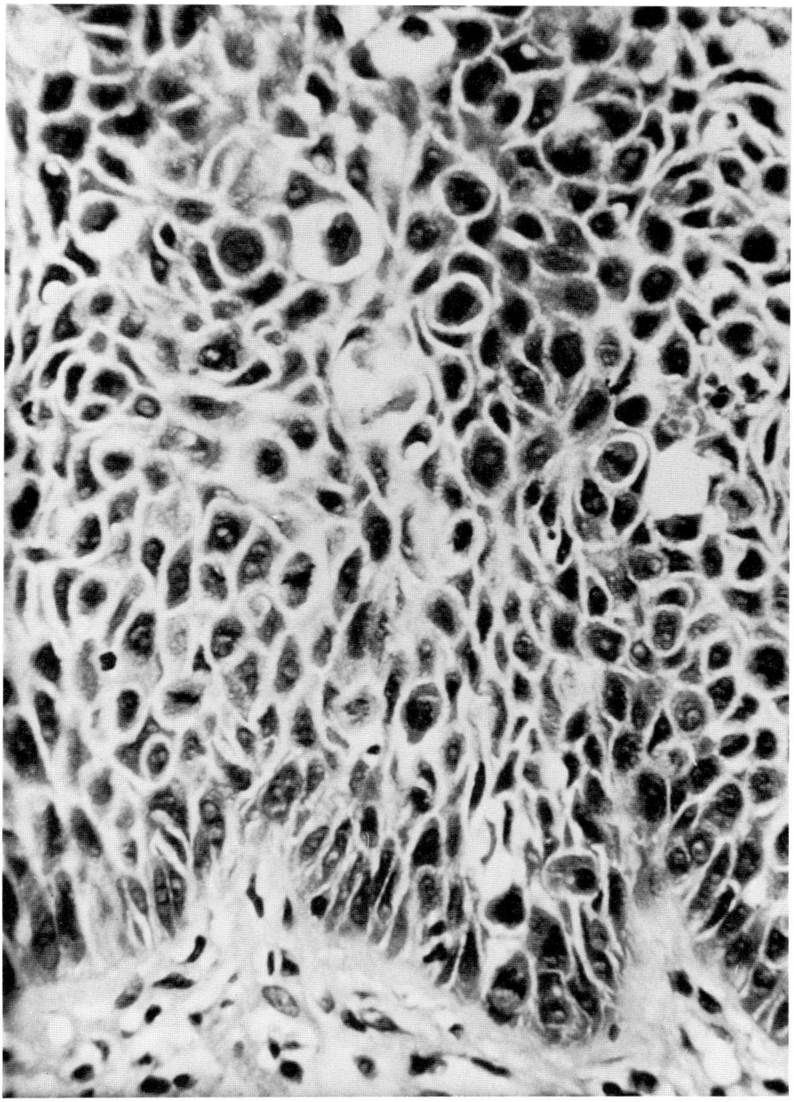

FIGURE 3. Disturbance of maturational sequence. Hematoxylin and eosin. X 410.

from Hillemanns et al. (1968a). In normal cervical epithelium, the nuclei are most closely packed in the basal cell layer, and they rapidly become fewer per unit area as the cells increase in cytoplasmic volume in the prickle cell and superficial layers. In a dysplastic epithelium, it is clear that the number of nuclei per unit area increases in the prickle cell and superficial layers—perhaps this could be equated with the concept of so-called basal cell hyperplasia.

In carcinoma in situ, the number of nuclei per unit area throughout the epithelium is approaching that of the basal cell layer—in the other terminology, there is a loss of the maturational sequence. Of special interest is the observation that, at the stage of drop-shaped rete processes, there may be almost the same number of nuclei per unit area throughout the whole thickness of the epithelium.

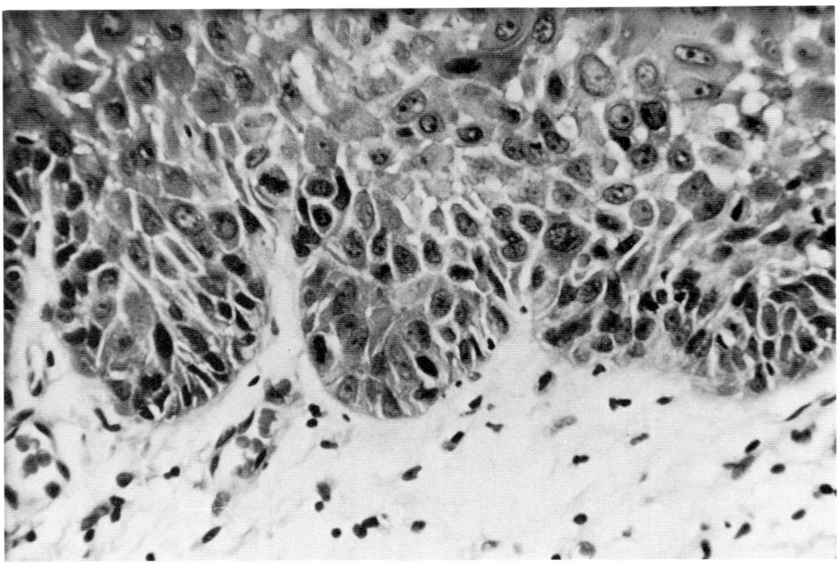

FIGURE 4. Increased nuclear: cytoplasmic ratio. Note also the slightly drop-shaped rete processes, and the evidence of reduced cell cohesion. Hematoxylin and eosin. X 310.

Mitotic activity in the oral epithelium is normally confined to the basal cell layer, except for the occasional mitosis in the suprabasal region (see chapter 9). In dysplastic epithelium, and indeed in an active epithelium that is not dysplastic, mitoses may be seen higher up in the epithelium than normal, and in greatly increased numbers (Fig. 8). Mitoses high up in the epithelium, and increased numbers of mitoses, are two of the generally accepted components of epithelial dysplasia. Hillemanns et al. (1968a)

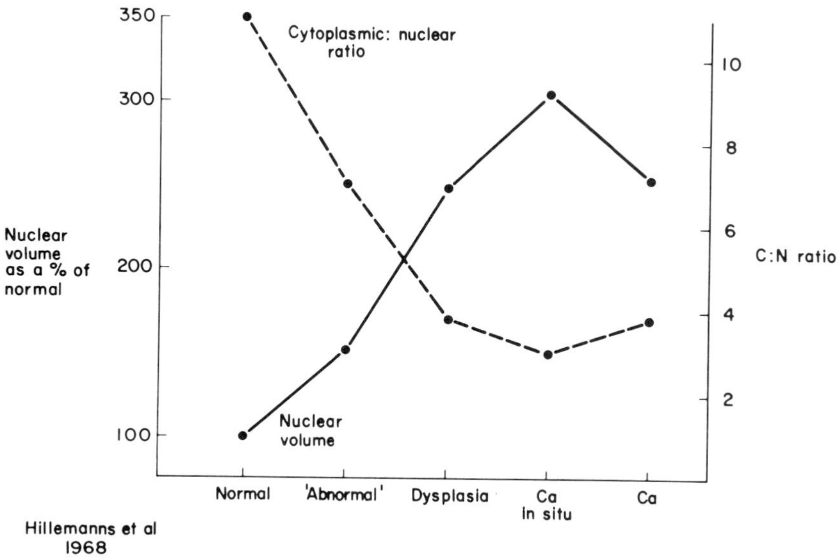

FIGURE 5. Nuclear volume expressed as a percentage of normal, and cytoplasmic: nuclear ratio, in cervical epithelium showing various degrees of dysplasia or carcinoma. Redrawn from data by Hillemanns et al. (1968b).

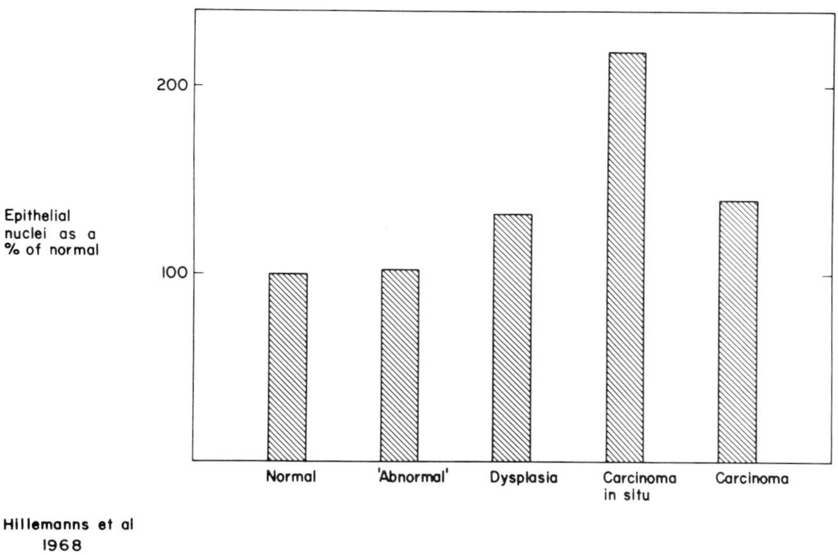

FIGURE 6. Numbers of cell nuclei per unit area, expressed as a percentage of normal, in cervical epithelia showing various degrees of dysplasia and carcinoma. Redrawn from data by Hillemanns et al. (1968b).

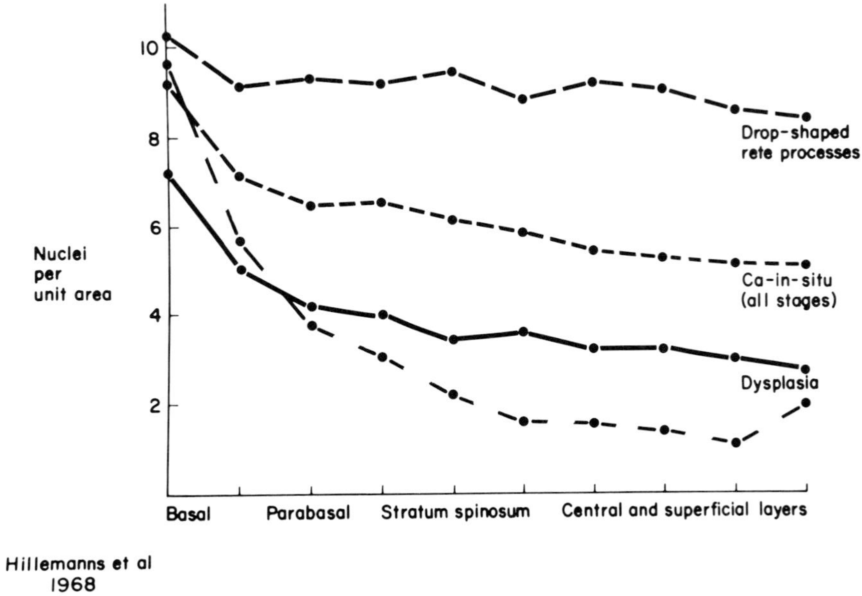

FIGURE 7. Numbers of nuclei per unit area at various levels of the epithelium in cervical epithelia showing dysplasia or carcinoma in situ. The unlabelled plot is for normal cervical epithelium. Redrawn from data by Hillemanns et al. (1968a).

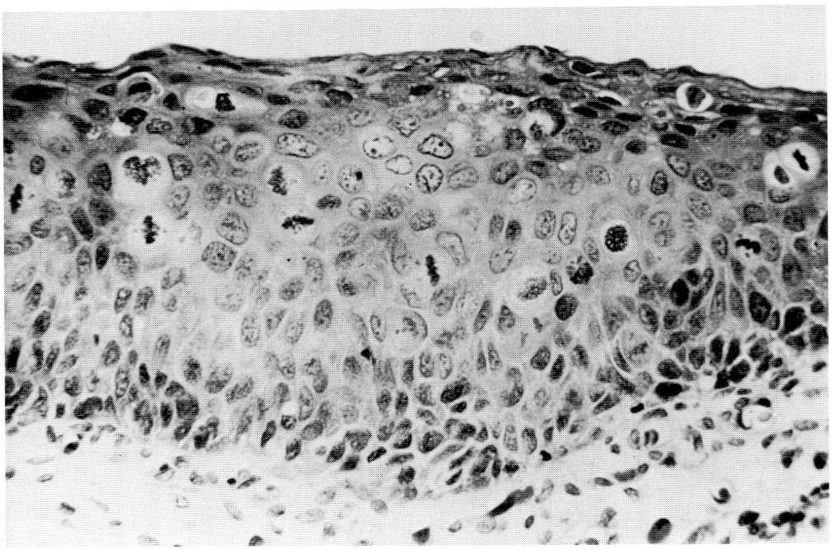

FIGURE 8. Numerous mitotic figures high in the epithelium. Hematoxylin and eosin. X 300.

have studied both the number of mitoses, and the levels at which they occur, in lesions of the cervix (Fig. 9), and although the cervical and oral epithelia obviously differ in some respects, their findings are probably in accord with those of oral epithelium.

In the normal cervical epithelium (and unlike the normal oral epithelium), most mitoses are in the parabasal or suprabasal layer and, as in oral epithelium, there is no mitotic activity at the higher levels. In dysplastic epithelium not only is the total mitotic activity increased; the mitotic activity is starting to spread into the higher levels of the epithelium. In severe dysplasia, mitotic activity in the higher layers becomes even more marked, and in carcinoma in situ there are many mitoses throughout the epithelium: indeed, at this stage, mitotic activity in the basal cell layer has dropped towards its normal value.

In this context, it is appropriate to sound a note of warning about the assessment of increased mitotic activity. El-Labban (unpublished data) has made a comparison of the subjective assessment of mitotic activity with actual mitotic counts made on the same sections. Sections with low mitotic counts were usually assessed as showing no increase in mitotic activity, and sections with very high counts were usually assessed subjectively as showing increased mitotic activity. However, there was a large middle group in which there was a poor correlation between the pathologist's impression and the actual count of mitotic figures. It thus appears that the pathologist, when he is asked to assess mitotic activity, is often influenced by factors other than the number of mitotic figures that he can see.

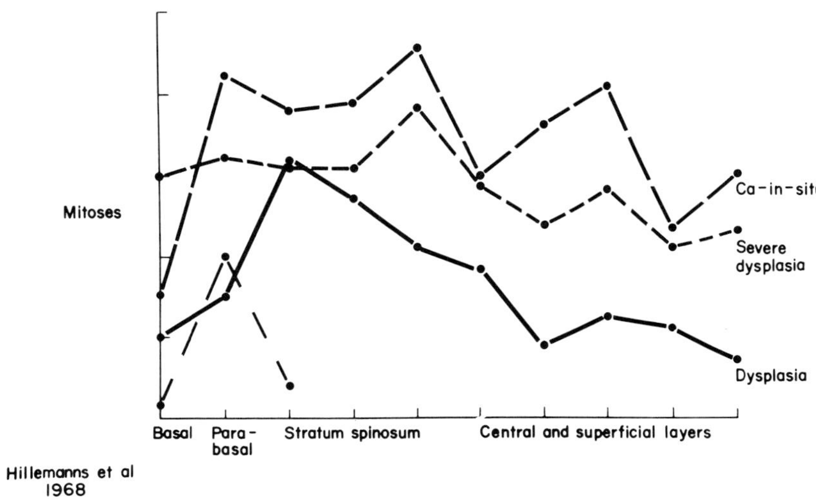

FIGURE 9. Numbers of mitoses at various levels in cervical epithelia showing dysplasia or carcinoma in situ. The unlabeled plot on the left is for normal cervical epithelium. Redrawn from data by Hillemanns et al. (1968a).

Another conventional component of epithelial dysplasia is the presence of abnormal mitoses (Fig. 10), and this again is more subjective than might readily be admitted. Looking at a metaphase spread preparation, quite small morphological abnormalities can be detected, but clearly it would be unwise to assume that anything approaching the same accuracy can be achieved from a section. Of course, given something as gross as a tripolar mitosis, there probably would be agreement, but all quantitative expressions of abnormal mitoses derived from tissue sections should be viewed with some suspicion. Before leaving the question of nuclear changes, it is worth referring to apparent changes in the nucleolus. In some dysplastic epithelia, and in some carcinomas, the nucleoli seem to become larger and denser, until they stand out like golf balls. Interestingly, one rarely sees such a change in basal cells: indeed, in normal basal cells nucleoli are hardly detectable in light microscope sections although they are readily seen in the electron microscope.

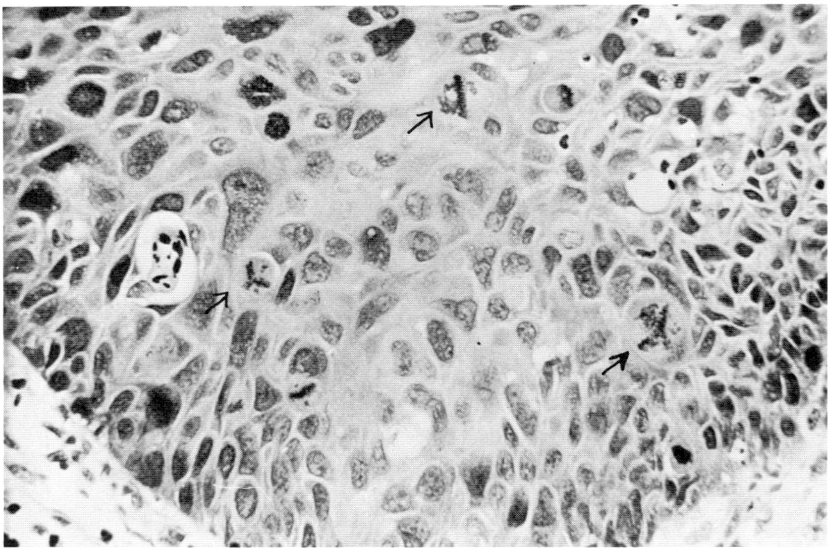

FIGURE 10. This epithelium shows several abnormal mitotic figures (arrows) together with other mitotic figures that are not obviously abnormal. Hematoxylin and eosin. X 300.

Intraepithelial keratinization may involve either cell groups or individual cells, and as a component of epithelial dysplasia individual cell keratinization is more likely to be seen. This change may affect the whole cytoplasm, or only limited areas. Sometimes, it is possible to actually see the bundles of tonofibrils even in a routine preparation.

A further component of epithelial dysplasia is usually called loss (or reduction) of cellular adherence or adhesion, although the term cohesion is more appropriate than adhesion or adherence. Cells can stick or adhere to all sorts of things: cohesion means to stick to one another, which is what is meant in the present context. Sometimes reduction in cohesion may be difficult to distinguish from spongiosis (where the cells are separated as a result of increased intercellular fluid, and the breaking of cell contacts is secondary), but in the field shown in Fig. 11 the cells are probably not losing their attachments because they are being forced apart: they are separating because their attachments are reduced or faulty. Morphometric studies on electron micrographs (see chapter 15) have shown that there really are desmosomal changes in the cells of a dysplastic epithelium, but the changes may have to be fairly gross before this effect is evident at the light microscopic level.

The generally listed components of epithelial dysplasia, together with some that are not always referred to by oral pathologists, are set out in Table 1. However, a list of the components of epithelial dysplasia is of little value unless there is agreement on what it means and how to use it.

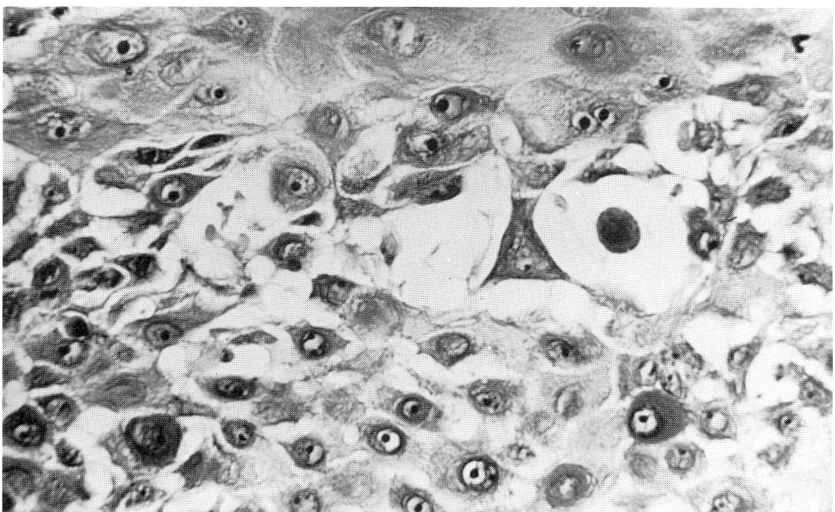

FIGURE 11. Reduction in cell cohesion in a dysplastic epithelium. Hematoxylin and eosin. X 300.

No single feature of epithelial dysplasia can be regarded as an absolute discriminator that will separate a lesion that is precancerous from one that is not, and this problem will be referred to in more detail later (chapter 19) in a discussion of the prognostic implications of what the light microscopist can see. At this point, however, it seems too simplistic to accept the statement that an epithelium shows dysplasia if it has any two or more of the components on the list—at least, if, by dysplasia, we mean a potentially precancerous change.

TABLE 1 Epithelial Dysplasia

Drop-shaped processes	Increased N:C ratio
Disturbed polarity	Cell crowding
"Basal cell hyperplasia"	Increased mitoses
Disturbed maturational sequence	Mitoses in upper layers
Pleomorphism/anisocytosis	Abnormal mitoses
Hyperchromatism	Reduced cohesion
Prominent nucleoli	Intra-epithelial keratinization

REFERENCES

Davidsohn, I., and Ni, L. Y. 1970. Immunocytology of cancer. *Acta Cytol.* **14**, 276–282.

Hillemanns, H. G., Fröhlich, D., and Prestel, E. 1968a. Zellzahl und Mitosefrequenz bei entstehung des Cervix-carcinoms (zum Carcinoma in situ und Mikrocarcinom der Cervix). *Arch. Gynaek.* **206**, 292–319.

Hillemanns, H. G., Sixtus-Klug, B., and Prestel, E. 1968b. Cytoplasma-Kernrelationen der Malignitätsstufen des Cervixepithels, gemessen mit dem Integrationsocular. I. Zum Carcinoma in situ und Mikrocarcinom der Cervix. *Arch. Gynaek.* **206**, 82–97.

Kramer, I. R. H., El-Labban, N. G., and Lee, K. W. 1978. The clinical features and risk of malignant transformation in sublingual keratosis. *Br. Dent. J.* **144**, 171–180.

MacDonald, D. G. 1975. Premalignant lesions of oral epithelium. In: *Oral Mucosa in Health and Disease.* (Edited by Dolby, A. E.), pp. 335–369. Blackwell Scientific Publications, Oxford.

Mühlbock, O. 1957. Karzinogenese, Endogenese und Exogenese. In: *Krebsforschung und Krebsbekämpfung.* Bd. 37S. 13–25. Urban and Schwarzenberg. Münschen u Berlin. (Quoted by Hillemanns, H. G., Fröhlich, D., and Prestel, E., 1968.)

Discussion

The discussion following the three papers on clinical and histopathological concepts of oral premalignancy was mainly related to four principal areas of concern:

(a) definition of specific premalignant lesions and of the general concept of premalignancy;
(b) the nature and importance of the clinical problem;
(c) practical problems associated with studies of oral premalignancy;
(d) the possible existence of several different, but as yet undefined, types of lesion and patient populations at risk.

In response to a question from Dr. Dabelsteen about definition of the term leukoplakia, Professor Pindborg pointed out that in Britain and Denmark, in conformity with discussions held under the auspices of the World Health Organization, leukoplakia is now often used as a purely clinical term. It provides a preliminary description prior to microscopic examination. Dr. Mashberg asked whether the definition of leukoplakia would include lesions with recognizable erythroplasia and whether carcinoma in situ would be included in the histological description "severe dysplasia." Professor Pindborg replied that subdivision of leukoplakias into homogeneous and nodular types would distinguish those lesions with erythroplastic areas. In his Indian study, lesions with an ulcerative red component that was clearly the result of trauma were also distinguished. He stated that differences between severe dysplasia and carcinoma in situ have been defined by the WHO study group, but pointed out that in making this distinction that there was often inconsistency between different pathologists.

Professor Johnson expressed concern that so much of the discussion of oral premalignancy was dominated by the term "leukoplakia." In his department the term is no longer used because its variable meaning leads to a risk of possible misinterpretation. He preferred to give a descriptive clinical account of the lesion instead. Dr. Wilbanks commented that in gynecological pathology, the use of terms such as red and white plaques had been discontinued some years ago. In response to a question from Dr. Binnie as to what such clinical lesions are called, Dr. Wilbanks replied that they are described as atrophic or hypertrophic.

Dr. Mashberg stated that the term "erythroplasia," used in a purely descriptive clinical sense, was of value because, in his experience, "erythroplasia" is the one component persistently observed to be associated with asymptomatic carcinoma. Dr. Shafer commented that, clinically, the progression of carcinoma in situ to frankly invasive cancer appeared to be faster when associated with a red lesion rather than a white lesion. As it is not possible to make this distinction histologically, it would be a mistake to discontinue the use of the clinical descriptive terms leukoplakia and erythroplakia.

Professor Pindborg asked whether it might not be better to be practical rather than too philosophical in the use of clinical terms. Previously the term leukoplakia has been used to imply a microscopic appearance. It had been used synonymously with "dyskeratosis" by some and with "hyperorthokeratosis" by others. Such variable use of a clinically descriptive term is obviously confusing. Nevertheless, there exist some well-defined clinical entities which could be briefly and conveniently described as leukoplakia or erythroplakia. However, such lesions observed through the microscope are seen as histological sections not as red or white patches! The pathologist, working at this level of examination, should therefore provide a descriptive diagnosis of what he sees microscopically rather than extend the use of a clinical term.

Dr. Binnie agreed with the need for clinically descriptive terms for premalignancy and pointed to the existence of a group of white lesions of the floor of the mouth which, as discussed by Professor Kramer, often progress to epidermoid carcinoma despite a perfectly benign histological appearance with virtually no atypia.

Dr. Pindborg was asked whether, in the definition of a premalignant lesion as "a morphologically altered tissue in which cancer is more likely to develop than in its normal counterpart" he referred to clinical or microscopic morphology. He replied that it had been intended to refer primarily to a histological change. Professor Johnson asked whether it might be useful to confine the description "premalignant" to lesions which, given adequate time, would inevitably become malignant and to use the description "potentially malignant" for lesions which, on a statistical basis, have a high probability of becoming malignant.

Dr. Mackenzie pointed to the subtitle used for the symposium "Epithelial changes prior to invasion" and asked whether the term "premalignant" as it was currently applied to a lesion had any meaning at the cellular level. Dr. Wilbanks replied that, as the biology of severely dysplastic cervical cells and the cells of carcinoma in situ indicate that the cells are altered and are indeed malignant, in gynecological pathology the term "preinvasive" is therefore preferred. This leads to a completely different concept, as in this sense carcinoma in situ and some dysplasias contain preinvasive malignant cells, which if left alone will eventually kill the patient. He was uncertain how classical concepts of initiation and promotion applied to such lesions, but he felt that the biology of such cells needed to be studied to provide quantitative criteria for defining preinvasive malignancy. At present, only subjective criteria are available.

With regard to the clinical significance of lesions exhibiting focal or mild atypias, Dr. Mashberg suggested that there may not be a great problem either ethically or practically. His clinical impression of the oral lesions referred to him for evaluation from a pool of about 5,000 patient examinations per year indicated that the asymptomatic lesions of significance were almost invariably found to be invasive carcinoma or carcinoma in situ at the time of histological examination. He found that few other lesions become carcinoma even if followed for long periods of time. Professor Pindborg pointed out that the data so far available are so limited that reliable subdivision of cases into slight, moderate, or severe atypia is not possible. He therefore questioned the evidence for the assumption that only severe atypias are dangerous. Dr. Mashberg, however, suggested that from the practical point of view the problem is not a difficult one. Early asymptomatic carcinoma or carcinoma in situ is almost totally curable by excision. There might therefore be no need to be overly concerned about moderate dysplasia as, with controlled follow-up, such lesions may be excised if they become carcinomas and rarely recur.

Professor Johnson indicated that it was his clinical impression that most cases of oral squamous cell carcinoma had no previous history of a long standing lesion (reviewed by MacDonald 1975). Most cases, perhaps as many as 80% (Johnson 1977), appear to be overtly invasive at presentation and are readily recognized as such histologically. Given the unknown, but probably extremely short, association of a recognizable premalignant phase in such cases, he felt that, in terms of the number of patients involved, prediction of what a premalignant lesion is going to do is a relatively small problem. He believed that if this were agreed upon, it should be stated and recognized if only to be set aside prior to going on to the discussion of premalignant lesions as such.

Professor Pindborg could not agree that many cases of oral carcinoma arose *de novo*. He thought that by far the majority arose in altered tissue. Professor Johnson agreed, but questioned whether the alteration was such that it produced a clinical lesion which brought the patient to seek attention. Dr. Mackenzie suggested that information about the rate of malignant transformation of normal mucosa did not appear to be available but would be of importance in considering the significance of premalignant oral lesions. Professor Kramer referred to MacDonald (1975) who pointed out that only a minority of oral squamous carcinomas appear to arise in clinically-detectable, preexisting lesions. This is a very important point, but did not in any way invalidate an attempt to recognize such clinical warning signs which do exist, such as leukoplakia and erythroplakia.

Dr. Wilbanks pointed out that if all invasive carcinoma of the mouth arose from normal epithelium, the whole discussion of premalignancy would be of little significance. However, he did not think that this would be true for the cervix. Although a few patients may show apparently normal cervical epithelium and yet develop an invasive malignancy some months later, he felt that even these cases would pass through a brief phase in which some sort of dysplastic change could be found.

Dr. Wilbanks asked whether "clinical recognition" might include exfoliative cytology. Professor Kramer stated that in this context several studies have suggested that exfoliative cytology is substantially less reliable for lesions of the oral cavity than for those of the cervix (see, for example, Dabelsteen et al. 1971).

Dr. Slavkin expressed some concern about the lack of agreement between different studies which had reported the prevalence or incidence of premalignant lesions. He asked whether Professor Pindborg would wish to comment further about what factors might be responsible for this variation. Professor Pindborg replied that there are many factors that could influence the reported figures in studies of oral premalignancy. Real differences in the incidence of oral premalignancy from one population to another may exist and, in fact, appear to do so. Clearly, however, there may be differences in the criteria used by groups of investigators for diagnosis of such lesions. The WHO group had attempted to standardize such criteria, but such standards are not universally applied. The population samples used in various studies, for example patients attending a particular hospital, do not always reflect a random sample of the local population as a whole. Although studies of a large random sample of a population are sometimes possible, for example in India, they are for a variety of reasons difficult to accomplish in many western countries. However, the Swedish study of Axéll (1976) was admirable in overcoming such problems. In addition to sampling problems there is probably a much higher rate of spontaneous or induced regression of leukoplakias than has hitherto been realized. This may be associated, for example, with cessation of smoking or interference with the natural course of the lesion by biopsy or other treatment. In general, therefore, the figures from epidemiological studies are only approximate, but at least give an indication of the size of the problem.

Dr. Waldron extended the discussion of variability of clinical diagnostic criteria to the question of the consistency of histological interpretation. For example, he referred to the circulation by Professor Pindborg of the histological sections and the clinical history of nineteen oral lesions. The participants in the study were all senior pathologists and were asked to classify each lesion as either free of dysplasia, showing mild, moderate, or severe dysplasia, or carcinoma in situ, and to estimate the degree of certainty with which they felt the classification could be made. There was total agreement in only four of the nineteen cases. Whereas one observer classified only three of the nineteen as showing severe dysplasia, another said that thirteen of the nineteen showed such changes. Such individual variation in classification would clearly influence the statistical data reported by different groups.

Dr. Dabelsteen referred to a comparable result obtained when a group of oral pathologists was asked to examine a histological preparation of a single lesion which he would describe as showing very early invasion. Good agreement was found between an initial and a subsequent examination, but the range of the description of the various examiners differed widely from nondysplastic epithelium to invasive carcinoma. Some of these differences could be explained by the varying degrees of experience of the examiners, and some was attributable to the increased differentiation, as observed by Shafer (1975), which occurs in an epithelium on progression from carcinoma in situ to invasive carcinoma. Nevertheless, the individual variation was disturbing and could account for much of the apparent lack of agreement in published reports of the rate of transformation of various types of lesion. In response to a comment by Professor Pindborg concerning the varying behavior of lesions of the labial mucosa and vermilion border of the lips, Dr. Waldron raised the further issue of the accuracy of the clinical description of the material seen by the pathologist. For example, tissue received at the pathological laboratory by mail might describe a lesion of the lip but fail to specify whether it was of the vermilion border or labial mucosa, regions in which the epithelium differs markedly in structure and behavior.

Professor Pindborg stated that, although the criteria for the basic diagnosis of dysplasia varied from one group of investigators to another, the way in which it varied was often known. This could therefore be taken into account to some extent when comparing the results of one study with another. A more important question, however, was which prognostic classification gives the best indication of actual cancer development at some later time. Were the pathologists who described many lesions as dysplastic overcautious, or were other pathologists overlooking changes which were in fact indicative of neoplastic change? As it often takes many years for cancer to develop in a lesion, this question could be answered only by long-term, follow-up studies. The WHO group had been following cases up to ten years, but even this period was inadequate to provide sufficient data to determine a common histological denominator in the cases becoming malignant.

Dr. Mashberg said that it appeared that Professor Pindborg and he were dealing with two rather different patient populations. Unlike Professor Pindborg, he rarely sees buccal carcinoma or carcinoma associated with homogeneous leukoplakic lesions. Professor Pindborg said that this is an aspect of the problem which clearly points to the need for comparative studies of populations from various parts of the world before any generalizations can be made about premalignant lesions. Dr. Waldron indicated that regional variations may be seen even within the United States. For example, he had been working closely with Dr. Shafer for about 25 years and, whereas Dr. Shafer continues to see a male predominance, he now sees a slight female predominance in his patient population. Dr. Waldron agreed that there are probably several ways in which oral cancer develops. He had seen low-grade carcinoma associated with leukoplakic lesions; others appeared to start in regions of erythroplakia, and yet others appeared to arise de novo. He felt that, for any particular lesion, the term precancerous is unsuitable and that perhaps "potentially malignant" is the description of choice. Professor Kramer suggested that "high risk lesion" and "low risk lesion" might form a more useful fundamental terminology and avoid the implications associated with terms such as premalignant and precancerous.

Dr. Waldron in closing the session commented that despite disagreement over a number of issues, two things appeared to be agreed upon: that there are probably several ways in which oral cancer can develop, and that there is very good evidence that there are in fact recognizable lesions of the oral mucosa which have a higher risk of developing cancer than normal mucosa.

REFERENCES

Axéll, T. 1976. A prevalence study of oral mucosal lesions in an adult Swedish population. *Odont. Din.* **27**, Suppl. 36, 1–103.

Dabelsteen, E., Roed-Petersen, R., Smith, C. J., and Pindborg, J. J. 1971. The limitations of exfoliative cytology for the detection of epithelial atypia in oral leukoplakias. *Br. J. Cancer* **25**, 21–24.

Johnson, N.W. 1977. Histological and histochemical studies of oral cancer. *Int. Dent. J.* **27**, 25–34.

MacDonald, D. G. 1975. Premalignant lesions of oral epithelium. In: *Oral Mucosa in Health and Disease*. (Edited by Dolby, A. E.), p. 364. Blackwell Scientific Publications, Oxford.

Shafer, W. S. 1975. Oral carcinoma in situ. *Oral Surg.* **39**, 227–238.

PART TWO
ETIOLOGY

4

Carcinogenesis in Selected Epithelia: General Biological Concepts

D. B. SOLT

Department of Pathology, University of Toronto, Toronto, Canada

1. INTRODUCTION

Although the development of malignancy is not yet understood at the molecular level, a large body of biological and clinicopathological evidence provides a conceptual basis for our understanding of the nature of preneoplasia and the evolution of malignancy. The following account is a brief consideration of some of the dominant concepts of the biological nature of carcinogenesis, as developed from a variety of in vivo systems and from observations in man. While most of these concepts are derived from animal experimentation and from clinicopathological observations in extraoral tissues, they should in theory be applicable to the oral cavity. Among the topics considered are the step-wise nature of carcinogenesis, the role of cell proliferation, the concept of tumor progression, and the phenomena of clonal selection and altered differentiation.

2. CARCINOGENESIS – A STEP-WISE PROCESS

The concept that cancer develops as a series of heritable cellular alterations is supported by observations in a variety of experimental systems and by clinicopathological observations in man (Foulds 1969, 1975; Farber 1973; Early lesions and the development of epithelial cancer, 1976).

Over 30 years ago, Rous and Kidd (1941) first called attention to the possibility that tumor formation proceeds in stages (Berenblum 1975). They based this inference on the observation that papillomas induced in rabbit skin by repeated applications of tar would regress when tarring was discontinued, but would reappear at the same site with the resumption of tarring or following a nonspecific irritant such as turpentine (Rous and Kidd 1941). Berenblum and Schubik (1947, 1949) identified two distinct stages of carcinogenesis using carcinogenic hydrocarbons and the cocarcinogen, croton oil, to induce skin cancer in mice. The application of a low dose of polycyclic hydrocarbon was shown to cause an irreversible alteration which, though not detectable by direct or microscopic examination, could be revealed by the development of visible tumors following subsequent applications of croton oil. The latter agent showed little carcinogenic potential, producing either no tumors or a negligible tumor yield, even after repeated administrations. When the sequence of administration was reversed, i.e., when application of croton oil preceded that of polycyclic hydrocarbon, the effect was comparable to the application of the polycyclic hydrocarbon alone in that no tumors were produced. Thus, a dose of polycyclic hydrocarbons which by itself failed to produce tumors had apparently "initiated" the carcinogenic process by converting normal cells to "potential tumor cells," which could undergo subsequent "promotion" to a visible tumor under the influence of a noncarcinogenic substance, croton oil.

A step-wise scheme of carcinogenesis is apparent during cancer development in tissues other than mouse skin. The cocarcinogenic activity of phenobarbital in hepatocarcinogenesis has recently been demonstrated in rats (Peraino et al. 1973). When the hepatocarcinogen 2-acetylaminofluorene was fed to young rats for 3 weeks (a period insufficient to induce a significant number of hepatic tumors with this carcinogen) and was followed by maintenance on a diet containing 0.05% phenobarbital, a high incidence of hepatic neoplasms developed over a period of several months. Administration of phenobarbital alone was insufficient to induce tumors in this species over the period of study. The cocarcinogenic action of saccharin has been demonstrated in the induction of bladder cancer following a single intravesicular administration of the carcinogen methylnitrosourea (Hicks et al. 1973). Man is undoubtedly a victim of cocarcinogenic agents. Tobacco tar and tobacco smoke appear to contain powerful promoting agents which may play a role in the development of carcinoma of the human bronchus (Wynder and Hoffman 1967). Other human malignancies, including colonic cancer, may also develop under the influence of combinations of carcinogens and cocarcinogens present in the intestinal lumen (Reddy et al. 1977).

Additional evidence for the step-wise nature of carcinogenesis, as demonstrated by a variety of animal models, is the early formation of hyperplastic lesions which develop prior to overt malignancy and which appear to serve as progenitor cell populations for the evolving cancers (Early lesions and the development of epithelial cancer, 1976). Perhaps the most convincing example is that of hyperplastic alveolar nodules which form spontaneously or following carcinogen exposure in the mammary gland of certain strains of mice. The tumorous potential of these lesions has been demonstrated by the tumor outgrowths formed following their transplantation into gland-free mammary fat pads (Slemmer 1974). Similarly, several lines of evidence support the belief that hyperplastic liver lesions developing during the course of chemical hepatocarcinogenesis are potential cancer precursors (Farber 1967). These hyperplastic liver lesions

(1) are formed prior to liver cancer formation with all known hepatocarcinogens, but are not formed during exposure to noncarcinogenic hepatotoxins, (2) contain marker compounds, including α-fetoprotein and γ-glutamyltranspeptidase—substances formed during fetal development and readily detectable in hepatocarcinomas, but not present in appreciable quantities in normal hepatocytes, and (3) occasionally contain populations of atypical cells which are indistinguishable from hepatocellular carcinomas.

While observations in several human tissues suggest that cancer in man may proceed through definable stages (Foulds 1975; Early lesions and the development of epithelial cancer, 1976), only two of the more convincing examples will be considered here. Carcinoma of the uterine cervix develops from normal cervical epithelium by successive stages of dysplasia, carcinoma in situ and finally, invasive cancer (Friedell 1976; Wilbanks, chapter 18). These lesions evolve in a time sequence which may span perhaps 20 or 30 years. The development of cytologic screening has made it possible to interrupt this process in many women at an early stage and has led to a significant decrease in morbidity and mortality in the female population as a whole from invasive cancer. Another example of well-established precursor lesions in the development of human cancer is exemplified by the adenomatous polyp, or adenoma, a precursor of colonic carcinoma (Lane and Fenoglio 1976). The dominant inherited disease, familial polyposis, is a natural human model which has availed pathologists of a wealth of tissue in which to study the progresion from adenomatous polyps to invasive carcinoma. Individuals with this disease develop innumerable adenomas throughout their colonic mucosa and, if left untreated, will invariably develop carcinoma of the colon at a relatively early age. Histopathologic study of colon specimens from individuals with familial polyposis has cast considerable doubt on the previous belief (Spratt and Ackerman 1962) that colonic cancer develops *de novo*, i.e., without passing through a precancerous state. While the morphology of adenomas forming in individuals with familial polyposis appears indistinguishable from that of adenomas seen in other individuals, the sheer concentration of lesions seen with familial polyposis greatly enhances the possibility of observing these lesions at the very earliest stages of neoplastic development. Consequently, neoplastic foci of microscopic size can be observed, some even as small as single crypts. These invariably prove to be adenomas, rather than carcinomas. Moreover, when microscopic foci of invasive cells are seen, they are always formed within the confines of a preexisting adenoma (Lane and Fenoglio 1976). Familial polyposis thus provides a clear demonstration of the step-wise nature of malignant development in man.

3. INITIATION IS RELATIVELY RAPID AND IRREVERSIBLE

Initiation of the carcinogenic process in skin can be accomplished either with a complete carcinogen, using a comparatively small dose acting for a brief period of time so that its potential promoting action is not manifest, or with a "pure" initiator such as urethane. Urethane, or ethyl carbamate, is an example of a compound which, on its own, lacks carcinogenic activity in mouse skin, but which can, following topical or systemic administration, initiate carcinogenesis in that tissue, as determined by the promoting action of subsequent applications of croton oil (Salaman and Roe 1953; Haran and Berenblum 1956).

Whether the initiating agent is a complete carcinogen or an incomplete carcinogen such as urethane, initiation appears to be accomplished rapidly. Mottram (1944a, 1944b) is credited with the first observation that a *single* application of a complete carcinogen (3,4 benzo(a)pyrene) and repeated applications of croton oil could lead to tumor formation. The observation that one application of a chemical carcinogen is sufficient to initiate skin carcinogenesis suggested that the initiation process is rapid and could occur during the limited period during which the carcinogen was presumed to act. This belief was supported by the observation that initiation could be effective, apparently over the whole surface of the mouse, by application of as little as 10 mg of urethane, a soluble substance that is rapidly eliminated (Haran and Berenblum 1956; Bryan et al. 1949). Attempts to determine the time required for completion of initiation have involved removing the carcinogenic hydrocarbon from the skin surface with appropriate solvents shortly after application (Ball and McCarter 1960), and inhibiting continued initiation action with actinomycin-D (Gelboin et al. 1965). While the results of such attempts are controversial, there seems little doubt that the time required for initiation in skin is of the order of hours rather than weeks or months (Berenblum 1975).

The evidence in chemical liver carcinogenesis also supports the contention that initiation is a rapid process. A single administration of several chemical hepatocarcinogens can induce liver cancer, either in intact animals or in animals subjected to a partial hepatectomy (Craddock 1976). Interestingly, in instances where partial hepatectomy is required to demonstrate this effect, the tumor induction seems to be most reliably accomplished when the carcinogen is administered during a brief period which coincides with the peak of hepatocyte DNA synthesis evoked by this surgical procedure (Craddock 1976). Although hepatomas induced by a single administration of carcinogen emerge only after a latent period of several months, the knowledge that these inducing carcinogens are rapidly metabolized in this organ and eliminated (Miller 1970; Heath 1962) is consistent with initiation in liver being completed in a brief period of time.

The relatively rapid initiation of liver carcinogenesis is further supported by enzyme histochemical studies. A single administration of the potent hepatocarcinogen diethylnitrosamine (DEN) results in microscopic nests of altered hepatocytes which persist for months and, under appropriate environmental conditions, proliferate to become grossly visible hyperplastic liver nodules—putative precursors of liver cancer (Solt et al. 1977). These focal populations can be detected as early as 7 days after administration of the carcinogen (Ogawa, Solt and Farber, unpublished observations) using enzyme histochemical staining for γ-glutamyl transpeptidase, a product of fetal liver and liver cancers.

The irreversible nature of the initiation phenomenon was demonstrated in skin by varying the interval between application of the initiating agent and that of the promoting agent. In this manner, Berenblum and Shubik (1949) noted persistence of initiated cells for at least 43 weeks in mice. A similar rationale has been used to demonstrate the persistence for 10 months of liver cells which have undergone initiation in response to a potent hepatocarcinogen (Solt and Farber 1976).

The rapid and irreversible nature of initiation suggests that this phenomenon is a mutation. This is further suggested by its relative rarity. Regardless of the nature or potency of the inducing carcinogen, the origin of the tumor is almost invariably a random phenomenon occurring in isolated cells or cell nests that initially comprise only a relatively small proportion of the target tissue. Evidence of the random focal nature of tumor origins has been obtained from studies in a variety of tissues, including skin (Berenblum 1954), breast (Pullinger 1952) and liver (Kitagawa and Pitot 1975; Solt et al. 1977).

4. PROMOTION IS SLOW AND PARTIALLY REVERSIBLE

In contrast to initiation, tumor promotion is a slow and at least partially reversible process. In two-stage skin carcinogenesis, croton oil or other promoting agents must be applied repeatedly (usually two or more times a week) for three or four months. Several observations indicate that the effect is reversible until a short time before tumors begin to emerge. The regression of rabbit skin papillomas which ensues when tarring is discontinued (Rous and Kidd 1941) may serve as one instance of the apparent reversibility of promotion. Another example is provided by work on mouse skin. By varying the dose and time interval between applications, Boutwell (1964) showed that the promoting effect of croton oil is cumulative only if given in sufficient amounts at each application and if the interval between applications is not unduly prolonged. He also provided data suggesting that promotion in mouse skin may be divided into demonstrable stages by initiating mouse skin with dimethylbenz(a)anthracene and promoting with either croton oil, turpentine, or a combination of both agents. In the latter instance, each agent was administered for half the promotion interval and in succession. The results showed that while turpentine alone was an inefficient promoting agent, it would result in tumor emergence when its application was preceded by that of croton oil (i.e., turpentine could finish the promotion process, but not start it). Boutwell proposed the term "conversion" for an early phase of promotion, indicating that potential tumor cells are converted to actual tumor cells, and "propagation" for a later phase which results in proliferation to a grossly visible tumor. Presumably, any hyperplastic agent could act as a propagator to complete the final stage of the carcinogenic process.

The partially reversible nature of tumor development is also evident in experimental liver carcinogenesis. Hyperplastic liver nodules, putative precursors for liver cancer, which form during the administration of chemical hepatocarcinogens, frequently undergo a type of regression when carcinogen treatment is discontinued (Goldfarb 1973; Farber 1976a). During this process, once pale nodules become mottled with the reddish-brown coloration characteristic of normal, mature liver. Microscopically, the hepatocytes in these remodelling nodules become smaller and reorganized into one-cell-thick plates (Farber 1976a) and simultaneously regain the histochemical properties of normal liver (Kitagawa and Pitot 1975). Some nodules slowly undergo this apparent regression process and blend almost imperceptibly with the surrounding liver, while other nodules seem to persist indefinitely. Using interrupted cycles of dietary carcinogen administration, Teebor and Becker (1971) have demonstrated a late conversion from regressing to persistent hyperplastic liver nodules. Three cycles of carcinogen exposure produced multiple liver nodules which regressed when the carcinogen feeding was discontinued. One additional cycle of carcinogen feeding resulted in a high proportion of persistent nodules and a highly significant increase in the number of liver cancers. Thus, the step-wise or divisible nature of tumor promotion previously recognized in skin may have a counterpart in liver carcinogenesis. Moreover, the evidence from both systems suggests that the reversible nature of the promotion phenomenon diminishes in the later stages of tumor development.

5. CELL PROLIFERATION ENHANCES RISK OF CARCINOGENESIS

Cell proliferation appears to play a major role in tumor development, both at the initiation step and during the promotion phase. The majority of human malignant tumors develop in epithelial surfaces which are engaged in continuous proliferative or physiological regeneration (Oehlert 1973). In nonproliferating or slowly proliferating tissues, malignant tumors frequently arise following a process of reparative growth. This is seen, for example, in liver cirrhosis, a condition in which cellular damage and nodular regeneration are accompanied by an increased risk of liver cancer development (Popper 1977). Evidence that cell proliferation can affect the initiation phase of skin carcinogenesis was provided by the work of Frei and Ritchie (1964). In confirmation of an earlier investigation (Mottram 1945), Frei and Ritchie demonstrated that more papillomas developed in mouse skin when the inducing carcinogenic hydrocarbon was given near midnight rather than near midday. They also observed that the numbers of epidermal cells synthesizing DNA was greater at night and suggested that replicating cells might be the principal targets of the inducing carcinogen. These conclusions were reinforced when croton oil was used as an inducer of DNA synthesis. In the classical experiments on initiation and promotion, the promoting agent always follows the initiating dose of the carcinogen. Administration of these agents in the reverse order does not result in enhancement of tumor yield if application of the initiator follows the promotor by three or more days (Berenblum 1941). However, croton oil and several other agents will increase tumor yield when administered during a period of one or two days prior to the application of the initiating dose (Pound 1968). A possible explanation for these observations is that the enhanced cell proliferation known to follow the application of croton oil and other skin irritants increases the risk of initiation.

This hypothesis was tested by applying a single initiating dose of urethane or 7,12-dimethylbenz(a)anthracene to mouse skin pretreated with croton oil (Shinozuka and Ritchie 1967). The initiators were applied to groups of mice either at 23 hr after croton oil administration, to coincide with the peak in DNA synthesis, or at 72 hr, by which time the phase of croton oil induced proliferation was completed. The results showed that application of urethane and 7,12-diethylbenz(a)anthracene during the peak of DNA synthesis resulted in an enhancement of initiation, as determined by papilloma formation after subsequent promotion. In addition to croton oil, other insults including scarification and acetic acid have been shown to enhance the risk of initiation with urethane by enhancing epidermal cell proliferation (Pound 1968).

Cell proliferation may also play a key role in the promotion phase of skin tumorogenesis. An impressive hyperplasia invariably accompanies the application of effective promoting agents to the epidermal surface (Shubik

1950). However, nonspecific proliferatory stimuli alone are not, except in the case of rabbit skin, sufficient to exert a promotional influence (Shubik 1950).

Extensive studies in chemical hepatocarcinogenesis reinforce the observations in skin that cell proliferation is an important factor in cancer development. In adult animals, the rate of liver cell proliferation is very low and a single treatment with hepatocarcinogen rarely induces liver cancer (Craddock 1976). However, a single treatment may be effective when given to animals in which the rate of liver cell replication is high, as in neonates or in animals in which reparative hyperplasia has been induced by partial hepatectomy, or by treatment with an hepatotoxin (Craddock 1976). Dimethylnitrosamine, for example, is a potent carcinogen which will induce liver cell cancer in adult rats when fed continuously in the diet, but will induce only kidney tumors when administered in a single administration. However, one injection of dimethylnitrosamine will cause liver cell tumors in newborn rats and in adult rats which have been subjected to partial hepatectomy, resulting in reparative hyperplasia (Craddock 1976). As a general rule, agents which induce liver cell cancer only when coupled with partial hepatectomy are most effective when given during the peak of DNA synthesis which, in rats, occurs at 24 hr after surgery.

An important observation on the possible role of cell proliferation in carcinogenesis was made by Maini and Stich (1961), who found that certain aminoazo compounds when fed in the diet induced replication of hepatocytes, while others given in association with partial hepatectomy produced chromosomal damage. Carcinogenic compounds caused both replication and damage to chromosomes. Thus, 2-Methyldimethylaminoazobenzene (2-MeDAB) was found to cause chronic chromosome damage, but when fed in the diet it did not induce cell proliferation or cancer. When 2-MeDAB administration was combined with partial hepatectomy, as an independent stimulus for mitosis, cancer of the liver was induced (Warwick 1967). These experiments lead one to suspect an important association between replication of damaged cells and the process of carcinogenesis. While the explanation of the increased sensitivity of replicating cells to carcinogenic action is by no means certain, it may result in part from DNA damage and aberrant replication which "fixes" a change and thereby serves as the essential event in initiation of carcinogenesis (Craddock 1976). This idea agrees with the concept that both genetic damage and cell replication may be essential for carcinogenesis (Borek and Sachs 1968) and with the observation that most carcinogens are mutagenic (Ames and McCann 1976).

6. TUMOR PROGRESSION AND CLONAL SELECTION

The rather rigid two-stage scheme of skin carcinogenesis is easily assimilated within the broader concept of tumor progression, as envisaged by Foulds (1965). Largely as a result of observations on the development of mouse mammary tumors, he defined characteristics of the progression of a neoplasm from its earliest detectable form, usually a benign lesion, to a rapidly growing, highly malignant, invasive neoplasm (Foulds 1965, 1969, 1975). Among the features of tumor progression defined were (1) the independent progression of tumors, and (2) the independent progression of characteristics. Tumors within the same host were thus believed to independently acquire individual characteristics of morphology, growth rate, hormone responsiveness, invasiveness and metastatic potential. In a similar fashion, it was recognized that individual tumors independently underwent qualitative changes in their characteristics with time.

The basic features of tumor progression are perhaps best defined in mouse mammary tumors which frequently develop focal lesions showing morphologic variations (Foulds 1969, 1976). These variant areas, because of their random distribution, their individual but homogeneous morphology, and their frequently spherical shape, present the striking impression to the observer that they represent proliferating subclones derived from the original neoplasm (Prehn 1976). The clonal nature of such variant areas developing both within malignant tumors and within preneoplastic mammary lesions (hyperplastic nodules) is further suggested by their relatively stable patterns of inheritance in the course of transplantation studies (Henderson and Rous 1962; Slemmer 1974).

There is considerable evidence that tumors undergo progression by a process of selection of clones of variant cells (Prehn 1976; Nowel 1976). Three lines of evidence indicate that most tumors are populations of cells originating from a single cell. Cytogenetic studies have demonstrated that many neoplasms in man are comprised of cells which share either the same abnormal karyotype or marker chromosome, suggesting a derivation from a common progenitor or "stem-line" (Nowell 1975). Studies of the isozymes of glucose-6-phosphate dehydrogenase in tumors of heterozygous females demonstrate a single isomeric form of the enzyme, indicating inactivation of the same member of a pair of x-chromosomes and thus providing evidence of descent from a single precursor cell (Fialkow 1972). Similarly, three squamous cell carcinomas of the palate were found to have predominantly single enzyme phenotypes, suggesting a clonal evolution for these tumors (Fialkow 1972). The third line of evidence for the clonal evolution of tumor cell populations is the homogeneity observed in the immunoglobulins produced by plasma cell tumors (Fialkow 1974).

The apparent clonal derivation of tumors, the long latent period associated with tumor development, and the morphological and biochemical evidence indicating a requirement for cell proliferation in the course of tumor development, lend considerable support to the notion that selective proliferation of variant cells is a dominant theme underlying the carcinogenic process. Evidence accrued from studies of chemical carcinogenesis provides some insight into the possible nature of the selection process.

It has long been known that chemically induced neoplasms are somewhat resistant to the toxic effects of chemical carcinogens (Haddow 1938; Prehn 1964). The recognition of this resistance and the general occurrence of cytotoxicity as a consequence of carcinogen exposure, provided the basis for the formulation of a clonal selection theory of chemical carcinogenesis (Prehn 1964). According to this theory, neoplasia occurs as a result of the selection by differential cytotoxicity of spontaneously occurring cellular variants. Although the concept of naturally occurring resistant variants has been discounted on the basis that chemical carcinogens transform (Heidelberger 1973) as well as select, the phenomenon of selective proliferation based on differential cytotoxicity appears to be an important factor in the evolution of chemically induced tumors. This is readily demonstrated in the case of chemical hepatocarcinogenesis.

The hyperplastic liver lesions which develop in response to chemical hepatocarcinogens are partially resistant to the toxic effects of these chemicals, such as their ability to induce liver cell necrosis and inhibit hepatocyte proliferation (Farber 1976b). This resistance may be a consequence of the decreased capacity on the part of hyperplastic liver nodules to take up and metabolize chemical carcinogens to their toxic intermediates (Cameron et al. 1976). In recognition of this fact, it was proposed that the initiating event in chemical hepatocarcinogenesis may be the induction of an altered metabolic pattern in some liver cells (similar to that seen in hyperplastic nodules), so that these cells become resistant and acquire a potential growth advantage over the other hepatocytes in a cytotoxic environment (Solt and Farber 1976). If this is the case, it should be possible to detect and quantitate the altered cells by creating an intense stimulus for their proliferation in the presence of a toxic growth inhibitor that depends on metabolic activation for its effect. Initiated cells with a decreased ability to take up or activate a carcinogen or other growth inhibitor should proliferate rapidly, whereas unaltered hepatocytes should metabolize the inhibitor normally and thereby generate a derivative which inhibits their proliferation.

An in vivo assay system designed to test this hypothesis provides a striking example of selective proliferation of carcinogen altered cells (Solt et al. 1977). The assay system devised consists of a one-week dietary administration of 2-acetylaminofluorene (2-AAF), followed by two-thirds partial hepatectomy. Using this system, resistant ("initiated") hepatocytes have been detected and quantitated in the liver of rats following a single administration of several hepatocarcinogens (Solt et al. 1977). Following partial hepatectomy, microscopic nests of carcinogen altered hepatocytes undergo selective proliferation and enlarge to become visible as greyish-white hyperplastic nodules on the capsular and cut surfaces of the unresected liver lobes within 7 days. These randomly distributed focal lesions are roughly spherical in shape, giving the impression that they are clonal in nature. That the focal lesions (or foci) may indeed represent clones of initiated hepatocytes is suggested by the following: (1) when the foci are induced by diethylnitrosamine (DEN), the number of foci formed is roughly proportional to the dose of DEN; (2) without selection, the foci have apparently not acquired the property of autonomous growth as a result of the inducing carcinogen, but will persist in a latent state for at least several months unless conditions for their selective proliferation are imposed; (3) whereas no cancer arises in unselected foci for at least 9 months, imposition of the conditions necessary for selective proliferation (2-AAF + partial hepatectomy) results in the emergence of hyperplastic liver nodules and a high incidence of liver cancer; (4) the precursor nature of the foci is revealed by the finding that hyperplastic nodules resulting from the selection procedure on rare occasions contain within their confines unequivocal liver cancer; (5) although the entire liver is presumably exposed to the initiating dose of DEN, only 10^3 foci are formed in the exposed liver. Assuming a clonal origin, the induction of resistant foci is thus a rare event, occurring in approximately one in 10^6 original hepatocytes. (6) The induction of foci is a relatively rapid event. Resistant cell populations can be seen as microscopic nests of cells as early as 7 days after administration of DEN, due to their positive histochemical staining for γ-glutamyltranspeptidase (Ogawa, Solt and Farber, unpublished observations), an enzyme characteristic of hyperplastic liver nodules and hepatomas.

The observed resistant qualities of preneoplastic as well as frankly malignant cell populations raises the intriguing possibility that neoplasia may have evolved as a type of protective adaptation to the hostile environment created by the inducing carcinogen. The formation of isolated cell populations able to thrive in a particular inimical environment may have survival value for the host organism. In the case of liver exposed to toxic chemical carcinogens, randomly distributed foci of altered hepatocytes serve as a reserve of resistant liver tissue for replacement of the damaged parenchyma. The evolution of a persistent, adaptive mechanism, which only rarely undergoes progression to malignancy and then only after a long latent period usually extending past the normal reproductive period of the host, would seem to be well suited for species preservation.

One might speculate that the recent association of a squamous cell carcinoma of the buccal mucosa resulting from chronic intra-oral exposure to PVC (polyvinyl chloride, a documented hepatocarcinogen) (Casterline et al. 1977) is an example of the role of cytotoxic selection in the development of an oral malignancy. In this instance, a cancer became clinically evident over a one-week period following a period of active recurrent aphthous stomatitis (stimulus for cell proliferation?) of the buccal mucosa. Perhaps the strongest suggestion that cytotoxic selection may operate in the development of human neoplasia is the well recognized occurrence of second primary neoplasms developing within two to three years after the institution of cancer chemotherapy (Chabner 1977; Reimer et al. 1977).

7. BASIS OF NEOPLASTIC VARIANTS: MUTATION vs ALTERED DIFFERENTIATION

Tumor progression involves a series of qualitative heritable changes in cell populations. A fundamental issue in tumor biology is whether the changes observed in the course of tumor progression require permanent alterations in the cellular genome or are epigenetic in nature and are concerned merely with the changes in the expression of the existing genetic information. The former concept is, of course, based primarily on the widely accepted though unproven belief that all chemical, physical, and biological carcinogenic stimuli are also mutagenic. An alternative view is held by many investigators who envisage carcinogenesis as a type of anomalous differentiation in which the basic cellular mechanisms underlying the neoplastic state are similar to those occurring during the course of development of all metazoan organisms (Pierce 1974; Markert 1968; Potter 1969). This concept gained impetus from the discovery that tumors frequently produce enzymes and other proteins which were previously expressed during normal fetal development (Uriel 1975). The nonmutational concept is further supported by observations that malignant cells can behave normally when placed in a different environment (Mintz and Illmensee 1975; Pierce and Wallace 1971). In one such study (McKinnel et al. 1969) nuclei isolated from frog kidney tumors and transplanted into enucleated frogs' eggs gave rise to functioning tadpoles. That the tumor nuclei had retained the information for a whole range of specialized functions required for tadpole development tends to discount mutation as a prerequisite for the expression of the malignant phenotype. In another study designed to test the "epigenetic" concept of tumorgenesis (Mintz and Illmensee 1975), mouse embryonal malignant carcinoma cells were injected into blastocysts of mice bearing genetic markers. The blastocysts developed into normal, fertile, mosaic mice, having tumor-derived cells in various tissues. This ability of malignant cells to participate in normal development and integrate into normal tissues argues against a simple mutational basis for malignant transformation.

A final argument frequently expressed in opposition to the mutational theory is that there has as yet been no single recognized biological or biochemical characteristic which is unique to cancer (Prehn 1971; Uriel 1975). Trophoblasts and melanoblasts in the course of embryogenesis and mature, functioning leukocytes tend to be "invasive" and/or capable of "metastasis." Probably no neoplasm exceeds the growth rate of the developing embryo or that of the residual liver following two-thirds partial hepatectomy. In addition, although tumors have frequently been shown to produce substances such as fetal antigens or trophic hormones, which seem inappropriate for the tissue of origin, the existence of *new* antigens, enzymes or other tumor products has never been demonstrated.

8. CONCLUSIONS

Carcinogenesis is a developmental process that usually requires several months in experimental animals and years or even decades in man. The process appears to begin as a rapid and irreversible alteration in isolated cells or cell populations. However, the subsequent changes in initiated cells which culminate in malignancy are not inevitable but may depend on other carcinogenic or cocarcinogenic factors operating in the environment. Advances in our basic understanding of the biology of premalignant lesions, including the development of practical techniques for the identification and eradication of premalignant lesions and/or the recognition of the environmental factors which lead to their formation or which encourage their progression to malignancy, could play a valuable role in the future control of oral cancer.

9. SUMMARY

Observations based primarily on in vivo models and on clinicopathological evidence in a variety of human tissues provide a conceptual picture of carcinogenesis which may be applicable to the development of malignancy in the oral cavity. The following concepts and observations, though not universally established as fact, have gained wide support among tumor biologists:

(1) Cancer formation is not a one-step phenomenon, but a multi-stage developmental process.

(2) While the initial event in carcinogenesis can be effected rapidly, the subsequent development of malignancy is invariably of long duration, requiring years or even decades in man. Even in laboratory animals exposed to optimal carcinogenic conditions, tumor evolution requires at least several months.

(3) Initiated cell populations, when detectable within tissues previously exposed to potent carcinogens, are frequently seen to be randomly distributed and clonal in nature. Their subsequent evolution to malignancy is not inevitable, but may depend on carcinogenic or cocarcinogenic environmental factors (dietary, hormonal, chemical, physical, biological, etc.). Such factors may act in part by causing the selective proliferation of variant clones of initiated cells.

(4) Although successive stages of carcinogenesis may be partially reversible, the initial event appears to be essentially irreversible and persistent throughout the normal lifespan of the individual.

(5) Although the initial event in carcinogenesis is mutational or "mutation-like," the subsequent alterations leading to malignant neoplasia may be similar to the process of differentiation in metazoan organisms, in that they proceed in the absence of any proven alteration in the genetic constitution of the participating cells.

REFERENCES

Ames, B. N., Lee, F. D., and Durston, W. E. 1973. An improved bacterial test system for the detection and classification of mutagens and carcinogens. *Proc. Natl. Acad. Sci. USA* **70**, 782–786.

Ames, B. N., and McCann, J. 1976. Carcinogens are mutagens: A simple test system. In: *Screening Tests in Chemical Carcinogenesis.* (Edited by Montesano, R., Bartsch, H. and Tomatis, L.), IARC Scientific Publications No. 12, pp. 493–502. International Agency for Research on Cancer, Lyon.

Ball, J. K. and McCarter, J. A. 1960. A study of dose and effect in initiation of skin tumors by a carcinogenic hydrocarbon. *Br. J. Cancer* **14**, 577–590.

Berenblum, I. 1941. Mechanism of carcinogenesis: A study of the significance of cocarcinogenic action and related phenomena. *Cancer Res.* **1**, 807-814.

Berenblum, I. 1954. Speculative review: Probable nature of promoting action and its significance in understanding of mechanism of carcinogenesis. *Cancer Res.* **14**, 471–477.

Berenblum I. 1975. Sequential aspects of chemical carcinogenesis: Skin. In: *Cancer.* (Edited by Becker, F. F.), Vol. 1, Chap. 10, pp. 323-344. Plenum Press, New York.

Berenblum, I. and Shubik, P. 1947. The role of croton oil application associated with a single painting of a carcinogen in tumour induction of the mouse's skin. *Br. J. Cancer* **1**, 379–391.

Berenblum, I., and Shubik, P. 1949. The persistence of latent tumour cells induced in mouse's skin by single application of 9:10 dimethyl-1:2-benzanthracene. *Br. J. Cancer* **3**, 384–386.

Borek, C., and Sachs, L. 1968. The number of cell generations required to fix the transformed state in X-ray-induced transformation. *Proc. Natl. Acad. Sci. USA* **59**, 83–85.

Boutwell, R. K. 1964. Some biological aspects of skin carcinogenesis. *Prog. Exp. Tumor Res.* **4**, 207–250.

Bryan, C. E., Skipper, H. E., and White, L., Jr. 1949. Carbamates in chemotherapy of leucemia; distribution of radioactivity in tissues of mice following injection of carbonyl-labeled urethane. *J. Biol. Chem.* **177**, 941–950.

Cameron, R., Sweeney, G. D., Jones, K., Lee, G., and Farber, E. 1976. A relative deficiency of cytochrome P-450 and aryl hydrocarbon (benzo(a)pyrene) hydroxylase in hyperplastic nodules induced by 2-acetylaminofluorene in rat liver. *Cancer Res.* **36**, 3888–3893.

Casterline, C. L., Casterline, P. F., and Jaques, D. A. 1977. Squamous cell carcinoma of the buccal mucosa associated with chronic oral polyvinyl chloride exposure: Report of a case. *Cancer* **39**, 1686–1688.

Chabner, B. A. 1977. Second neoplasm: A complication of cancer chemotherapy. *N. Engl. J. Med.* **297**, 213–215.

Craddock, V. M. 1976. Cell proliferation and experimental liver cancer. In: *Liver Cell Cancer*. (Edited by Cameron, H. M., Linsell, D. A., and Warwick, G. P.), Chap. 8, p. 163. Elsevier, Amsterdam.

Early lesions and the development of epithelial cancer. 1976. Symposium. Sponsored by the Carcinogenesis Program, Division of Cancer Cause and Prevention, National Cancer Institute. *Cancer Res.* **36**, 2475–2706.

Farber, E. 1973. Carcinogenesis: Cellular evolution as a unifying thread: Presidential address. *Cancer Res.* **33**, 2537–2550.

Farber, E. 1976. The pathology of experimental liver cancer. In: *Liver Cell Cancer*. (Edited by Cameron, H. M., Linsell, D. A., and Warwick, G. P.), Chap. 10, p. 243. Elsevier/North Holland, Amsterdam.

Farber, E., Parker, S., and Gruenstein, M. 1976. The resistance of putative premalignant liver cell populations, hyperplastic nodules, to the acute cytotoxic effects of some hepatocarcinogens. *Cancer Res.* **36**, 3879–3887.

Fialkow, P. J. 1972. Use of genetic markers to study cellular origin and development of tumors in human females. *Adv. Cancer Res.* **15**, 191–226.

Fialkow, P. J. 1974. The origin and development of human tumors studied with cell markers. *N. Engl. J. Med.* **291**, 26–35.

Foulds, L. 1965. Multiple etiologic factors in neoplastic development. *Cancer Res.* **25**, 1339–1347.

Foulds, L. 1969. *Neoplastic Development*. Vol. 1. Academic Press, London.

Foulds, L. 1975. *Neoplastic Development*. Vol. 2. Academic Press, London.

Frei, J. V., and Ritchie, A. C. 1964. Diurnal variation in the susceptibility of mouse epidermis to carcinogen and its relationship to DNA synthesis. *J. Natl. Cancer Inst.* **32**, 1213–1220.

Friedell, G. H. 1976. Carcinoma, carcinoma in situ, and "early lesions" of the uterine cervix and the urinary bladder: Introduction and definitions. *Cancer Res.* **36**, 2482–2484.

Gelboin, H. V., Klein, M., and Bates, R. R. 1965. Inhibition of mouse skin tumorigenesis by actinomycin D. *Proc. Natl. Acad. Sci. USA* **53**, 1353–1360.

Goldfarb, S. 1973. A morphological and histochemical study of carcinogenesis of the liver in rats fed 3-methyl-4-dimethylaminoazobenzene. *Cancer Res.* **33**, 1119–1128.

Haddow, A. 1938. Cellular inhibition and origin of cancer. *Acta Unio. Internat. Contre Cancer* **3**, 342–352.

Haran, N., and Berenblum, I. 1956. The induction of the initiating phase of skin carcinogenesis in mouse by oral administration of urethane (ethyl carbamate). *Br. J. Cancer* **10**, 57–60.

Heath, D. F. 1962. The decomposition and toxicity of dialkylnitrosamines in rats. *Biochem. J.* **83**, 72–91.

Heidelberger, C. 1973. Chemical oncogenesis in culture. *Adv. Cancer Res.* **18**, 317–366.

Henderson, J. S., and Rous, P. 1962. The plating of tumor components on the subcutaneous expanses of young mice. Findings with benign and malignant epidermal growths and with mammary carcinomas. *J. Exp. Med.* **115**, 1211–1230.

Hicks, R. M., Wakefield, J. St. J., and Chownaiec, J. 1973. Co-carcinogenic action of saccharin in the chemical induction of bladder cancer. *Nature* **243**, 347–349.

Kitagawa, T., and Pitot, H. C. 1975. The regulation of serine dehydratase and glucose-6-phosphatase in hyperplastic nodules of rat liver during diethylnitrosamine and N-2-fluorenylacetamide feeding. *Cancer Res.* **35**, 1075–1084.

Lane, N., and Fenoglio, C. M. 1976. I. Observations on the adenoma as precursor to ordinary large bowel carcinoma. *Gastrointest. Radiol.* **1**, 111–119.

Linder, D. and Gartler, S. M. 1965. Glucose-6-phosphate dehydrogenase mosaicism: Utilization as a cell marker in the study of leiomyomas. *Science* **150**, 67–69.

Maini, M. M., and Stich, H. F. 1961. Chromosomes of tumor cells. II. Effect of various liver carcinogens on mitosis of hepatic cells. *J. Natl. Canc. Inst.* **26**, 1413–1427.

Markert, C. L. 1968. Neoplasia: A disease of cell differentiation. *Cancer Res.* **28**, 1908–1914.

McKinnell, R. G., Deggins, B. A., and Labat, D. D. 1969. Transplantation of pluripotential nuclei from triploid frog tumors. *Science* **165**, 394–396.

Miller, E. C., and Miller, J. A. 1971. The mutagenicity of chemical carcinogens: Correlations, problems, and interpretations. In: *Chemical Mutagens.* (Edited by Hollaender, A.), Vol. I, Chap. 3, pp. 83–119. Plenum Press, New York.

Miller, J. A. 1970. Carcinogenesis by chemicals: An overview. G. H. A. Clowes Memorial Lecture. *Cancer Res.* **30**, 559–576.

Mintz, B., and Illmensee, K. 1975. Normal genetically mosaic mice produced from malignant teratocarcinoma cells. *Proc. Natl. Acad. Sci. USA* **72**, 3585–3589.

Mottram, J. C. 1944a. Developing factor in experimental blastogenesis. *J. Path. and Bact.* **56**, 181–187.

Mottram, J. C. 1944b. Sensitising factor in experimental blastogenesis. *J. Path. and Bact.* **56**, 391–402.

Mottram, J. C. 1945. A diurnal variation in production of tumours. *J. Path. and Bact.* **57**, 265–267.

Nowell, P. C. 1975. Cytogenetics. In: *Cancer.* (Edited by Becker, F. F.), Vol. 1, Chap. 1, pp. 3–31. Plenum Press, New York.

Nowell, P. C. 1976. The clonal evolution of tumor cell populations. *Science* **194**, 23–28.

Oehlert, W. 1973. Cellular proliferation in carcinogenesis. *Cell. Tissue Kinet.* **6**, 325–335.

Peraino, C., Fry, R. J., Staffeldt, E., and Kisieleski, W. E. 1973. Effects of varying the exposure to phenobarbital on its enhancement of 2-acetylaminofluorene-induced hepatic tumorigenesis in the rat. *Cancer Res.* **33**, 2701–2705.

Pierce, G. B. 1974. The benign cells of malignant tumors. In: *Developmental Aspects of Carcinogenesis and Immunity*. (Edited by King, T. J.), pp. 3–33. Academic Press, New York.

Pierce, G. B., and Wallace, C. 1971. Differentiation of malignant to benign cells. *Cancer Res.* **31**, 127–134.

Popper, H. 1977. Pathologic aspects of cirrhoses. A review. *Am. J. Pathol.* **87**, 228–264.

Potter, V. R. 1969. Recent trends in cancer biochemistry. The importance of studies of fetal tissue. *Canad. Cancer Conf.* **8**, 9–30.

Pound, A. W. 1968. Carcinogenesis and cell proliferation. *New Zeal. Med. J.* **67**, 88–99.

Prehn, R. T. 1964. A clonal selection theory of chemical carcinogenesis. *J. Natl. Cancer Inst.* **32**, 1–17.

Prehn, R. T. 1971. Immunosurveillance, regeneration and oncogenesis. *Prog. Exp. Tumor Res.* **14**, 1–24.

Prehn, R. T. 1976. Tumor progression and homeostasis. *Adv. Cancer Res.* **23**, 203–236.

Pullinger, B. D. 1952. Spontaneous mammary adenoma and carcinoma in RIIIb mice deprived of milk agent. *Br. J. Cancer* **6**, 69–77.

Reddy, B. S., Watanabe, K., Weisburger, J. H., and Wynder, E. L. 1977. Promoting effect of bile acids in colon carcinogenesis in germ-free and conventional F344 rats. *Cancer Res.* **37**, 3238–3242.

Reimer, R. R., Hoover, R., Fraumeni, J. F., Jr., and Young, R. C. 1977. Acute leukemia after alkylating-agent therapy of ovarian cancer. *N. Engl. J. Med.* **297**, 177–181.

Rous, P., and Kidd, J. G. 1941. Conditional neoplasms and subthreshold neoplastic states: A study of tar tumors of rabbits. *J. Exp. Med.* **73**, 365–390.

Salaman, M. H., and Roe, F. J. 1953. Incomplete carcinogens: Ethyl carbamate (urethane) as an initiator of skin tumour formation in the mouse. *Br. J. Cancer* **7**, 472–481.

Shinozuka, H., and Ritchie, A. C. 1967. Pretreatment with croton oil, DNA synthesis, and carcinogens followed by croton oil. *Int. J. Cancer* **2**, 77–84.

Shubik, P. 1950. Studies on promoting phase in stages of carcinogenesis in mice, rats, rabbits, and guinea pigs. *Cancer Res.* **10**, 13–17.

Slemmer, G. 1974. Proceedings: Interactions of separate types of cells during normal and neoplastic mammary gland growth. *J. Invest. Dermatol.* **63**, 24–47.

Solt, D., and Farber, E. 1976. New principle for the analysis of chemical carcinogenesis. *Nature* **263**, 701–703.

Solt, D. B., Medline, A., and Farber, E. 1977. Rapid emergence of carcinogen-induced hyperplastic lesions in a new model for the sequential analysis of liver carcinogenesis. *Am. J. Path.* **88**, 595–618.

Spratt, J. S., Jr., and Ackerman, L. V. 1962. Small primary adenocarcinomas of the colon and rectum. *JAMA* **179**, 337–346.

Stich, H. F., and San, R. H. C. 1971. Reduced DNA repair synthesis in xeroderma pigmentosum cells exposed to the oncogenic 4-nitroquinoline-1-oxide and 4-hydroxy-aminoquinlin-1-oxide. *Mutat. Res.* **13**, 279–282.

Teebor, G. W., and Becker, F. F. 1971. Regression and persistence of hyperplastic hepatic nodules induced by N-2-fluorenylacetamide and their relationship to hepatocarcinogenesis. *Cancer Res.* **31**, 1–3.

Uriel, J. 1975. Fetal characteristics of cancer. In: *Cancer*. (Edited by Becker, F. F.), Vol. 3, Chap. 2, pp. 21–55. Plenum Press, New York.

Warwick, G. P. 1967. The covalent binding of metabolites of tritiated 2-methyl-4-dimethylaminoazobenzene to rat liver nucleic acids and proteins, and the carcinogenicity of the unlabelled compound in partially hepatectomized rats. *Eur. J. Cancer* **3**, 227–233.

Wynder, E. L., and Hoffman, D. 1967. *Tobacco and Tobacco Smoke: Studies in Experimental Carcinogenesis*. Academic Press, New York.

5

Candida Leukoplakia and Carcinoma: A Possible Relationship

R. A. CAWSON and W. H. BINNIE

Department of Oral Medicine and Pathology, Guy's Hospital Medical School, London, England

1. INTRODUCTION

Chronic infection of the oral mucous membrane by *Candida albicans* can give rise to persistent, firm white lesions justifying the clinical title of leukoplakia and appearing clinically similar to other varieties. It is accepted that leukoplakia in general is a precancerous condition, but the magnitude of the risk for specific etiologic types of leukoplakia remains in doubt. Studies to determine the rate of transition to carcinoma vary widely in their findings and no extensive study has concentrated on a single histological or etiological type of leukoplakia (see chapters 1 and 2).

2. ORAL LEUKOPLAKIA AS A PRECANCEROUS LESION

The reputation of oral leukoplakia as a precancerous disease depends upon reports of series of cases showing a higher incidence of carcinoma in association with leukoplakia than in normal patients, i.e., the evidence is essentially epidemiological in character (see chapter 1). In addition, varying degrees of epithelial dysplasia are seen on histological examination of leukoplakias, but, inevitably, no large series exists where histologically benign lesions have been followed stage by stage and a progressive change to carcinoma shown. There is virtually no direct evidence of a cause and effect relationship between any of the known causes of leukoplakia and carcinoma.

Estimates of the incidence of carcinoma in leukoplakias vary widely and are discussed in chapters 1 and 2.

3. CHRONIC CANDIDIASIS AS A CAUSE OF LEUKOPLAKIA

While accepting that leukoplakia in general (as defined by Pindborg et al. 1968) is a precancerous lesion, there may still be lingering doubts as to whether candida infection is in fact a cause of leukoplakia or is, as stated by Jepsen and Winther (1965), Pindborg et al. (1968), and others, a "superimposed" infection. This concept, however, requires *first* that evidence be found of preexistence of an earlier lesion which has become infected by candida. *Second*, it ignores longstanding evidence that chronic candidiasis can cause leukoplakia lesions even in children, i.e., in an age group not otherwise subject to leukoplakia. Accounts of these lesions in mucocutaneous candidiasis, by Thorpe and Handley (1929) for instance, extend back for nearly half a century.

4. CANDIDA LESIONS

4:1 CLINICAL ASPECTS

Candidal leukoplakia cannot be recognized by its clinical features alone, but the plaque is usually irregular in thickness and texture and is speckled in character.

In a study that will be discussed in this chapter, a group of 30 patients showing histological evidence of candida leukoplakia was examined. There was a high incidence (i.e., 15 out of 30) of speckled lesions consisting of many firm white flecks or nodules on an erythematous velvety background, while the remainder showed a more or less continuous plaque of variable thickness.

The extent of the lesions was somewhat related to age. All those with mild lesions, i.e., of about 1 sq. cm total extent or less, were 40 years of age or younger. All those with more extensive lesions and who subsequently developed carcinoma (see section 5) were over 50.

In Jepsen and Winther's 1965 series (notwithstanding the interpretation they placed upon their finding), all 11 of the speckled leukoplakias examined histologically showed the features of chronic candidiasis. Of 23 speckled leukoplakias, 21 yielded *Candida albicans* on culture, and treatment with nystatin caused these lesions to lose their speckled character.

4:2 HISTOLOGICAL FEATURES

The diagnosis of candidiasis was made where there was clear evidence of invasion of the epithelium by hyphae of *Candida albicans* with a hyperplastic epithelial response and characteristic inflammatory changes. The essential findings were as follows (Figs. 1–3):

Hyphae.

These were rarely visible in hematoxylin and eosin stained sections, but showed up clearly by the periodic acid Schiff method. The hyphae grew more or less at right angles to the surface and penetrated the epithelial plaque to the glycogen-rich zone. Deeper penetration was not seen.

Epithelial reaction.

The plaque was always parakeratotic in character and well-nucleated cells were apparent even in the most superficial layers.

Superficial inflammatory reaction.

A superficial (intraepithelial) inflammatory reaction is characteristic and was usually most intense at the base of the plaque, that is between the parakeratotic zone and the deeper layers. Polymorphonuclear leukocytes were numerous and edema appeared as beads of fluid which tended to coalesce along the junction between the two zones, causing some separation between them. In some cases, collections of leukocytes produced microabscesses at the base of the plaque.

Deeper epithelial reaction.

All grades of reaction were seen from mild acanthosis to dysplasia and frank squamous cell carcinoma. The epithelium was hyperplastic in all cases.

Connective tissue.

There was a subepithelial inflammatory reaction. The chronic inflammatory infiltrate was mixed in character; occasionally there were follicular aggregations of lymphocytes, but no consistent pattern was apparent.

5. INCIDENCE OF DYSPLASIA AND CARCINOMA IN ASSOCIATION WITH CHRONIC CANDIDIASIS

Pindborg et al. (1963) emphasized the importance of speckled leukoplakias as showing an abnormally high incidence of malignant change. In their later study, Pindborg et al. (1968) again noted that a majority of their patients who had speckled lesions developed carcinoma. Renstrup (1970) found no fewer than 61% of speckled leukoplakias showed candida invasion and of these, 71% were characterized by epithelial atypia. Only 3% of the "homogeneous" leukoplakias showed candida and in none was atypia present. Roed-Petersen et al. (1970) found that 40% of leukoplakias invaded by candida showed atypia and that in 67% of leukoplakias showing atypia, candida was present, but these workers still had reservations about the relationship of the fungus to the epithelial changes.

In the present series an attempt was made to follow all patients from whom histological material was available but, partly due to the lapse of some years since the initial biopsy, a high proportion, particularly among those with mild lesions, was lost to follow-up. Of the 30 patients with chronic hyperplastic candidiasis (candida leukoplakia), 9 (i.e., 30%) are known to have developed carcinoma. Of 153 other (non-candida) leukoplakias only 16 (i.e., 10%) were known ultimately to have developed carcinoma.

All of the candida leukoplakias where carcinoma developed within the period of observation had a speckled appearance. This suggests that speckled plaques are more likely to be due to candidiasis than other causes and are more likely to show dyskeratosis or to undergo malignant change.

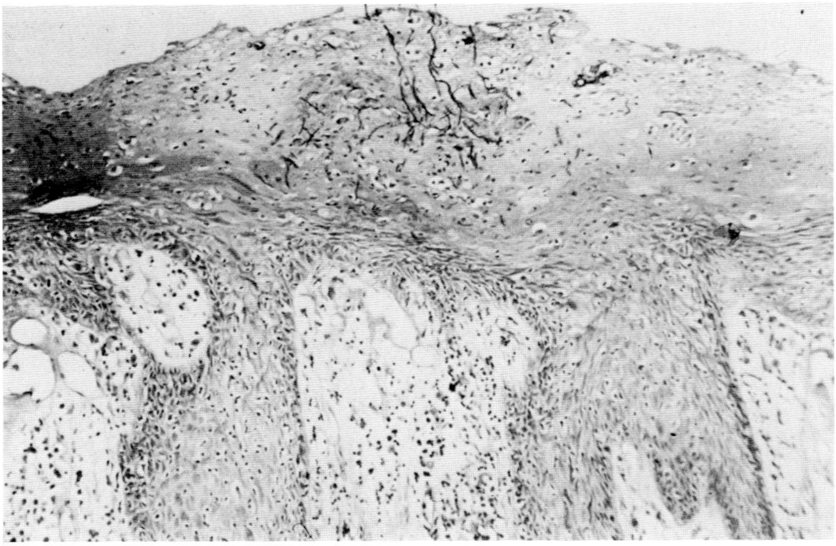

FIGURE 1. Section showing invasion of candidal hyphae through the superficial parakeratinized plaque as far as the glycogen rich layer. There is mild acanthosis and the dermal papillae are inflamed and edematous. Periodic acid–Schiff. X 70.

6. SYSTEMIC FACTORS IN CANDIDA LEUKOPLAKIA

Higgs and Wells (1972) have established that the most consistent metabolic abnormality associated with chronic mucocutaneous candidiasis is iron deficiency. Earlier, Rose (1968) had shown that there was a significant association between angular cheilosis and iron deficiency, and suggested that iron deficiency impaired the metabolism of the epithelial cells and favored the growth of *Candida albicans* or other organisms. There is no doubt as to the effects of severe iron deficiency on the oral mucosa, as evidenced by the characteristic sign of atrophic glossitis. On the other hand, iron deficiency has also been associated with oral cancer in the Paterson-Kelly (Plummer Vinson) syndrome; Ahlbom (1936), Wynder and Fryer (1958), Shamma'a and Benedict (1958), Watts (1961), and others have reported series of patients with Paterson-Kelly syndrome who developed single or multiple oral cancers. The relationship between candida and oral cancer may thus be multifactorial and if there ultimately proves to be a significant association between chronic candidiasis and cancer, this may be mediated by way of a defect of iron metabolism. Joynson et al. (1972) have demonstrated an impairment of cell-mediated immunity in iron deficient patients and, in their words, "this condition carries important implications with regard to the pathogenesis of malignant disease and chronic infections such as candidiasis." However the relation between immunity and cancer is complex and is discussed in chapters 16, 17, and 21.

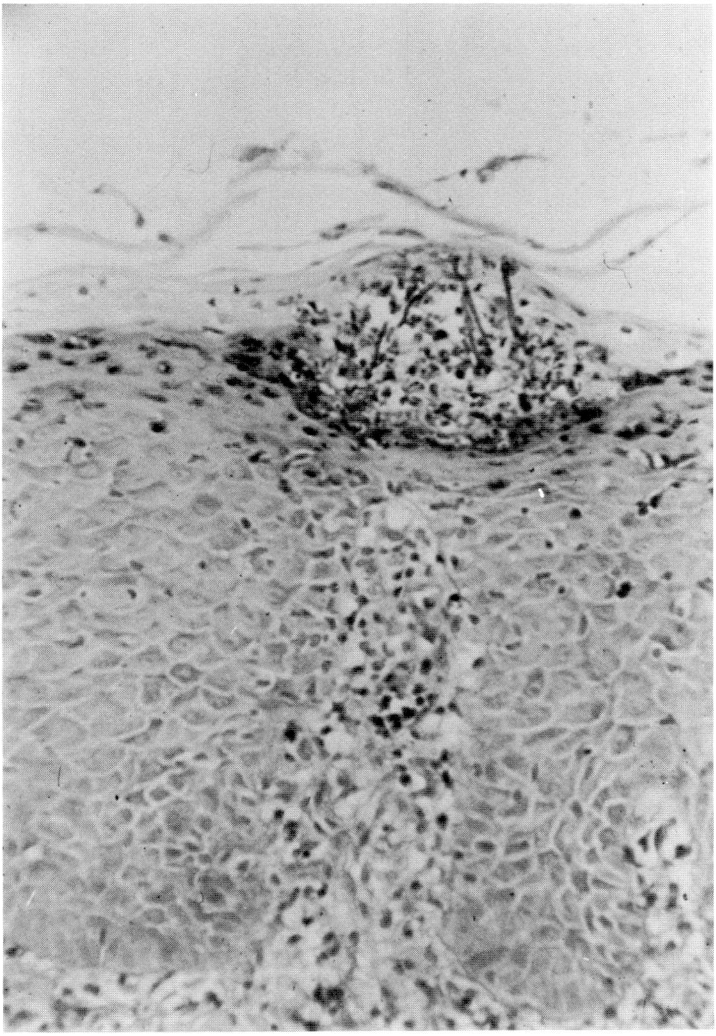

FIGURE 2. Superficial inflammatory reaction. A micro-abscess with hyphae in the parakeratinized layer. Periodic acid–Schiff. X 170.

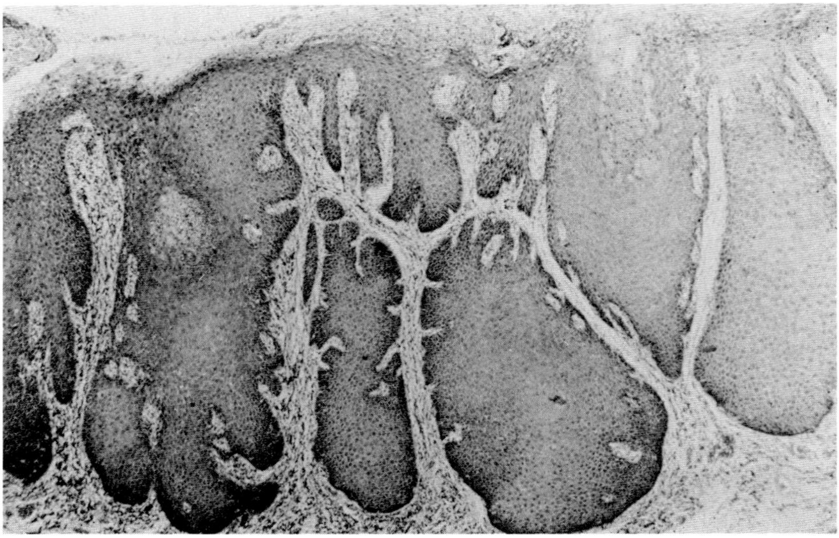

FIGURE 3. Epithelial hyperplasia. There is severe acanthosis with moderate cell atypia. The dermal papillae extend close to the surface and there is a diffuse mixed mononuclear cell infiltrate in the corium. Hematoxylin and eosin. X 30.

7. EXPERIMENTAL FINDINGS RELEVANT TO THE BEHAVIOR OF CANDIDA LEUKOPLAKIA

Experimental infection of the chick embryo chorioallantoic membrane shows a uniform response characterized by epithelial hyperplasia and formation of plaque invaded by candida hyphae (Cawson 1973). Russell and Jones (1973) have also shown that essentially similar hyperplastic lesions can be induced in the rat.

Ultrastructural investigation has established that the hyperplastic lesions of mucosal candidiasis are characterized by intracellular parasitization of the epithelial cell by the hyphae of candida. Hyphae of candida also undergo considerable changes in ultrastructural organization of cytoplasmic organelles following the transition from extracellular to intracellular habitat (Cawson and Rajasingham 1972). This mode of growth of *Candida albicans* suggests a means whereby it can affect the metabolism and behavior of the epithelial cell in fundamental fashion. Proliferation of the epithelium is clearly one of the consequences (see chapter 4).

8. CONCLUSION

It would be quite unjustifiable on present evidence to state categorically that chronic candidiasis per se is a precancerous condition. Nevertheless, data from the present paper and earlier reports indicate that there is a relationship between chronic candidiasis and squamous cell carcinoma. This relationship is based on the following findings:

(a) Chronic candidiasis itself is a cause of leukoplakic lesions and as such must be regarded as having possible premalignant potential.

(b) Clinically, candida leukoplakias are frequently "speckled" in character and these lesions have been shown to be especially likely to show epithelial dysplasia or carcinoma.

(c) On the basis of the cases described both here and in earlier papers, there is evidence of at least an association between chronic candidiasis and cancer and this association seems to be somewhat stronger than for many other types of leukoplakia.

(d) Unlike other types of leukoplakia, a possible mechanism can be demonstrated as to how chronic candida infection might disturb epithelial cellular activity in a way that could lead to neoplastic change, in that:

(1) in experimental candidal infection, chick embryo ectoderm undergoes squamous metaplasia and proliferative activity and produces hyperplastic plaques;

(2) ultrastructural investigation shows that *Candida albicans* is an intracellular parasite of epithelial cells and might affect the behavior of epithelia.

(e) Iron deficiency has for long been known to have profound effects on the oral mucosa and also to have associations both with oral and pharyngeal cancer (Paterson-Kelly Syndrome) and with chronic candidiasis.

REFERENCES

Ahlbom, H. E. 1936. Simple achlorhydric anaemia, Plummer-Vinson syndrome, and carcinoma of the mouth, pharynx and oesophagus in women. Observations at Radiumhemmet, Stockholm. *Br. Med. J.* **2**, 331–333.

Cawson, R. A. 1973. Induction of epithelial hyperplasia by Candida albicans. *Br. J. Dermatol.* **89**, 497–503.

Cawson, R. A., and Rajasingham, K. C. 1972. Ultrastructural features of the invasive phase of Candida albicans. *Br. J. Dermatol.* **87**, 435–443.

Einhorn, J., and Wersäll, J. 1967. Incidence of oral carcinoma in patients with leukoplakia of the oral mucosa. *Cancer* **20**, 2189–2193.

Higgs, J. M., and Wells, R. S. 1972. Chronic muco-cutaneous candidiasis: Associated abnormalities of iron metabolism. *Br. J. Dermatol.* **86**, Suppl. 8, 88–102.

Jepsen, A., and Winther, J. E. 1965. Mycotic infection in oral leukoplakia. *Acta Odont. Scand.* **23**, 239–256.

Joynson, D. H., Walker, D. M., Jacobs, A., and Dolby, A. E. 1972. Defect of cell-mediated immunity in patients with iron-deficiency anaemia. *Lancet* **2**, 1058–1059.

Pindborg, J. J., Renstrup, G., Poulsen, H. E., and Silverman, S., Jr. 1963. Studies in oral leukoplakias. V. Clinical and histologic signs of malignancy. *Acta Odont. Scand.* **21**, 407–414.

Pindborg, J. J., Jolst, O., Renstrup, G., and Roed-Petersen, B. 1968. Studies in oral leukoplakia: A preliminary report on the period prevalence of malignant transformation in leukoplakia based on a follow-up study of 248 patients. *J. Am. Dent. Assoc.* **76**, 767–771.

Renstrup, G. 1970. Occurrence of Candida in oral leukoplakia. *Acta Pathol. Microbiol. Scand.* **78**, 421–424.

Roed-Petersen, B., Renstrup, G., and Pindborg, J. J. 1970. Candida in oral leukoplakias: A histologic and exfoliative cytologic study. *Scand. J. Dent. Res.* **78**, 232–328.

Rose, J. A. 1968. Aetiology of angular cheilosis: Iron metabolism. *Br. Dent. J.* **125**, 67–72.

Russell, C., and Jones, J. H. 1973. Effects of oral inoculation of Candida albicans in tetracycline-treated rats. *J. Med. Microbiol.* **6**, 275–279.

Shamma'a, M. H., and Benedict, E. B. 1958. Esophageal webs: A report of 58 cases and an attempt at classification. *N. Engl. J. Med.* **259**, 378–384.

Thorpe, E. S., Jr., and Handley, H. E. 1929. Chronic tetany and chronic mycelial stomatitis in a child aged 4½years. *Amer. J. Dis. Child.*, **38**, 328–338.

Watts, J. M. 1961. The importance of the Plummer-Vinson syndrome in the aetiology of carcinoma of the upper gastro-intestinal tract. *Postgrad. Med. J.* **37**, 523–533.

Wynder, E. L., and Fryer, J. H. 1958. Etiologic considerations of Plummer-Vinson (Paterson-Kelly) syndrome. *Ann. Intern. Med.* **49**, 1106–1128.

Discussion

Dr. Slavkin said he understood that work with transplanted nuclei argued against the existence of permanent nuclear change in malignant or teratocarcinoma cells, and asked whether there is any biochemical evidence for structural alterations in the DNA of malignant cells. He was aware of the work of John Gurdon, A. J. MacGillivray, John Paul, and many others (see Paul 1974), who have not been able to find such changes. Dr. Solt replied that while there is some biochemical evidence that the alkylation patterns in chromatin and DNA of carcinogen treated cells are both nonrandom and persistent, such evidence is difficult to interpret in terms of ultimate cancer production (Sarma et al. 1975). On the one hand present techniques may not be sufficiently sensitive to detect changes at the level of the single gene, while on the other hand, the concept that the phenotype of a cancer cell, or for that matter a normal cell, might be dependent on extragenomic factors did not exclude the possibility of coexisting mutations. A further factor which may be of importance is the possibility of DNA repair. Dr. Mackenzie asked about the consistency of the association between hyperplasia and carcinogenesis. Dr. Solt referred to work described in his paper and replied that work indicating that application of carcinogens has greater effect at a peak in tissue DNA synthesis suggested a relationship between carcinogenesis and cell replication. However, the association between hyperplasia and carcinogenesis is not always consistent. For example, a nonspecific irritant which could act as a promoting agent in the rabbit might not act this way in the mouse. Extrapolation of an effect from one tissue to another or extrapolation from animal experiments to the human situation is therefore of uncertain reliability. In response to a question from Dr. Slavkin concerning systemic effects on promotion, Dr. Outzen replied that there is a considerable literature indicating that starvation depressed the rate of epithelial tumor production (see Berenblum 1954 for a review of factors influencing carcinogenesis). Professor Johnson commented that whereas earlier work had associated the higher prevalence of cancer in old age with a higher rate of epithelial proliferation, more recent data indicated that the mitotic rate in aged tissues is in fact reduced (reviewed by Squier et al. 1975).

Professor Pindborg asked Dr. Binnie whether he considered candidal infection to be causal or only superimposed on preexisting leukoplakic conditions. In his experience although nodular leukoplakic lesions associated with Candida invariably become homogeneous leukoplakias following antifungal therapy; they do not regress completely unless an associated habit, such as smoking, is controlled. Dr. Binnie agreed that following antifungal therapy many nodular lesions became homogeneous but added that in his experience they became erythroplakic not leukoplakic. Professor Kramer, commenting on the suggested oncogenic activity of candidal infections, pointed out that the Candida itself never appeared to penetrate to the progenitor compartment of the epithelium and asked Dr. Binnie how it might act. Dr. Binnie commented that no mechanism has been postulated but it is known that Candida could quickly produce epithelial hyperplasia under experimental conditions. Dr. Mackenzie asked whether an apparent relationship between candidal infection and oral cancer could be explained by candidal infection acting as a promoter. As Dr. Solt had explained, it is clear that the two stages of initiation and promotion are required for carcinogenesis in skin. Could it be that leukoplakic lesions represent initiated regions of oral epithelium which require promotion to progress to carcinoma? The candidal infection, by inducing hyperplasia or by some other mechanism, serves to promote such lesions. This could explain a relationship between malignant transformation and candidal infection and yet not rule out the possibility of promotion of uninfected lesions by other mechanisms such as continued smoking.

Dr. Dabelsteen asked Dr. Binnie how reliably a diagnosis of candidal hyperplasia could be made on clinical and histopathological grounds. Dr. Binnie replied that clinical impressions are not particularly reliable. A number of features visible on routine hematoxylin and eosin sections, for example an inflammatory infiltrate, acanthosis, parakeratosis, and occasionally microabscesses, lead to the suspicion of candidal infection. However, demonstration of hyphae by a paS reaction is the only reliable method. Dr. Waldron commented that from the histological appearance of a lesion he had often suspected a candidal infection which he had been unable to demonstrate by paS. He asked whether there were any quantitative data about the frequency of candidal infection of lesions showing the type of histological appearance Dr. Binnie had described. Dr. Binnie indicated that such quantitative data are not available but added that the clinical history of the patient is particularly important in such cases because antifungal therapy appears to eradicate the Candida well before there is a change in the histological appearance of the lesion.

Dr. Wilbanks referred to the possibility of depressed cell-mediated immunity in patients infected with Candida. He asked whether such a depression might account for a relationship between candidal infection and cancer. Dr. Binnie replied that he was unaware of any increased frequency of other types of malignant disease in candidal patients studied.

Professor Johnson asked about the relationship between therapy for iron deficiency and candidal infection. Dr. Binnie agreed that a relationship between iron deficiency and Candida is often observed, and that it is often difficult to get such patients to retain iron. Dr. Wilbanks stated that candidal infection of the vagina and cervix is very common and that many of the infected female population are iron deficient. However, he was unaware that any association had ever been made between Candida and the carcinomatous process at the cervix. Trichomonal infection could produce cellular abnormalities in Papanicolaou smears but, even though 30–50% of women have a candidal infection at some time during pregnancy, change associated with Candida has not been reported. The clinical appearance of candidal infection of the cervical mucosa is similar to that of thrush, forming a loosely adherent white patch. Dr. Binnie felt that perhaps the type of chronic hyperplastic candidal infection to which he was referring is a specific clinical-pathological entity and differs from the more common manifestations of thrush or denture sore mouth.

Dr. Slavkin stated that chick embryos are immunodeficient until about day 17 (Hamilton 1952) and asked Dr. Binnie the age of the chorioallantoic membranes that had shown a hyperplastic response to the Candida and whether he thought the response was mediated by the immune system. Dr. Binnie replied that the hyperplastic changes described by Professor Cawson occurred in chorioallantoic membranes of less than 17 days of age and that an immune relationship is therefore unlikely. Ideally one would like to leave Candida-infected epithelium for an extended period of time to see if dysplasia developed but this is not possible with the chick system. Dr. Outzen added that the response to fungal infections is for the most part thought to be T-cell-dependent. Of general interest to the topic of the symposium was the observation that very little growth is observed in tumor cells grafted to the chorioallantoic membrane until the time of T-cell activation at which time angiogenic responses are seen.

Professor Smith pointed out that, in terms of present concepts of the cellular mechanisms of carcinogenesis, little seems to be known about the precise etiology of human oral lesions. Professor Kramer commented that there was however nothing to suggest that the general concepts do not apply to the oral mucosa. Professor Pindborg thought that if particular etiological factors could be identified for specific oral lesions there might be a prognostic significance. For example, in India the leukoplakias produced by hookli smoking are found on the labial mucosa and have not been observed to develop into carcinoma even in a 10-year observation period. On the other hand, lesions of the buccal mucosa caused by tobacco chewing often become malignant. The lesions of snuff dippers in the southern United States are typically associated with low-grade malignancies. Dr. Waldron said that he had observed the existence of a type of leukoplakic lesion of particularly high risk in older women who had used neither tobacco nor alcohol and asked Professor Pindborg to comment about the existence of such a high risk group of lesions in female patients. Professor Pindborg agreed with Dr. Waldron's observation and said that the highest risk of malignancy in the group of patients observed in Copenhagen was apparently found in tongue lesions in women of late middle age who had no history of using either tobacco or alcohol. He felt that this type of lesion might be associated with the sideropenic dysphagia found in Scandinavian women and which is associated with a very atrophic epithelium. Dr. Waldron commented that he had been unable to find any hematological or other systemic abnormalities in his group of female patients. Dr. Van Scott pointed to the problem of knowing what type of proprietary products such individuals may have used and, as an example of such a relationship in dermatology, mentioned that basal cell carcinoma of the scalp has been associated with previous use of hair tonics containing arsenic. Dr. Binnie supported the comments of Drs. Pindborg and Waldron and pointed to the sublingual keratoses as lesions of particularly high risk even if the histological appearance is not suggestive of dysplasia. Only one of 12 patients with such lesions that he had examined had any history of use of tobacco or alcohol. As Einhorn and Wërsall (1967) pointed out, it appears that white lesions in patients without a history of smoking or alcohol consumption are a particularly high risk.

REFERENCES

Berenblum, I. 1954. Carcinogenesis and tumor pathogenesis. *Adv. Cancer Res.* **2**, 144–147.

Einhorn, J., and Wërsall, J. 1967. Incidence of oral carcinoma in patients with leukoplakia of the oral mucosa. *Cancer* **20**, 2189–2193.

Hamilton, H. L. 1952. *Lillie's Development of the Chick.* Henry Holt, New York.

Paul, J. 1974. *Biochemistry of Cell Differentiation.* Butterworth, London.

Sarma, D. S. R., Rajalakshmi, S., and Farber, E. 1975. Chemical carcinogenesis: Interactions of carcinogenes with nucleic acids. In: *Cancer. A Comprehensive Treatise.* Vol. 1. Etiology: Chemical and Physical Carcinogenesis. (Edited by Becker, Fredrick, F.), Chap. 8, pp. 235–287. Plenum Press, New York.

Squier, C. A., Johnson, N. W., and Hackemann, M. 1975. Structure and function of normal human oral mucosa. In: *Oral Mucosa in Health and Disease.* (Edited by Dolby, A. E.), pp. 1–112. Blackwell Scientific Press, Oxford.

PART THREE
MODELS FOR STUDYING CHANGES IN ORAL PREMALIGNANCY

6

Skin As a Model for Studying Oral Premalignancy

E. J. VAN SCOTT

The Skin and Cancer Hospital of Philadelphia, Temple University
School of Medicine, Philadelphia, Pennsylvania

1. INTRODUCTION

Several important events have accounted for the major role of the skin in contributing to our present understanding of the nature of cancer, its development and its control. As the skin has been of great value in the study of epithelial cancer in particular it may enable us now to reach certain conclusions and to make some proposals in regard to the potential value of skin as a model in studying oral malignancy. Pathogenic patterns of squamous cell cancer and basal cell cancer in the epidermis suggest these may have relevance to an understanding of carcinogenic events in oral epithelial malignancy.

However, the value of skin as a model for studying oral premalignancy or malignancy has limitations. As is the case with many pathologic processes involving a given tissue or organ, the validity and predictability of phenomena found in other apparently similar systems are not necessarily applicable to the system or organ under scrutiny.

2. LESSONS LEARNED FROM THE SKIN

Some of the more relevant lessons on cancer, carcinogenesis, prevention, and treatment today have come principally from analysis of the skin of man. The following are illustrative.

2:1 ENVIRONMENTAL CARCINOGENS

The importance of carcinogens encountered in man's changing technological environment was heralded over 200 years ago by Percival Pott's clinical observations of scrotal cancer in chimney sweeps (Pott 1775). Since that original recognition of soot as a potent carcinogenic material, the role of tar products and their constituents as major carcinogenic burdens have become well established. With the exception of scrotal cancer, however, tar has not been the greatest cause of skin cancer in humans, but has had a more important role in carcinogenesis of organs with epithelial linings, notably the lungs.

Actinic radiation, in the ultraviolet wavelengths, has in fact proved to be the predominant carcinogenic stimulus to the skin. This single natural carcinogenic factor has made skin cancer today the most prevalent of all cancers. Skin cancer is nevertheless more controllable than most cancers, as a result of the progress made in comprehending the essentials of the problem, i.e., etiology, prevention, early detection, and adequate treatment. This state has been reached for the most part because of direct studies of the disease in the skin of man.

2:2 IATROGENIC CARCINOGENS

Two agents, inorganic arsenic and ionizing radiation, administered for the treatment of skin diseases and other disorders, are classic examples of carcinogenic hazards that can inadvertently attend therapy. While animal models provide an understanding of the problem of ionizing radiation, this is not so with arsenic. Only after centuries of the use of arsenic as a popular therapeutic agent was it realized, on the basis of clinical observations alone, that this drug was in fact substantially carcinogenic. It is instructive that repeated studies of arsenic in laboratory animals have failed to identify its carcinogenic potential for humans.

2:3 MONITORING OF NEW CUTANEOUS CARCINOGENS

Lessons learned from the skin serve as reminders for clinical investigators today concerned with the application of new or old dermatologic therapies. Several pharmacologic agents intended for long term dermatologic use are under scrutiny for their carcinogenic potential. These include topical nitrogen mustard for therapy of the lymphoma mycosis fungoides (Vonderheid et al. 1977), topical tar preparations for a multiplicity of skin disorders (Rook et al. 1956), and the combination of psoralens and long wave ultraviolet radiation for the treatment of psoriasis and other dermatologic disorders (Van Scott 1976). Because of the phenomenon of latency, extended intervals of monitoring are required to determine the actual degree of carcinogenicity of agents such as these.

2:4 THE CHARACTERISTIC OF LATENCY IN CARCINOGENESIS

The characteristic of latency has become soundly established both from laboratory experiments and clinical experience (see chapter 4). Impressive indeed is the emergence of carcinomas in individuals decades after exposure to a carcinogen such as arsenic, or in the instance of diethylstilbestrol, in the offspring of mothers who received this hormone during pregnancy. The cumulative aspects of carcinogenic stimuli is perhaps best illustrated in the skin where it has been determined that long term exposure to sunlight determines the probability of skin cancer in lightly pigmented individuals (O'Beirn et al. 1970).

2:5 REALITY OF EARLY DETECTION, EARLY TREATMENT AND PREVENTION

Even though skin cancer is the most common of cancers today, it is the most controllable and curable, a state due to the ease of early clinical and histologic detection, the adequacy of treatment, and means of prevention. Means of prevention, discovered and developed during the past quarter century, have added substantially to what appears to be complete resolution of skin cancer as a serious problem. One example was the discovery that topical application of 5-fluorouracil can destroy precancerous actinic keratoses and prevent their progression into actual cancers (Dillaha et al. 1963; Klein 1968). Another has been the development of topically applied chemical sunscreens which limit the transmission of carcinogenic ultraviolet radiation into the skin. While actual reduction of skin cancers by the use of sunscreen preparations has not yet been quantified, it would seem to be substantial if widespread use of such preparations by light-skinned populations is consistently adopted.

Important questions remaining that are amenable to exploration in the skin are whether malignant transformation of cells is reversible, and whether the malignant behavior of cells, after transformation, can be restrained or modified. Delineation of post-transcriptional events at the cellular level may be an important first step in exploring these questions (see chapter 10).

3. COMPARISON BETWEEN CANCER OF SKIN AND ORAL TISSUES

The problem of cancer, i.e., the disruption or destruction of body functions or parts, is fundamentally a problem of cell behavior. Some cancers, relatively benign in behavior, histologically appear highly malignant while others may appear histologically benign but behave in a severely malignant fashion. Lack of differentiation is usually a reliable measure of degree of malignant behavior in skin. Therefore, a first step in attempting to understand better the problem for a given type of cancer would seem to be an appreciation of the normal differentiated functions of the cells involved, as might be obtained from clinical, cytologic, and experimental evidence.

Epithelial cells of the skin surface or its appendages are highly differentiated. In each location, these cells are engaged in synthesis of highly specific products, e.g., keratin proteins or sebaceous lipids, by processes that require programmed death or destruction of the cells themselves. Thus the cells of the epidermis upon migration from the basal germinative layer immediately embark upon a process of maturation by the synthesis of filaments which aggregate into tonofibrils (Fig. 1). This is the first event of the keratinization process that includes the formation of keratohyalin granules (the nature and function of which are still far from clear), loss of nuclei, and fabrication of a stratum corneum that is relatively impermeable, consisting of a tough meshwork of structural protein formed by the keratinocyte (Fig. 2). Malignant transformation of epidermal cells resulting in nondifferentiated cells involves a disturbance of the highly specific system of synthesis and cytolysis.

Many oral epithelial cells, on the other hand, do not show the pattern of maturation seen in epidermis (see chapter 9). In buccal and alveolar mucosa comparatively little keratinization occurs and cells are shed at the surface with nuclei still evident. Malignant transformation of such epithelial cells to an undifferentiated state might require a lesser degree of change than in epidermal cells and the greater degree of malignancy of oral squamous cell cancers (Binnie 1975) suggests that this degree of malignant transformation is often achieved.

The almost complete absence in oral mucosa of basal cell cancer, which is so common to the skin, may be better explained if we have a more precise understanding of the nature of this tumor. In earlier publications (Van Scott 1964; 1966), it has been proposed that basal cell tumors arise in skin as a result of a loss of the ability to keratinize, this loss seeming to represent a post-transcriptional defect since the reacquisition of the potential for keratinization can be demonstrated in transplantation experiments (Van Scott and Reinertson 1961; Flaxman and Van Scott 1968; Cooper and Pinkus 1977). Within the intact tumor, the nonkeratinizing cells continue to replicate but, unable to participate in the process of keratinization, are trapped beneath overlying normally keratinizing cells and accumulate as tumors of germinative cells. Such entrapment might not occur in oral epithelium because there is frequently little or no keratin.

4. RELEVANCE OF SKIN AS A MODEL FOR STUDIES OF ORAL MALIGNANCY

The foregoing account is intended to illustrate some similarities and differences of the integument *vis a vis* the oral lining. Clearly studies on the former may have direct relevance to the latter because of their similarities. In regard to the problem of development of malignancy, an area such as the lips is similar to the skin in the structure of its epithelium, in its relative impermeability, and in sharing a common carcinogenic agent, ultraviolet radiation. Other areas however may be dissimilar in a number of characteristics (e.g., such as permeability, ambient humidity, and pH) and will show a corresponding modification in behavior when exposed to carcinogenic stimuli. Insofar as advances in understanding and control of epithelial cancer of the skin in man have come primarily from studies directly on the skin in man, it would seem reasonable to advocate that the problem of oral epithelial cancer be best studied directly on oral epithelium, and preferably in humans.

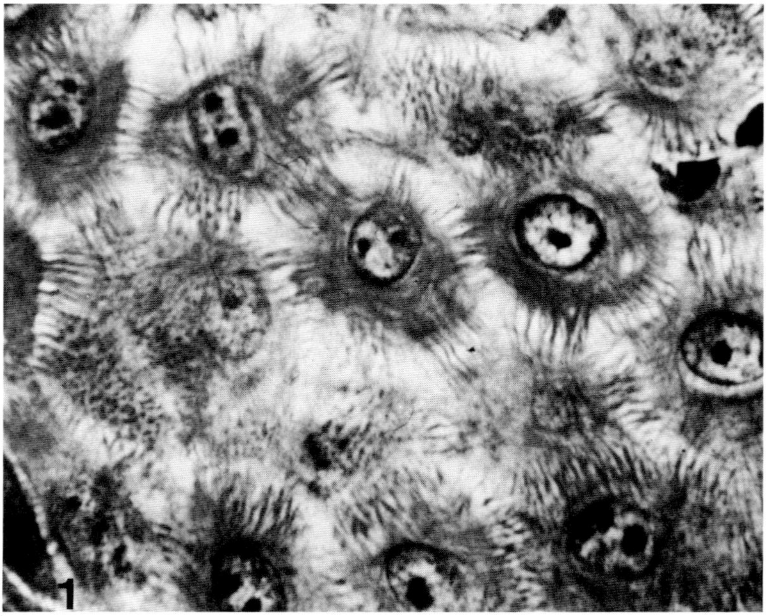

FIGURE 1. Epidermal cells filled with tonofibrils. Gomori trichrome x 1200.

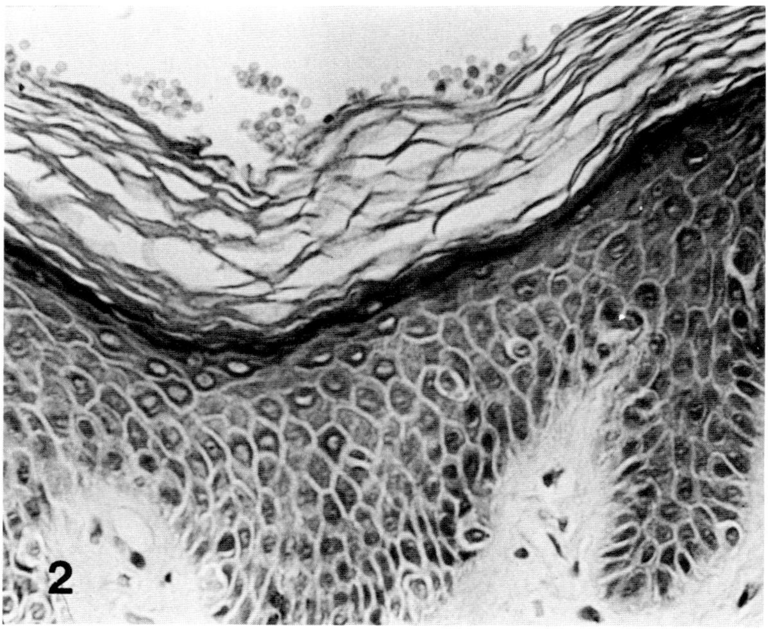

FIGURE 2. Epidermis; keratinization complete. Hematoxylin and eosin x 300.

REFERENCES

Binnie, W. H. 1975. Oral Cancer. In: *Oral Mucosa in Health and Disease.* (Edited by Dolby, A. E.), Chap. 6, pp. 301–334. Blackwell Scientific Publications, Oxford.

Cooper, M., and Pinkus, H. 1977. Intrauterine transplantation of rat basal cell carcinoma as a model for reconversion of malignant to benign growth. *Cancer Res.* **37**, 2544–2552.

Dillaha, C. J., Jansen, G. T., Honeycutt, W. M., and Bradford, A. C. 1963. Selective cytotoxic effect of topical 5-fluorouracil. *Arch. Dermatol.* **88**, 247–256.

Flaxman, B. A., and Van Scott, E. J. 1968. Keratinization in vitro of cells from a basal cell carcinoma. *J. Nat. Cancer Inst.* **40**, 411–422.

Klein, E. 1968. Tumors of skin. IX. Local cytostatic therapy of cutaneous and mucosal premalignant and malignant lesions. *New York J. Med.* **68**, 886–889.

O'Beirn, S. F., Judge, P., Urbach, F., MacCon,C. F., and Martin, F. 1970. Skin cancer in County Galway, Ireland. In: *National Cancer Conference. Proceedings, sixth.*, pp. 489–500. J. B. Lippincott, Philadelphia.

Pott, P. 1775. *Chirurgical observations relative to the cataract, the polypus of the nose, the cancer of the scrotum, the different kinds of ruptures and the mortification of the toes and feet.* Hawes, Clarke, and Collins, London.

Rook,A., Gresham, G. A., and Davis, R. A. 1956. Squamous epithelioma possibly induced by the therapeutic application of tar. *Br. J. Cancer* **10**, 17–23.

Van Scott, E. J. 1964. Definition of epidermal cancer. In: *The Epidermis.* (Edited by Montagna, W., and Lobitz, W. C., Jr.), Chap. 29, pp. 573–586. Academic Press, New York.

Van Scott, E. J. 1966. Reaction patterns of normal and neoplastic epithelium. In: *Advances in Biology of the Skin.* Vol. 7. (Edited by Montagna, W., and Dobson, R. L.), Chap. 4, pp. 75–87. Pergamon Press, Oxford.

Van Scott, E. J. 1976. Therapy of psoriasis, 1975. *JAMA* **235**, 197–198.

Van Scott, E. J., and Reinertson, R. P. 1961. The modulating influence of stromal environment on epithelial cells studied in human autotransplants. *J. Invest. Derm.* **36**, 109–131.

Vonderheid, E. C., Van Scott, E. J., Johnson, W. C., Grekin, D. A., and Asbell, S. O. 1977. Topical chemotherapy and immunotherapy of mycosis fungoides. *Arch. Dermatol.* **113**, 454–462.

7

Experimental Animal Models for Oral Premalignancy

C. J. SMITH

Department of Oral Pathology, University of Sheffield, Sheffield, England

1. INTRODUCTION

Animal models of human oral premalignant lesions enable not only more controlled investigations into the pathogenesis of these lesions, but they may also be of value in studies of etiological factors, diagnostic and prognostic criteria, and the evaluation of methods for treatment and prevention. One of the main problems requiring resolution in this respect is the comparability between human oral premalignant lesions and any animal counterpart.

Reports of spontaneous oral cancer or precancer in animals are rare (for brief review see Navia 1977) and the prospects for studying these diseases in such occurrences are extremely unfavorable. Recourse is therefore made to experimental models, about which it must be said that by far the greatest effort has been expended for the production of oral cancer rather than precancer. Most of the information concerning oral premalignant lesions has therefore been derived from these experiments largely coincidentally. For the most part it is apparent that the experimental lesions have a built-in capacity to progress to malignancy from their outset, though much work remains to be done to ascertain the veracity of this belief; however, it is only a relatively small proportion of so-called premalignant lesions in human oral mucosa that actually achieves this transformation. Thus, experimental approaches to the subtle clinical and biological problems of oral premalignancy are still relatively crude.

There would appear to be two approaches by which to develop models of oral premalignancy. The first depends upon the use of known carcinogenic agents to produce mucosal changes which can be shown by a variety of methods to be comparable to those in human lesions. The second depends upon attempts to produce lesions in animals through the action of agents believed to play an etiological role in the production of oral precancer or cancer in humans.

The history of experimental oral carcinogenesis reflects similar difficulties and frustrations to those experienced by earlier workers in the field of skin carcinogenesis. Through the unlucky or inappropriate choice of carcinogen, experimental animal species, site of application, or duration and frequency of application of the carcinogen, many attempts to produce oral cancer have been unsuccessful; it was not until 1954 that Salley described the first reasonably acceptable and reproducible method for the production of experimental oral cancer in the cheek pouch mucosa of golden Syrian hamsters. As this particular model has been chosen by many other workers for their investigations into different aspects of experimental oral cancer, it will be described and discussed first and in some detail. There then follow sections on carcinogenesis in other oral sites, in the hamster, and in other animals, and another section dealing with animal experiments employing agents believed to be, directly or indirectly, etiological factors in human oral cancer. Consideration is then given to the influence exerted on experimental carcinogenesis by factors believed to be implicated in human oral carcinogenesis. A final section deals with certain problems of control procedures.

2. HAMSTER CHEEK POUCH CARCINOGENESIS WITH KNOWN CARCINOGENS

Hamster cheek pouches are blindly ending sacs that arise from immediately inside the commissures of the lips and extend almost as far as the clavicles, passing lateral to the "buccinator" muscle; they are capable of great distension and eversion, having food storage as their main function. Histologically, the pouch comprises a deep layer of voluntary muscle and loose areolar tissue that supports fibrous connective tissue and a surface of stratified squamous epithelium, 4–6 cells thick, with an orthokeratinized superficial layer (Fig. 1). The junction between epithelium and connective tissue is relatively smooth, there being no rete-ridge formation and no accessory appendages such as salivary glands. It is a simple matter to paint the surface of the cheek pouch with the carcinogenic solution, no anesthesia being required if the animal is handled correctly. Some workers use the anterior vein passing vertically down the medial wall of the pouch as a marker for the site of application of the carcinogen.

Salley (1954) produced squamous cell carcinomas by applying the potent carcinogen 9, 10-dimethyl- 1, 2-benzanthracene (DMBA) to the cheek pouch mucosa of golden Syrian hamsters. Development of this method by Salley (1957) and Morris (1961) showed that young animals (3–9 weeks old) were more susceptible than old animals (18 months old), and that carcinogen was best applied thrice weekly as a 0.5% solution in high-grade mineral oil. Smith (1968) later found that liquid paraffin (B.P.) was a suitable substitute for the mineral oil vehicle.

After about six to nine applications of DMBA, the carcinogen most commonly used, the normally smooth and pink pouch surface exhibits slight roughening, occasional ulceration, and reddening. This is due to an inflammatory reaction that subsides within a week or two ("inflammatory stage"). There then follows a short period of apparent return to normality ("recovery stage") that gives way to a sequence of events passing microscopically from epithelial hyperplasia and hyperkeratosis (Fig. 2) through increasingly severe epithelial dysplasia (Fig. 3), occasionally with carcinoma in situ, to invasive well-differentiated squamous cell carcinoma (Fig. 4). To the naked eye, these changes are manifest in young animals from approximately the seventh week of painting onwards, first of all as rough pink or white patches on the surface, then as raised pedunculated papillomatous lesions that are red, pink, or white in color, and finally from 10–12 weeks as large, fleshy, exophytic nodules with partially red, ulcerated, and pink mucosa covering their surface (Fig. 5). It is within the latter outgrowths that most of the invasive carcinomas are found, though not exclusively, and these eventually penetrate through the stroma to involve the muscle of the pouch wall proper. Metastases to local lymph nodes, though rare, have been seen in our own experiments (Fig. 6) and were described by Salley (1954). Morris and Reiskin (1965) discovered that application of 0.5% DMBA to cheek pouch mucosa for four weeks at thrice-weekly intervals would lead to the development of carcinomas after only a slightly increased latent period compared with persistent regular applications. The value of this observation is that it enables the important premalignant phase to be studied in the absence of immediate side effects that might be due to recent local action of the carcinogen solution. Only the most meager histological evidence of any effect of the carcinogen, as slight hyperplasia and hyperkeratosis, is present at the end of this 4-week period.

Criticisms concerning the acceptability of this system as a model for human oral cancer and precancer can be levelled on several grounds—anatomical, histological, physiological, and pathological (Kolas 1955; Stormby and Wallenius 1964). Salley has defended its use, however, on the grounds that, although the pouch may serve a physiological function (food storage) different from the rest of the oral mucosa, it is derived embryologically from the primitive buccal cavity and its histology, apart from the absence of salivary glands, is similar to that of the remainder of the hamster's oral mucosa. As Salley has further pointed out, the pouch is susceptible over its whole surface, including the part adjacent to the oral opening where it is subjected to similar salivary, microbiological, and traumatic influences as the oral cavity proper. Neither anatomically nor histologically, however, does the hamster cheek pouch mucosa have a strict counterpart in human oral mucosa. No information appears to be recorded concerning permeability barriers in hamster cheek pouch epithelium compared with other sites; it is known, however, that topically applied carcinogens soon reach the connective tissue (Salley 1961; Meskin and Woolfrey 1964).

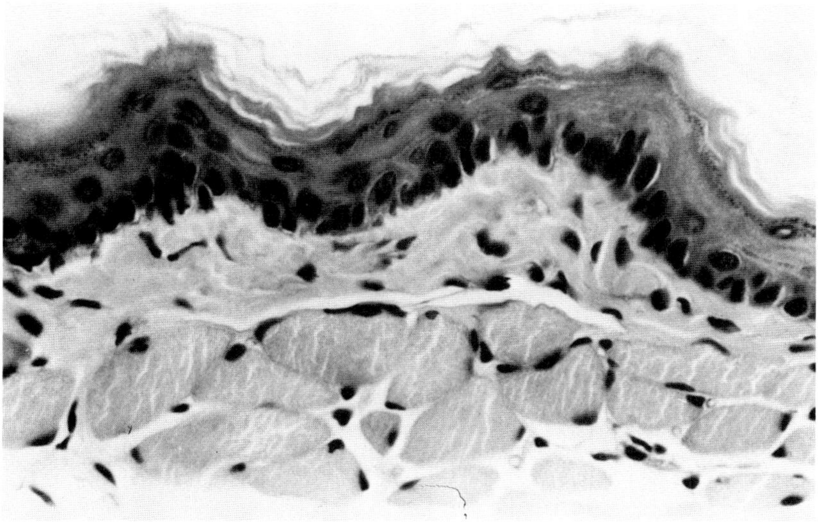

FIGURE 1. Normal hamster cheek pouch mucosa. Hematoxylin and eosin. X 520.

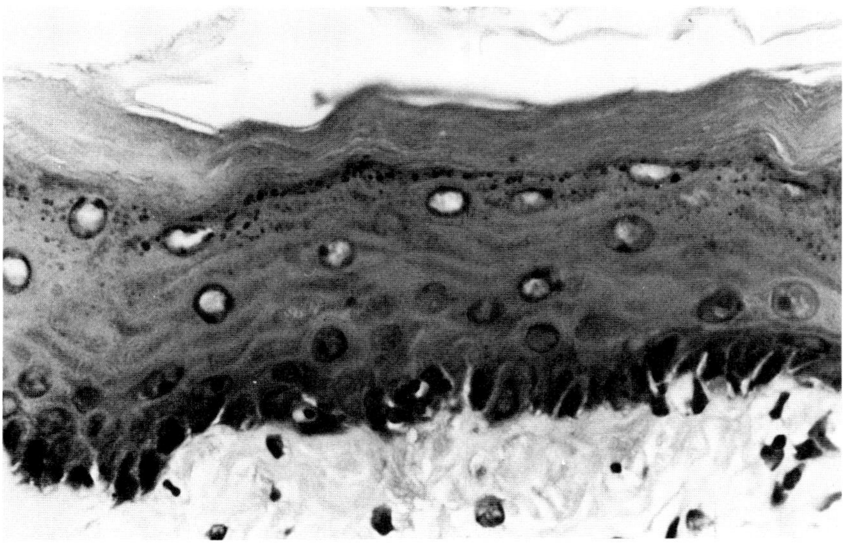

FIGURE 2. Hamster cheek pouch mucosa painted with DMBA, showing epithelial hyperplasia and hyperkeratosis. Hematoxylin and eosin. X 550.

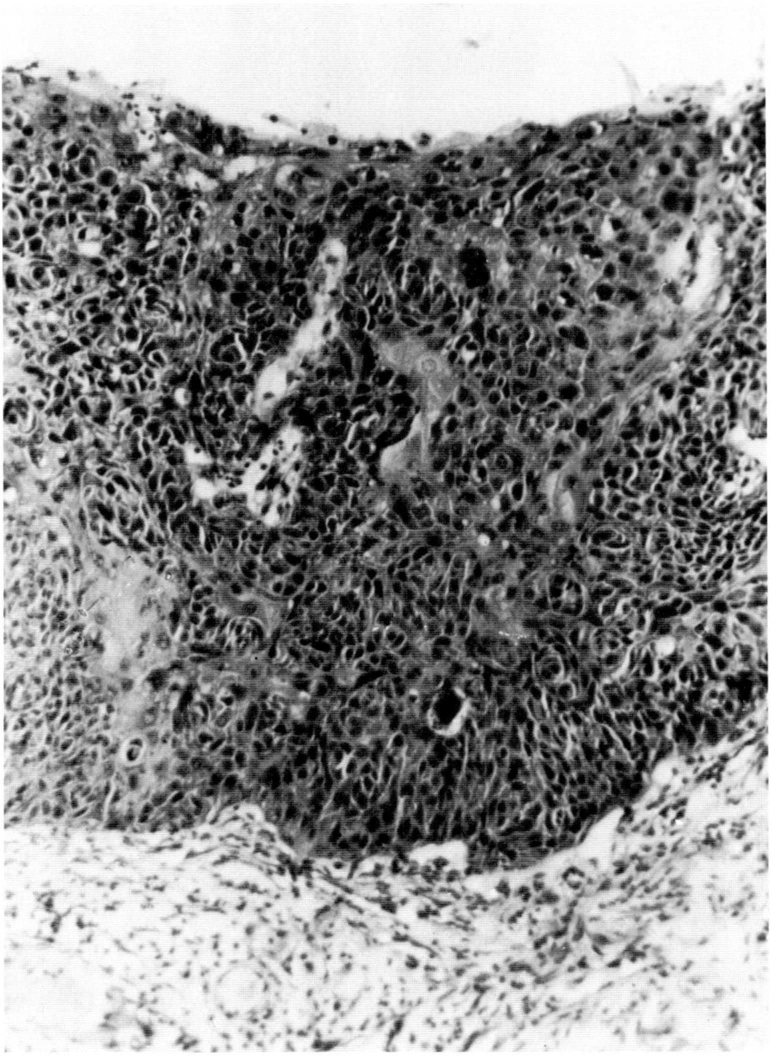

FIGURE 3. Hamster cheek pouch mucosa painted with DMBA, showing severe epithelial dysplasia. Hematoxylin and eosin. X 180.

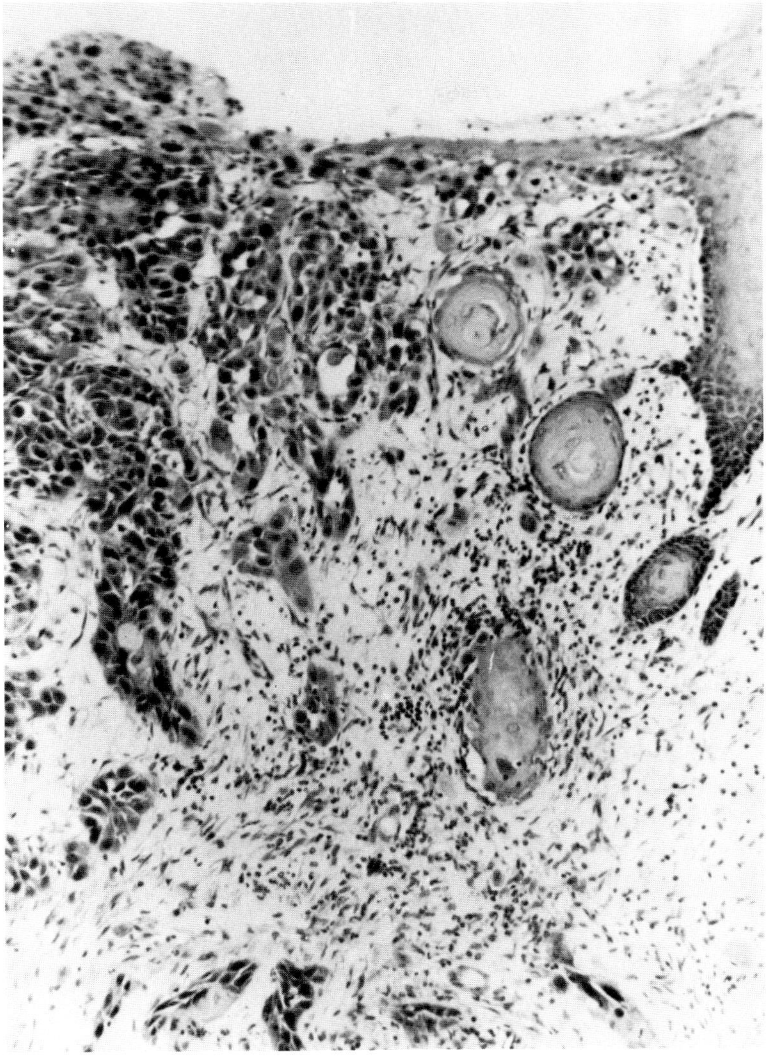

FIGURE 4. Hamster cheek pouch mucosa painted with DMBA, showing invasive well-differentiated squamous cell carcinoma. Hematoxylin and eosin. X 140.

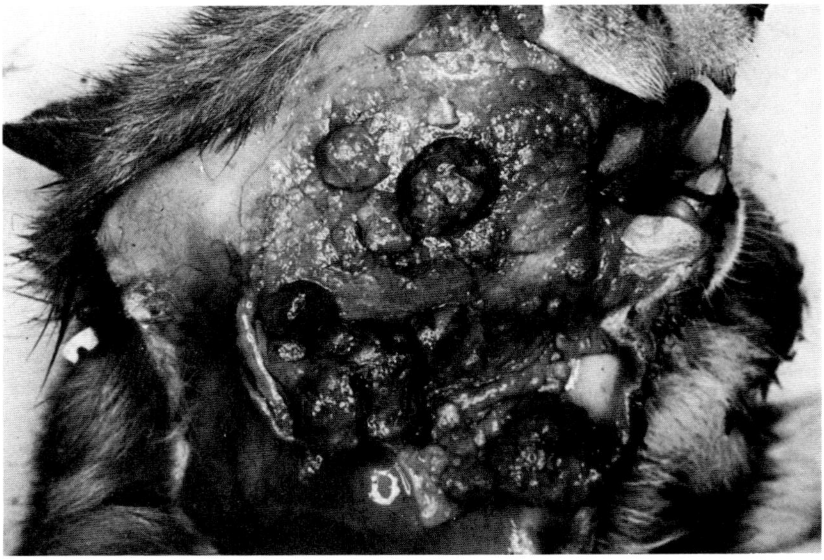

FIGURE 5. Gross appearance of hamster cheek pouch mucosa after several weeks' painting with DMBA, showing variety of fleshy nodules and plaque-like lesions. (By courtesy of Dr. C. D. Franklin.)

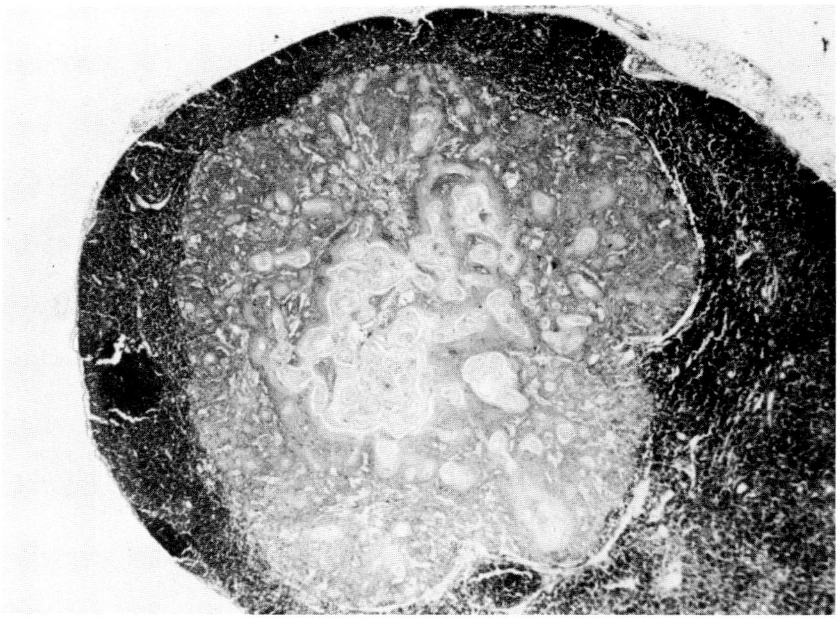

FIGURE 6. Metastatic deposit of experimental squamous cell carcinoma from hamster cheek pouch mucosa located in cervical lymph node. Hematoxylin and eosin. X 30.

One of the most interesting and unusual biological properties of the hamster cheek pouch is its behavior as an immunologically privileged site. Heterografts and homografts of normal and neoplastic tissue are accepted and continue to grow without rejection following their transplantation to submucosal sites in the cheek pouch (Lutz et al. 1951; Lemon et al. 1952; Billingham et al. 1960). This tolerance of the cheek pouch towards the acceptance of antigenically foreign tissues has been largely ignored by previous workers on hamster cheek pouch carcinogenesis, though it could theoretically be highly influential in the susceptibility of the pouch to carcinogenesis and the subsequent behavior of the carcinomas produced. If the hamster cheek pouch has reduced immunocompetence, this may influence development of the tumors (see chapters 16, 17, and 21). However, it would then remain to be explained why there is no increased susceptibility to naturally occurring neoplasms in the cheek pouch.

Although no work appears to have been done specifically on the humoral immune reactions associated with pathological or physiological events in hamster cheek pouch, there is an accumulating body of information to show that cell-mediated immune reactions are not impaired in this site. Immunosuppressive agents of various types all have the reported effect of enhancing chemical carcinogenesis in the cheek pouch by allowing the earlier emergence of malignant tumors that are more numerous, larger, or more anaplastic than usual; this applies to work with specific antilymphocyte serum (Woods 1969; Giunta and Shklar 1971), methotrexate (Shklar et al. 1966), and azathioprine (Sheehan et al. 1971). Furthermore, retardation of the carcinogenic process, with later development of smaller tumors, has been reported following treatment with levamisole, which is thought to have a stimulating effect on cell-mediated immunity (Eisenberg and Shklar 1977). On the other hand, immunosuppression produced by thymectomy is associated with a reduced yield of premalignant and malignant tumors in this model (Polliack et al. 1972). None of these studies, however, was subject to control monitoring procedures on the immunological competence of test animals and the antigenicity of the tumors produced. This apparent conflict of evidence regarding the effect of immunosuppression may make sense when the recent work of Outzen and Prehn (see chapter 16) is considered; they have demonstrated that immunological reactions in some circumstances may stimulate tumor growth. When DMBA is painted on the surface of cheek pouch mucosa there is a detectable general suppression of immunological responses in the animal (Gould 1976); furthermore, one of the effects of regular DMBA applications is enlargement of the draining cervical lymph node (Craig 1977). Both of these observations would seem to indicate that there is no substantial impairment of the mechanisms whereby a carcinogen applied to the pouch surface can influence the local and general immunological system. From experiments involving application of dinitrochlorobenzene and dinitrofluorobenzene to skin and the pouch surface (Mohammed and Mincer 1976; Craig and Clark 1978), contact hypersensitivity reactions can be detected in the pouch within the normal timespan for such events. Although further work is required on this phenomenon, it provides another piece of circumstantial evidence to suggest that the mucosal tissues of hamster cheek pouch may not be much affected by the immunologically privileged reputation of the organ as a whole. It would seem likely that transplants inserted into the areolar connective tissue in the pouch wall are not immunologically rejected (Billingham and Silvers 1964; Lindenmann and Strauli 1968); this tissue may possess particular properties favoring their growth (Walker et al. 1970), and the mucosal lining may not be involved in immunological protection. Of course, should this prove to be the case then whilst early stages of carcinogenesis may be unaffected by considerations of immune privilege, there may still be implications for the invasive stage of tumor growth.

Pertinent objections that can be made against the cheek pouch model of oral cancer on pathological grounds are mainly concerned with the exophytic nature of the tumors and the rarity of metastases. There can be no doubt that the neoplasm eventually produced is usually a well-differentiated squamous cell carcinoma; examination of these tumors by exfoliative cytology, histology, histochemistry, and electron microscopy has so far failed to show significant differences when the epithelial component is compared with that of human oral cancers (Camilleri and Smith 1965; Smith 1972a, 1972b; Woods and Smith 1969). These squamous cell carcinomas are sometimes found to be only moderately or poorly differentiated, a property that can be encouraged by various treatments to the animals, some of which have been mentioned above. Although some of the carcinomas appear to invade directly from the epithelial lining of the pouch, the majority arise within fleshy pedunculated outgrowths that possess loose fibromucoid stromal tissue differing in character from that seen beneath the epithelium in the normal pouch. In both the latter respects, the carcinomas are dissimilar from most human oral cancers, though to what degree this may be significant has yet to be determined.

The relative freedom of hamsters from metastatic spread of tumor is often quoted as an example of the unsuitability of the model. For example, Sheehan and his colleagues (1971) have found no metastases in over 1,000 animals subjected to cheek pouch carcinogenesis. Discrete cervical lymph node metastases have been found in our own experiments, however, and were also described in the early reports from Salley (1954). Although it might be argued that various local factors such as the chemical or physical nature of the tumor stroma, a scarcity of lymphatics, or immunological protection mechanisms may all hinder metastatic spread, the most significant reasons are likely to be found elsewhere. The first of such reasons is related to the fact that a large majority of carcinogenesis experiments in hamster cheek pouch have been terminated soon after carcinomas have developed, this being the main purpose of most of the experiments, and few have allowed animals to survive with a tumor burden for long enough so that metastases might be reasonably anticipated. A second point worthy of mention is that the capacity to produce readily-metastasizing carcinomas is a relatively rare feature of most chemical carcinogenesis experiments in any other species and site.

Examples of the use of the hamster cheek pouch model of oral precancer and early cancer for the purposes of evaluating diagnostic and treatment possibilities are few in number. The use of exfoliative cytology for diagnosis has been explored by Camilleri and Smith (1965) and an investigation into the effectiveness of toluidine blue applications for determining biopsy site has been reported by Sabes et al. (1972). Poswillo (1971) has described the results of treatment of hamster cheek pouch lesions by cryosurgery and Shklar (1966) and Sheehan et al. (1971) recorded the effects of methotrexate and azathioprine respectively.

A different consideration when contemplating criticisms of this model concerns the concentration of carcinogen traditionally used. The reasons for selecting 0.5% DMBA in thrice-weekly doses mainly relate to the short latent period before malignancy ensues (approximately 3 months) and bear no known relationship to the dose or time exposure of human oral mucosa to environmental carcinogenic agents.

Carcinogenic nitroso compounds, dimethylnitrosamine (DMNA), and diethylnitrosamine (DENA), applied in 0.1 mg amounts to the cheek pouch mucosa twice-weekly for 9 months, resulted in only slight hyperkeratosis and epithelial atrophy (Milievskaja and Kiseleva 1976); the same authors found that similar applications of N-methyl-N-nitrosourea (MNU) produced only one carcinoma in 25 animals.

3. OTHER EXPERIMENTAL ANIMAL MODELS OF ORAL CARCINOGENESIS USING KNOWN CARCINOGENS

3:1 CHEMICAL CARCINOGENS

Although Bonne (1927) had reported the production of three squamous cell carcinomas in the palatal mucosa of fifty mice after application of coal tar for fifty weeks, and Oyama (1935) described lingual carcinomas in two rabbits developing from the injection of crude coal tar into an ulcerated area, it was not until several years later that more reproducible results were obtained from the selection of more suitable experimental animals, test sites, and potent carcinogens.

3:1:1 *Hamsters*

Apart from the susceptibility of their cheek pouch mucosa, hamsters have been shown to develop carcinomas in response to DMBA in palatal mucosa (Salley and Kreshover 1959; Stormby and Wallenius 1964), in gingival mucosa (Al-Ani and Shklar 1966; Mesrobian and Shklar 1969), and in lingual mucosa (Stormby and Wallenius 1964; Fujita et al. 1973). Almost all portions of the tongue appear to be susceptible to the action of DMBA, in periods ranging from 15 weeks to one year, if the surface is scratched before each application of carcinogen. The nodular or ulcerated lesions that develop occasionally metastasize to local lymph nodes (Fujita et al. 1973). Widespread oral preneoplastic and neoplastic changes have followed the administration of a different carcinogen, the alkyl nitrosamide N-methylnitrosourea (NMU or MNU), by intragastric or intravenous routes (Herrold 1968; Kohgo 1972; Suzuki 1976). The mandibular gingival region appears to be the most prone to develop carcinomas, though some doubt has been expressed on histological grounds about their comparability with oral squamous carcinomas in man (Suzuki 1976); it has been suggested that the keratotic lesions of palatal epithelium may prove a more satisfactory model of premalignancy (Edwards 1978). Of special interest in the experiments with NMU is the development of oral mucosal changes without direct application of the carcinogen to oral sites.

3:1:2 *Mice*

These animals have not proved to be particularly susceptible to oral applications of chemical carcinogens, though van Prohaska et al. (1939) reported some success with methylcholanthrene and Goldhaber (1957) with dimethylbenzanthracene. Levy et al. (1951) studied the effects of single applications of methylcholanthrene to the labial mucosa and compared the effects with those produced on skin. The injection of an aqueous suspension of 0.3 mg of methylcholanthrene into the tongue was followed, in 15 out of 18 instances, by the development of lingual carcinomas (Levy 1958), a more effective method in these animals than straightforward painting on the tongue surface. A different carcinogen, 4-nitroquinolone-N-oxide, however, is effective in producing carcinomas on local application to both labial and lingual mucosal surfaces in mice (Fujino et al. 1965).

3:1:3 *Rats*

Although the yield of malignant and premalignant oral lesions is small, single and multiple doses of NMU have been found effective by several workers (Druckrey et al. 1964; Druckrey 1967; Leaver et al. 1969; Ebling et al. 1973). DMBA, however, produced carcinomas in rat oral mucosa only if salivary flow was inhibited (Wallenius 1966) (see chapter 9). The surgical creation of artificial pouches in the lower lip mucosa (Yamamura et al. 1975) enabled the production of squamous cell carcinomas through the action of both DMBA and methylcholanthrene. A new development of some promise is the discovery that the water-souble carcinogen 4-nitroquinoline N-oxide (4NQO) has a potent effect on the palatal mucosa of rats (Wallenius and Lekholm 1973a; Philipsen et al. 1977). A 0.5% solution of 4NQO in propylene glycol applied thrice-weekly to the palatal mucosa of Wistar rats will cause the development of infiltrating squamous cell carcinomas from approximately the twentieth week. Philipsen et al. (1977) have described the sequence of histological changes, including epithelial hyperplasia, hyperorthokeratosis, focal acantholytic dyskeratosis and features of epithelial dysplasia, that precede malignancy. Wallenius and Lekholm (1973a) refer also to the carcinomas that developed at the base of the tongue and in the mandibular gingival mucosa in some of their experimental animals.

3:1:4 *Monkeys*

Monkey oral mucosa appears from limited experience to be completely resistant to the action of DMBA; two animals painted in various oral sites for long periods, one for more than four years, resulted in minimal gross and histological changes (Cohen and Smith 1967).

3:2 PHYSICAL AND VIRAL CARCINOGENS

Experimental oral carcinomas arising from the action of nonchemical carcinogens are extremely rare. One, reported by Melnikov (1963), resulted in a carcinoma of the tongue in a monkey in whom a radioactive source of cobalt or silver had been implanted into the maxillary antrum. The only other example that could be gleaned from the literature is the description of gingival carcinomas induced in mice by the action of polyoma virus (Stanley et al. 1964).

4. EFFECTS OF SUSPECTED HUMAN ORAL CARCINOGENS ON EXPERIMENTAL ANIMAL ORAL MUCOSA

Roffo (1930) produced "oral leukoplakia" in rabbits through subjecting them to the persistent effects of cigarette smoke, but the more precise nature of these lesions is unknown. Epidemiological evidence incriminating certain forms of tobacco or betel quid ingredients as causative agents for human oral cancer and precancer (see chapters 1 and 2) has fueled interest in the effects of these substances on experimental animals' oral mucosa.

Not surprisingly, the hamster cheek pouch has been chosen for many of these investigations, both for its convenience and its known susceptibility to proven carcinogens. Dunham and Herrold (1962) were unable to produce significant changes in hamster cheek pouch mucosa subjected to snuff and various components of the betel quid made up into beeswax pellets. Later, Dunham et al. (1966) applied powdered forms of slaked lime, gambier (a resinous substance from a Malayan vine, used for chewing with betel nut), snuff, and cornstarch, alone or in various combinations, to the cheek pouch mucosa on five consecutive days each week for the entire lifetime of hamsters. Those animals receiving slaked lime applications, whether alone or mixed with other substances, showed the most pronounced gross and microscopical changes; three out of 29 animals treated with lime were described as possessing epithelial changes suggestive of a preneoplastic condition, comprising small foci of atypical cells with loss of cellular polarity and basal cells that were hyperchromatic and fusiform. Chang (1966) has claimed the production of cheek pouch precancerous lesions by the action of betel quid juice which included lime, but not by betel quid juice alone; a solution of lime alone produced similar precancerous lesions. Lime, snuff, and betel quid components were found to be ineffective in producing significant changes in hamster cheek pouch when tested in 1974 by Dunham et al., although in the same series of experiments a plant extract believed to be carcinogenic to man produced one "spreading superficial squamous carcinoma" and one example of "advanced epithelial atypia" from 64 animals after a lifetime's exposure of the cheek pouches. Kandarkar and Sirsat (1977) have described epithelial hyperplasia, alterations in keratinization patterns, and epithelial dysplasia, in hamster cheek pouch mucosa following thrice-weekly applications of lime, or lime plus tobacco, over a 24-week period or more. Snuff, chewing tobacco, and cigarette smoke tar obtained from Western sources, have produced at most only minimal histological changes in hamster cheek pouch mucosa (Tabah et al. 1957; Kreshover and Salley 1957; Moore and Miller, 1958; Peacock et al. 1960; Peacock and Brawley 1959; Kendrick 1964; Protzel et al. 1964). Nas, a tobacco-containing mixture common in Central Asia where it is believed to be implicated in the etiology of oral cancer, has been applied daily to cheek pouch mucosa both as a dry powder and as a 50% solution in sunflower oil; no significant effects were observed (Kiseleva et al. 1976). Nas was not found to be cocarcinogenic when regularly applied following a single application of 0.1% DMBA to the pouch surface (Milievskaja and Kiseleva 1976).

It is of interest to note that carcinomas have been reported following the application to mouse skin of extracts obtained from the tobacco component of betel quids (Muir and Kirk 1960; Ranadive et al. 1963).

Little work has been done on the assessment of the effects of putative human oral carcinogenic agents on sites other than hamster cheek pouch mucosa. In view of the known variability in response that is observed between sites and species when exposed to various carcinogens, it is perhaps a pity that more diversity in choice of test site has not been shown by those involved in the investigation of these substances. Epithelial dysplasia has been described, however, as one of the results obtained following the application of lime to rat oral mucosa (Sirsat and Kandarkar 1968). Also, investigations employing the exposure of surgically isolated monkey cheek pouches, which in several important respects are different from hamster cheek pouches, to long-term contact with Mainpuri tobacco have led to the development of hyperplastic epithelium containing "shrivelled" and "ballooned" cells in the stratum spinosum (Cohen and Smith 1967; Cohen et al. 1971). Electron microscopy has revealed changes in the monkey cheek pouch epithelium, where it adjoins connective tissue, that are similar to the effects produced by known chemical carcinogens (Cohen et al. 1971). Although these changes are not considered to be a component of epithelial dysplasia, similar counterparts were found in human leukoplakias from individuals exposed to Mainpuri tobacco. This tobacco, which contains other substances including lime, is a common constituent of the betel quid chewed in Uttar Pradesh, India.

In recent years interest has arisen concerning the possible carcinogenic attributes of intraoral infection by *Candida* organisms (see chapter 5), although it is pertinent to note that recently developed animal models of intraoral *Candida* infection have failed to reveal progression of involved epithelium to malignancy and have not appeared to produce histological changes markedly suggestive of premalignancy (Jones and Adams 1970; Budtz-Jorgensen 1971; Jones and Russell 1973).

5. MODIFYING LOCAL AND SYSTEMIC INFLUENCES

Certain factors thought to be of significance in the etiology of human oral cancer have been tested by either systemic or local applications for their modifying effect on experimental oral carcinogenesis.

5:1 LOCAL FACTORS

For many years chronic irritation in various forms has been considered to act on some occasions in either a carcinogenic or cocarcinogenic capacity. Some slight shortening of the latent period was obtained by Renstrup et al. (1962) when chronic mechanical trauma was superimposed on hamster cheek pouch carcinogenesis with DMBA. Likewise, croton oil, a known carcinogen and chemical irritant, can reduce the latent period in the same experimental model (Silberman and Shklar 1963). Tattooing the mucosa at the same time as carcinogen solution was being applied had no effect on overcoming the resistance of monkey oral mucosa to the action of DMBA (Cohen and Smith 1967), and it is not clear whether scarification of the lingual mucosa in hamsters exposed to topical applications of DMBA (Fujita et al. 1973) had any significant enhancing effect.

The possible influence of saliva on oral carcinogenesis has been the subject of investigations by Wallenius (1966) and Wallenius and Lekholm (1973b), who have concluded that the action of water-soluble carcinogens may be potentiated by the presence of saliva whereas fat-soluble ones may be retarded (see chapter 9). There is a need for further experimentation with appropriate controls in this area, largely to investigate further species and site variations, the effects of carcinogen concentration, the role of the vehicle, and the simple dilution effect of saliva.

5:2 SYSTEMIC FACTORS

Alcohol appears to be taking on increasing significance as an etiological factor in human oral cancer (see chapter 18), although there is little to suggest whether this effect is exerted through local or systemic mechanisms. In this context it is of interest that Protzel et al. (1964) found that alcohol and other liver intoxicants potentiated the effects of benzpyrene and tobacco tar on the oral mucosa of mice; the substances producing liver damage were administered without coming into contact with the oral mucosa and a systemic action must therefore be implicated.

Although Poswillo and Cohen (1971) observed that excess dietary zinc markedly inhibited hamster cheek pouch carcinogenesis, Edwards (1976) was unable to confirm this effect.

The role played by Vitamin A in carcinogenesis is somewhat confused, with some reports indicating that topical or systemic Vitamin A can retard carcinogenesis or bring about resolution of neoplastic conditions whereas other workers have found a potentiating effect, or at best no action, on carcinogenesis (for references see Brown et al. 1977). Some of these reports have concerned oral lesions and Ibrahim et al. (1977) have found deficient levels of Vitamin A and carotene in oral cancer patients as compared with age- and sex-matched controls. The possible etiological role of Vitamin A has yet to be ascertained, though at a cellular level an effect on membrane systems would be most probable. Vitamin A appears to enhance DMBA-induced carcinogenesis in the hamster cheek pouch, malignant tumors appearing earlier and in greater numbers than usual (Rowe and Gorlin 1959; Polliack and Levij 1969), and also potentiates the action of lime and tobacco on the same site (Kandarkar and Sirsat 1977). Vitamin A deficiency, however, had no effect on the development of hamster cheek pouch carcinomas (Rowe and Gorlin 1959).

With regard to the possible influence of hormones, perhaps one of the most important points to be made is that no work known to the author has demonstrated a significant difference in the response between male and female animals in any aspects of experimental oral carcinogenesis. Shklar (1966) and Sabes et al. (1959, 1963) found that systemic cortisone and prednisolone reduced the latent period in hamster cheek pouch carcinogenesis; however, Polliack et al. (1970) discovered that topical application of cortisone inhibited tumor development.

Single large doses of irradiation proved not to be cocarcinogenic for hamster cheek pouch mucosa subsequently treated regularly with DMBA (Hamner 1966). Immunological mechanisms and their manipulation have already been discussed in the section dealing with immune privilege in the hamster cheek pouch.

6. CONTROL PROCEDURES

Appropriate experimental controls are essential for the correct interpretation of cellular and tissue effects arising as a result of chemical carcinogenesis. These substances have other properties in addition to a capacity to induce malignant tumors and their irritant action alone may produce toxic, inflammatory, or hyperplastic responses not necessarily related to their carcinogenicity. The effects of the solvent or vehicle for the carcinogen must also not be overlooked if topical agents are applied to the mucosa; any possible dilution effect should always be borne in mind in an assessment of their influence on carcinogenesis. Furthermore, ingestion or local toxicity of the carcinogen, solvent, or indeed tumors, may lead to interference with nutritional or immunological mechanisms that could produce changes in cheek pouch mucosa unrelated to the carcinogenic process.

In connection with the property of chemical carcinogens to produce epithelial hyperplasia en route to carcinoma, it is clearly important to clarify which features of such tissue are essentially premalignant and which are common to an epithelial hyperplasia that does not possess the inherent capacity to become malignant (i.e., whether they are tumor specific or tumor associated). Models of epithelial hyperplasia in the latter category may therefore be suitable as controls for some studies on carcinogenesis. In oral mucosa, these include epithelial hyperplasia produced by chronic mechanical irritation to hamster cheek pouch mucosa (Mackenzie and Miles 1973) and to rat lingual mucosa (Shteyer et al. 1976), as well as turpentine-induced epithelial hyperplasia in hamster cheek pouch (Craig and Franklin 1977; Franklin and Craig 1978; chapter 15).

CONCLUSIONS

Oral premalignant lesions can apparently be produced in several different species of experimental animal by the action of various carcinogens. No single model is ideal and though most is known about the effects of chemical carcinogens on hamster cheek pouch mucosa, there is a need not only to learn more about this system but also to investigate other alternatives. It is of as much fundamental interest to know why some animals and certain oral sites should be resistant to particular carcinogens as it is why others prove so susceptible. Negative results obtained from such experiments should, therefore, be reported in addition to positive ones so that a profile can be built up across a range of species and sites for the various types of carcinogens.

Despite the objections that can be raised to the hamster cheek pouch mucosa as a site in which to study oral premalignant lesions, there are good reasons for its continued use. Confining applications of carcinogen to the pouch mucosa for an initial four-week period provides a potentially valuable model; it offers the hope of studying premalignant tissue changes in the absence of short-term toxic side effects from recent applications of the carcinogen and should be used more often.

Just as resistance and susceptibility to various carcinogens are observed amongst experimental animals, so human oral mucosa has to be considered within the same context. If an agent suspected on good evidence to be involved in the etiology of human oral cancer is found not to produce tumors (or even premalignant lesions) in animals, then it does not necessarily follow that the agent has been proved noncontributory towards human oral cancer; perhaps the species chosen as the test animal is among those resistant to that agent. Conversely, substances that induce premalignant or malignant changes in experimental animals' oral mucosa may be completely innocuous if applied to human oral mucosa. Where experiments are mounted to test suspected human oral carcinogens under experimental conditions, however, it would seem a wise precaution that the substances under test should be prepared for application to the animals' oral mucosa in a manner as similar as possible to their human use. Study of experimental oral carcinogenesis teaches the lesson, even more obviously than examination of human lesions, that for probably the greater part of the latent period following initial carcinogenic exposure there are no morphological or other recognizable changes in the tissue that can be identified as indicators of future malignancy. If, as is believed to be the case for human lesions, only a proportion of epithelial dysplasias and carcinomas in situ progress to invasive malignancy, and of the remainder some persist in a stable state and others regress, two further questions require to be asked. What makes potentially malignant lesions develop the microscopical characteristics of premalignancy and, if progression to premalignancy and malignancy is not inevitable, how may initiated epithelium in the premalignant or morphologically unaltered state be made to stabilize or regress? (See also chapter 4.) These are potentially fruitful fields for further investigation.

When morphological changes can be observed microscopically there are still many opportunities for confusion. Because the descriptions of cellular and tissue changes are almost all based on subjective impressions, and as several investigators have been inexperienced in histopathological interpretation, terms such as atypia and dysplasia have either not often been carefully defined or have been defined variably. Consequently, it is seldom possible to compare accurately the results of one worker or group with those of others. This applies especially to experimental animal work involving potential human oral carcinogens but also affects experiments with known carcinogens.

It is difficult to understand the logic behind descriptions of "precancerous" changes in, for example, animal mucosa treated with slaked lime when no progression to malignancy has ever been produced by this substance. It is dangerous to assume that because the changes seen are in some ways similar to those observed in more certain premalignant lesions, they imply a similar outcome. A solution to these problems can be found only by adopting stated rigid criteria for the definition of histopathological states in the premalignant sequence and by pursuing a progressively more objective approach to the analysis of morphological changes; this is discussed further in chapter 15.

REFERENCES

Al-Ani, S., and Shklar, G. 1966. Effects of a chemical carcinogen applied to hamster gingiva. *J. Periodontol.* **37**, 36–42.

Billingham, R. E., Ferrigan, L. W., and Silvers, W. K. 1960. Cheek pouch of the Syrian hamster and tissue transplantation immunity. Abstract. *Science* **132**, 1488.

Billingham, R. E., and Silvers, W. K. 1964. Studies on homografts of foetal and infant skin and further observations on the anomalous properties of pouch skin grafts in hamsters. *Proc. Roy. Soc.* **161**, 161–190.

Bonne, C. 1927. Ueber Geschwülste bei Teertieren. *Z. Krebs-forsch.* **25**, 1–22.

Brown, I. V., Lane, B. P., and Pearson, J. 1977. Effects of depot injections of retinyl palmitate on 7, 12-dimethylbenz (α) anthracene-induced preneoplastic changes in rat skin. *J. Natl. Cancer Inst.* **58**, 1347–1355.

Budtz-Jorgensen, E. 1971. Denture stomatitis. IV. An experimental model in monkeys. *Acta Odont. Scand.* **29**, 513–526.

Camilleri, G. E., and Smith, C. J. 1965. Exfoliative cytology of the early lesions of experimental oral cancer in the hamster. *Arch. Oral Biol.* **10**, 465–470.

Chang, K. M. 1966. Experimental production of lesions on cheek pouch of the hamster by betel quid. *J. Formosan Med. Assoc.* **65**, 125–131. (Abstract in: *Oral Res. Abstr.* **1**, 667–668, 1966.)

Cohen, B., Poswillo, D. E., and Woods, D. A. 1971. The effects of exposure to chewing tobacco on the oral mucosa of monkey and man. A histological and ultrastructural study. *Ann. R. Coll. Surg. Engl.* **48**, 255–273.

Cohen, B., and Smith, C. J. 1967. Aetiological factors in oral cancer: Experimental investigation of early epithelial changes. *Helv. Odont. Acta* **11**, 112–124.

Craig, G. T. 1977. Local lymph node response to solutions of turpentine and of a chemical carcinogen applied to hamster cheek pouch epithelium. Abstract. *J. Dent. Res.* **56**, Special issue D, D116.

Craig, G. T., and Clark, A. 1978. Contact hypersensitivity responses to DNFB in hamster cheek pouch and skin. Abstract. *J. Dent. Res.*, in press.

Craig, G. T., and Franklin, C. D. 1977. The effect of turpentine on hamster cheek pouch mucosa: A model of epithelial hyperplasia and hyperkeratosis. *J. Oral Pathol.* **6**, 268–277.

Druckrey, H. 1967. Quantitative aspects of chemical carcinogenesis. In: *Potential Carcinogenic Hazards from Drugs.* (Edited by Truhaut, R.), UICC Monograph Vol. 7, pp. 62–77. Springer-Verlag, Berlin.

Druckrey, H., Steinhoff, D., Preussmann, R., and Ivankovic, S. 1964. Erzeugung von Krebs durch eine einmalige Dosis von Methyl-nitroso-Harnstoff und verschiedenen Dialkylnitrosamininen an Ratten. *Z Krebsforsch.* **66,** 1–10.

Dunham, L. J., and Herrold, K. M. 1962. Failure to produce tumors in the hamster cheek pouch by exposure to ingredients of betel quid; histopathologic changes in the pouch and other organs by exposure to known carcinogens. *J. Natl. Cancer Inst.* **29**, 1047–1067.

Dunham, L. J., Muir, C. S., and Hamner, J. E. 1966. Epithelial atypia in hamster cheek pouches treated repeatedly with calcium hydroxide. *Br. J. Cancer* **20**, 588–593.

Dunham, L. J., Sheets, R. H., and Morton, J. F. 1974. Proliferative lesions in cheek pouch and esophagus of hamsters treated with plants from Curaçao, Netherland Antilles. *J. Natl. Cancer Inst.* **53**, 1259–1269.

Ebling, H., Barbachan, J. J., Castro do Valle, J. G., and De Oliveira, L. Y. 1973. N-methyl-N-nitrosourea-induced odontogenic neoplasms in rats. *J. Dent. Res.* **52**, 177.

Edwards, M. B. 1976. Chemical carcinogenesis in the cheek pouch of Syrian hamsters receiving supplementary zinc. *Arch. Oral Biol.* **21**, 133–135.

Edwards, M. B. 1978. Some effects of N-methylnitrosourea on the oral and odontogenic tissues of the Syrian golden hamster. *Arch. Oral Biol.* **23**, 515–524.

Eisenberg, E., and Shklar, G. 1977. Levamisole and hamster pouch carcinogenesis. *Oral Surg.* **43**, 562–571.

Franklin, C. D., and Craig, G. T. 1978. Stereological quantification of histological parameters in turpentine-induced hyperplasia of hamster cheek pouch epithelium. *Arch. Oral Biol.* **23**, 347–353.

Fujino, H., Chino, T., and Imai, T. 1965. Experimental production of labial and lingual carcinoma by local application of 4-nitroquinoline N-oxide. *J. Natl. Cancer Inst.* **35**, 907–918.

Fujita, K., Kaku, T., Sasaki, M., and Onoe, T. 1973. Experimental production of lingual carcinomas in hamsters: Tumor characteristics and site of formation. *J. Dent. Res.* **52**, 1176–1185.

Goldhaber, P. 1957. The role of saliva and other local environmental factors in oral carcinogenesis. *J. Amer. Dent. Assoc.* **54**, 517–524.

Giunta, J. L., and Shklar, G. 1971. The effect of antilymphocyte serum on experimental hamster buccal pouch carcinogenesis. *Oral Surg.* **31**, 344–353.

Gould, A. R. 1976. DMBA and immunosuppression in the Syrian golden hamster. *J. Dent. Res.* **55**, Special issue D, D98–D102.

Hamner, J. E. 1966. Co-carcinogenesis in the hamster cheek pouch. *J. Dent. Res.* **45**, 46–51.

Herrold, K. M. 1968. Odontogenic tumors and epidermoid carcinomas of the oral cavity. An experimental study in Syrian hamsters. *Oral Surg.* **25**, 262–272.

Ibrahim, K., Jafarey, N. A., and Zuberi, S. J. 1977. Plasma vitamin 'A' and carotene levels in squamous cell carcinoma of oral cavity and oro-pharynx. *Clin. Oncol.* **3**, 203–207.

Jones, J. H., and Adams, D. 1970. Experimentally induced acute oral candidosis in the rat. *Br. J. Dermatol.* **83**, 670–673.

Jones, J. H., and Russell, C. 1974. The histology of chronic candidal infection of the rat's tongue. *J. Pathol.* **113**, 97–100.

Kandarkar, S. V., and Sirsat, S. M. 1977. Changes in vitamin A conditioned hamster cheek pouch epithelium on exposure to commercial shell lime (calcium hydroxide) and tobacco. I. Optical histopathology. *J. Oral Pathol.* **6**, 191–202.

Kendrick, F. J. 1964. Some effects of a chemical carcinogen and a cigarette smoke condensate upon hamster cheek pouch mucosa. *Health Sci.* **24**, 3698–3699.

Kiseleva, N. S., Milievskaja, I. L., and Caklin, A. V. 1976. Development of tumours in Syrian hamsters during prolonged experimental exposure to nas. *Bull. WHO* **54**, 597–605.

Kohgo, T. 1972. An experimental study of odontogenic tumors in hamsters by N-nitrosomethylurea. *Kokubyo Gakkai Zassh.* **39**, 191–212.

Kolas, S. 1955. Investigation of normal human saliva for possible anticarcinogenic action and chemical carcinogenesis in mucous membranes. *Oral Surg.* **8**, 1192–1203.

Kreshover, S. J., and Salley, J. J. 1957. Predisposing factors in oral cancer. *J. Amer. Dent. Assoc.* **54**, 509–514.

Leaver, D. D., Swann, P. F., and Magee, P. N. 1969. The induction of tumours in the rat by a single oral dose of N-nitrosomethylurea. *Br. J. Cancer* **23**, 177–187.

Lemon, H. M., Lutz, B. R., Pope, R., Parsons, L., Handler, A. H., and Patt, D. I. 1952. Survival and growth of human tissue transplanted to the hamster cheek pouch. *Science* **115**, 461–465.

Levy, B. M., Gorlin, R. J., and Gottsegen, R. 1951. Histology of early reactions of skin and mucous membrane of the lip of the mouse to a single application of a carcinogen. *J. Natl. Cancer Inst.* **12**, 275–285.

Levy, B. M. 1958. The experimental production of carcinoma of the tongue in mice. *J. Dent. Res.* **37**, 950.

Lindenmann, R., and Sträuli, P. 1968. Lymphatic vessels in the cheek pouch of the golden hamster. *Transplantation* **6**, 557–561.

Lutz, B. R., Fulton, G. P. Patt, D. I., Handler, A. H., and Stevens, D. F. 1951. The cheek pouch of the hamster as a site for the transplantation of a methylcholanthrene-induced sarcoma. *Cancer Res.* **11**, 64–66.

Mackenzie, I. C., and Miles, A. E. W. 1973. The effect of chronic frictional stimulation on hamster cheek pouch. *Arch. Oral Biol.* **18**, 1341–1349.

Melnikov, R. A. 1963. The induction of tumors in monkeys and rabbits by chemical and radiation agents. *Acta Un. Int. Cancr.* **19**, 708–709.

Meskin, L. H., and Woolfrey, B.F. 1964. Radiographic localisation of labeled carcinogen. Carbon 14 labeled dimethylbenzanthracene in the hamster cheek pouch. *Arch. Path.* **78**, 643–647.

Mesrobian, A., and Shklar, G. 1969. Gingival carcinogenesis in the hamster, using tissue adhesives for carcinogen fixation. *J. Periodont.* **40**, 603–606.

Milievskaja, I. L., and Kiseleva, N. S. 1976. Comparative study of the carcinogenic activities of nas and some chemical carcinogens when introduced into the buccal pouch of the Syrian hamster. *Bull. WHO* **54**, 607–614.

Mohammad, A. R., and Mincer, H. H. 1976. Dinitrochlorobenzene contact hypersensitivity in the hamster cheek pouch. *J. Oral Pathol.* **5**, 169–174.

Moore, C., and Miller, A. J. 1958. Effect of cigarette smoke tar on the hamster pouch. *A.M.A. Arch. Surg.* **76**, 786–793.

Morris, A. L. 1961. Factors influencing experimental carcinogenesis in the hamster cheek pouch. *J. Dent. Res.* **40**, 3–15.

Morris, A. L., and Reiskin, A. B. 1965. Hamster cheek pouch response to varying lengths of carcinogen exposure. *J. Dent. Res.* **44**, 664–667.

Muir, C. S., and Kirk, R. 1960. Betel, tobacco, and cancer of the mouth. *Br. J. Cancer* **14**, 597–608.

Navia, J. M., and Baker, H. J. 1977. Experimental oral neoplasia. In: *Animal Models in Dental Research.* (Edited by Navia, J. M.), pp. 338–362. University of Alabama Press, University, Alabama.

Oyama, S. 1935. Experimentelle Studien über die Entstehung des Zungenkrebses. *Mitt. Med. Akad. Kioto* **15**, 861–880. (Cited by Fujita et al., 1973.)

Peacock, E. E., and Brawley, B. W. 1959. An evaluation of snuff and tobacco in the production of mouth cancer. *Plast. Reconstr. Surg.* **23**, 628–635.

Peacock, E. E., Greenberg, B. G., and Brawley, B. W. 1960. The effect of snuff and tobacco on the production of oral carcinoma: An experimental and epidemiological study. *Ann. Surg.* **151**, 542–550.

Philipsen, H. P., Fisker, A. V., and Stage, I. 1977. Experimental production of palatal carcinoma in rats by local application of 4-nitroquinoline N-oxide (4NQO). Abstract. *J. Dent. Res.* **56**, Special Issue A, A101.

Polliack, A., and Levij, I. S. 1969. The effect of topical vitamin A on papillomas and intraepithelial carcinomas induced in hamster cheek pouches with 9, 10-dimethyl-1, 2-benzanthracene. *Cancer Res.* **29**, 327–332.

Polliack, A., Levij, I. S., and Rwomushana, J. W. 1970. 9,10-dimethyl-1, 2-benzanthracene carcinogenesis in the hamster cheek pouch. Inhibitory effect of topically administered cortisone acetate. *Arch. Pathol.* **90**, 494–498.

Polliack, A., Levij, I. S., and Pfefferman, R. 1972. Observations on the effect of thymectomy on chemical carcinogenesis in the hamster cheek pouch. *Br. J. Cancer* **26**, 368–372.

Poswillo, D. E. 1971. Cryosurgery and electrosurgery compared in the treatment of experimentally induced oral carcinoma. *Br. Dent. J.* **131**, 347–352.

Poswillo, D. E., and Cohen, B. 1971. Inhibition of carcinogenesis by dietary zinc. *Nature* **231**, 447–448.

Protzel, M., Giardina, A. C., and Albano, E. H. 1964. The effect of liver imbalance on the development of oral tumors in mice following the application of benzpyrene or tobacco tar. *Oral Surg.* **18**, 622–635.

Ranadive, K. J., Gothoskar, S. V., and Khanolkar, V. R. 1963. Experimental studies on the etiology of cancer types specific to India. *Acta Un. Int. Cancr.* **19**, 634–639.

Renstrup, G., Smulow, J. B., and Glickman, I. 1962. Effect of chronic mechanical irritation on chemically induced carcinogenesis in the hamster cheek pouch. *J. Amer. Dent. Assoc.* **64**, 770–777.

Roffo, A. H. 1930. Leucoplasie expérimentale produite par le tabac. *Rev. Sudamér. Méd. Chir.* **1**, 321–330.

Rowe, N. H., and Gorlin, R. J. 1959. The effect of vitamin A deficiency upon experimental oral carcinogenesis. *J. Dent. Res.* **38**, 72–83.

Sabes, W. R., Chaudhry, A. P., and Gorlin, R. J. 1959. The effects of Tween-80 and prednisilone acetate on chemical carcinogenesis in the hamster cheek pouch. Abstract. *J. Dent Res.* **38**, 713.

Sabes, W. R., Chaudhry, A. P., and Gorlin, R. J. 1963. Effects of cortisone on chemical carcinogenesis in hamster pouch and submandibular salivary gland. *J. Dent Res.* **42**, 1118–1130.

Sabes, W. R., Singer, R. E., and Kuhn, T. 1972. Effectiveness of toluidine blue as an aid to biopsy in the diagnosis of DMBA-induced hamster pouch dysplasia and carcinoma. *Cancer* **29**, 1584–1589.

Salley, J. J. 1954. Experimental carcinogenesis in the cheek pouch of the Syrian hamster. *J. Dent. Res.* **33**, 253–262.

Salley, J. J. 1957. Experimental oral carcinogenesis. In: *Proceedings: 25th Year Celebration* (of the University of Rochester Dental Research Fellowship Program), pp. 132–140. University of Rochester, Rochester, New York.

Salley, J. J. 1961. Penetration of carcinogenic hydrocarbons into oral tissues as observed by fluorescence microscopy. *J. Dent. Res.* **40**, 177–184.

Salley, J. J., and Kreshover, S. J. 1959. The effect of topical application of carcinogens on the palatal mucosa of the hamster. *Oral Surg.* **12**, 501–508.

Sheehan, R., Shklar, G., and Tennenbaum, R. 1971. Azathioprine effects on the development of hamster pouch carcinomas. *Arch. Pathol.* **91**, 264–270.

Shklar, G. 1966. Cortisone and hamster buccal pouch carcinogenesis. *Cancer Res.* **26**, 2461–2463.

Shklar, G., Cataldo, E., and Fitzgerald, A. L. 1966. The effect of methotrexate on chemical carcinogenesis of hamster buccal pouch. *Cancer Res.* **26**, 2218–2224.

Shteyer, A., Greenman, S., and Lewin-Epstein, J. 1976. The effect of long standing chronic mechanical irritation on the tongue of rats. *J. Oral Pathol.* **5**, 287–294.

Silberman, S., and Shklar, G. 1963. The effect of a carcinogen (DMBA) applied to the hamster's buccal pouch in combination with croton oil. *Oral Surg.* **16**, 1344–1355.

Sirsat, S. M., and Kandarkar, S. V. 1968. Histological changes in the oral mucosa of the Wistar rat treated with commercial lime (calcium hydroxide). An optical and submicroscopic study. *Br. J. Cancer* **22**, 303–315.

Smith, C. J. 1968. Experimental carcinogenesis in the hamster cheek pouch: An histochemical investigation. Ph.D. dissertation, University of London.

Smith, C. J. 1972a. Variations in histochemical properties of hydrolytic enzymes in oral precancerous conditions. *J. Dent. Res.* **51**, 308–318.

Smith, C. J. 1972b. The epithelial-connective tissue junction in the pathogenesis of human and experimental oral cancer. In: *Tissue Interactions in Carcinogenesis.* (Edited by Tarin, D.), Chap. 7, pp. 191–225. Academic Press, London.

Stanley, H. R., Dawe, C. J., and Law, L. W. 1964. Oral tumors induced by polyoma virus in mice. *Oral Surg.* **17**, 547–558.

Stormby, N. G., and Wallenius, K. 1964. Effect of reduced salivation on oral tumour induction in hamsters by 9, 10-dimethyl-1, 2-benzanthracene. *Odont. Revy* **15**, 186–209.

Suzuki, M. 1976. Histological studies on early changes of the hamster gingival epithelium by N-nitrosomethylurea. *Bull. Tokyo Med. Dent. Univ.* **23**, 115–134.

Tabah, E. J., Gorecki, Z., Ritchie, A. C., and Skoryna, S. C. 1957. Effects of saturated solutions of tobacco tars and of 9, 10-dimethyl-1,2-benzanthracene on the hamster's cheek pouch. Abstract. *Proc. Am. Assn. Cancer Res.* **2**, 254.

Van Prohaska, J., Brunschwig, A., and Wilson, H. 1939. Oral administration of methycholanthrene to mice. *Arch. Surg.* **38**, 328–333.

Walker, F., Carter, J., Crawford, G. P., Laird, H., Lessels, A. M., and Pollet, J. E. 1970. Hamster cheek pouch mucosubstances and immunological privilege. *Br. J. Exp. Pathol.* **51**, 379–384.

Wallenius, K. 1966. Experimental oral cancer in the rat with special reference to the influence of saliva. *Acta Path. Microbiol. Scand.*, Suppl. 180, 1–91.

Wallenius, K., and Lekholm, U. 1973a. Oral cancer in rats induced by the water-soluble carcinogen 4-nitrochinoline N-oxide. *Odontol. Revy* **24**, 39–48.

Wallenius, K., and Lekholm, U. 1973b. Influence of saliva on epidermal cancer in rat induced by water- or fat-soluble carcinogens. *Odontol. Revy* **24**, 115–126.

Woods, D. A. 1969. Influence of antilymphocyte serum on DMBA induction of oral carcinomas. *Nature* **224**, 276–277.

Woods, D. A., and Smith, C. J. 1969. Ultrastructure of the dermal-epidermal junction in experimentally induced tumors and human oral lesions. *J. Invest. Derm.* **52**, 259–263.

Yamamura, T., Nishida, Y., Eda, S., Shimono, M., Yamane, H., Tachikawa, T., Koike, H., Ichikawa, T., Yoshida, M., Watanabe, O., and Matsuyama, H. 1975. An experimental study of intraoral carcinogenesis in rats. *Oral Surg.* **39**, 87–102.

8

Cervical Intraepithelia Neoplasia: A Model for Studying Oral Premalignancy

G. D. WILBANKS

Department of Obstetrics and Gynecology, Rush Medical College, Chicago, Illinois

1. INTRODUCTION

The "mouth of the womb" and the "mouth" of the alimentary tract, although quite distant anatomically, have many similarities in relation to early neoplastic epithelial lesions. They both have a mucocutaneous junction. Both the oral and vaginal epithelia are exposed to various foreign products and microorganisms, some of which are carcinogenic. This exposure is subject to cultural influences. Both areas are readily available to visible inspection and cell sampling. Finally, there is a rather high incidence of early lesions which should allow statistical analysis and encourage support for study from a public health standpoint.

This paper will be a short and simplified summary of a large and growing collection of data, both clinical and basic, from many investigators, regarding early cervical neoplasia. This data indicates strongly that the carcinogenic process in the cervix is a continuum beginning with mild dysplasia, usually progressing through more severe grades of dysplasia and carcinoma in situ (CIS), but remaining an intraepithelial neoplasm (hence the term cervical intraepithelial neoplasia, i.e., CIN). The end of the spectrum occurs when the basement membrane is breached initially with "microinvasion," then finally invasive carcinoma (Fig. 1). Not all the pieces of the puzzle are complete, but the hypothesis seems quite plausible.

2. HISTOLOGY

The human uterine cervix is composed of three types of epithelia, the native or original squamous epithelium, the columnar mucous epithelium of the endocervix, and the transformation zone (Fig. 2). The transformation zone is the area of the exposed endocervical mucous epithelium that eventually becomes squamous epithelium. This change usually occurs after puberty and is influenced by the hormonal, microbial, pH, and probably other changes in the milieu. The process has been classically described as a "squamous metaplasia," however the exact source of the cells that become these new squamous cells is debated at the present time. Some observers are able to find "reserve cells" beneath the columnar epithelium that possibly are the source of the new squamous epithelium (Johnson 1969). Others suggest that certain undifferentiated cells in the stroma are the source (Coppleson and Reid 1975). Finally, there are the proponents of the replacement occurring by the growing in of cells from the original squamous epithelium (Richart 1973). Whatever the source of these new cells in the transformation zone, this is the area in which the early neoplastic lesions of the cervix develop. It is postulated that it is these active, changing cells that are susceptible to the venereally transmitted carcinogen(s) as implicated by epidemiologic and other studies to be discussed later in this paper.

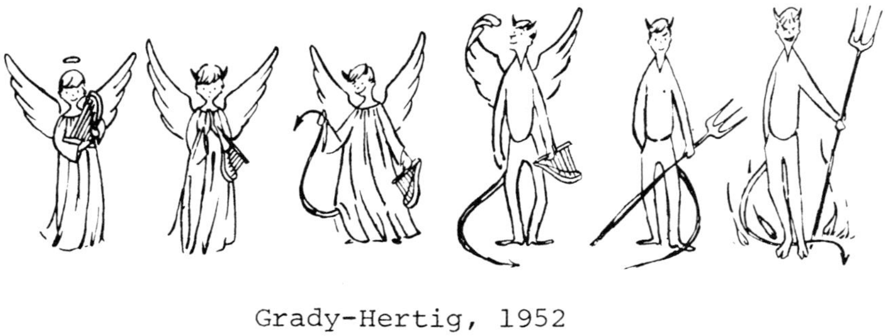

FIGURE 1. The metamorphosis of the angel to the devil depicts the theory of the pathogenesis of cervical neoplasia; i.e., from left to right: the normal cell, the "initiated" cell, dysplasia (early CIN), CIS (advanced CIN), microinvasion, and frank invasive cancer (see text for details). (Reproduced from McKelvey, J. L. 1952. Carcinoma in situ of the cervix: A general consideration. *Am. J. Obstet. Gynecol.* **64**, 816–832, by permission.)

Cervical carcinoma in situ has traditionally been defined as a lesion consisting of undifferentiated neoplastic cells extending throughout the full thickness of the epithelium. There obviously can be no penetration of the basement membrane. This definition differs from that of similar precursor states in other organ systems in that it requires that the cells not only fulfill the cytologic requirements for the diagnosis of neoplasia, but that the entire thickness be undifferentiated. Those lesions composed of cytologically abnormal cells but which failed to meet the criterion of full thickness dedifferentiation had many names until an international committee on terminology agreed on the term dysplasia (Stafl and Mattingly 1973). Dysplasia was defined as "all other disturbances of differentiation in the squamous epithelium lining the glands or covering the surface." This definition is so broad that almost any change from the completely normal cervical epithelium has been included under this term, without rigid cytologic criteria or consideration of other biologic parameters of the lesion. Currently, most cervical pathologists reserve the term dysplasia to define the earliest stage of the preinvasive neoplastic lesion of the cervix and the beginning of this continuum. In order to stress this continuum that is supported by much clinical and basic data, Richart (1973) has utilized the term cervical intraepithelial neoplasia (CIN) to encompass the true neoplastic lesions of dysplasia and carcinoma in situ (CIS). This is not a new concept, as Richart quotes Arthur Purdy Stout who wrote in 1957: "In the cervix the diagnosis of carcinoma in situ is generally not made if the surface is covered by a single layer of flattened cells that are not obviously anaplastic even though all of the surface beneath the flattened layer are anaplastic. This has always seemed to me to be a very arbitrary decision. If the anaplastic cells are in fact cancer cells, then a cancerous process is present whether or not it has involved the full thickness of the mucous membrane" (Richart 1973).

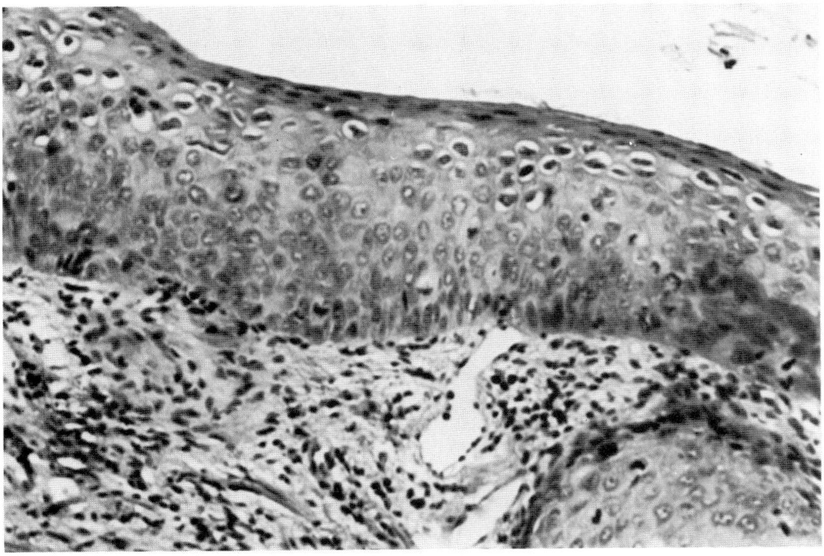

FIGURE 2. CIN 1 or mild dysplasia. There are undifferentiated cells with the characteristics of malignancy only in the lower ⅓ of the epithelium, but the cytologic atypia and disorderliness of maturation extend throughout the entire epithelium. Hematoxylin and eosin. X 160.

Therefore, the histologic diagnosis of CIN implies that even the earliest or mildest changes from the normal so diagnosed has the potential to become an invasive carcinoma. The continuum is broad so CIN has been divided into three grades. Grade I describes the earliest changes usually involving only the lower one-third of the epithelium appearing as undifferentiated neoplastic cells (Fig. 3). This would correspond to mild dysplasia in the older terminology. Grade 2 is utilized for those lesions previously described as "moderate dysplasia" in which the undifferentiated neoplastic cells constitute the lower two-thirds of the epithelium (Fig. 4). Grade 3 encompasses the lesions previously described as "severe dysplasia" and "carcinoma in situ" (Fig. 5). In these lesions essentially the entire thickness of the epithelium is involved.

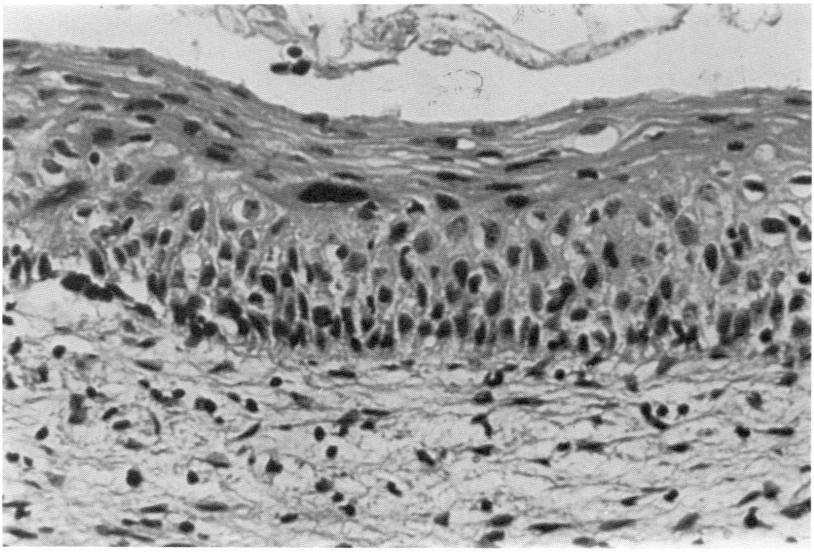

FIGURE 3. CIN 2 or moderate dysplasia. The lower ⅔ of the epithelium is composed of undifferentiated cells. The cytologic atypia and disorderly maturation is marked. Mitoses are seen in the middle epithelium. Hematoxylin and eosin. X 160.

The histologic definition of these lesions is dependent on the evaluation of the individual cell cytology of the involved epithelium and the overall assessment of the organizational pattern. Richart (1973) has described this nicely: "These lesions have in common a disorderliness in the epithelial maturation process and a degree of cytologic pleomorphism that are not seen in the non-neoplastic lesions of abnormal maturation which are confused with CIN. The CIN lesions have an 'irregularly irregular' pattern as opposed to the 'regularly irregular' pattern that is seen in the mimics." It is beyond the scope of this paper to discuss the details of the histologic nuances of these diagnoses, however Figures 3 to 5 illustrate the grades of CIN and an area of active squamous metaplasia with which early CIN is commonly confused.

The usual histologic criteria have been expanded by the electron microscope. With the transmission electron microscope, the cells of CIN lesions have an increase in microvilli and a decrease in the number of desmosomes, with many of the desmosomes present being abnormal and/or poorly formed (Shingleton and Wilbanks, 1974). The surface of a CIN lesion seen with the scanning electron microscope is characteristically different from normal cervical epithelium, both in standard biopsy specimens (Murphy et al. 1974) and in membrane filter "biopsy" specimens (the latter may be obtained without trauma to underlying cells) (Murphy et al. 1975). The cells of CIN are more rounded and variable in size and shape than are the normal squamous cells. Normal squamous epithelium has orderly ridges, whereas the cells of CIN have microvilli that vary in size, shape, and direction (Aurelian et al. 1971; Williams et al. 1973).

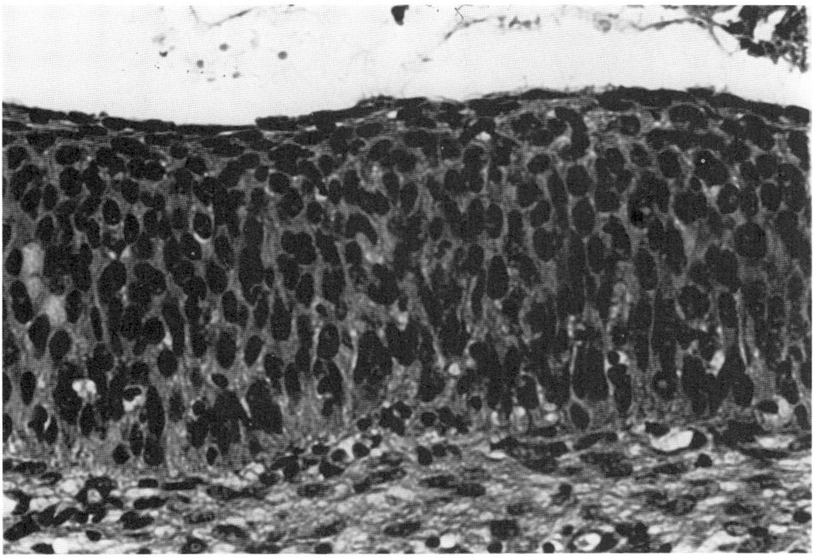

FIGURE 4. CIN 3 or severe dysplasia/CIS. The entire epithelium is composed of undifferentiated neoplastic cells. There is virtually no attempt at maturation. Mitoses are seen throughout the epithelium. Hematoxylin and eosin. X 160.

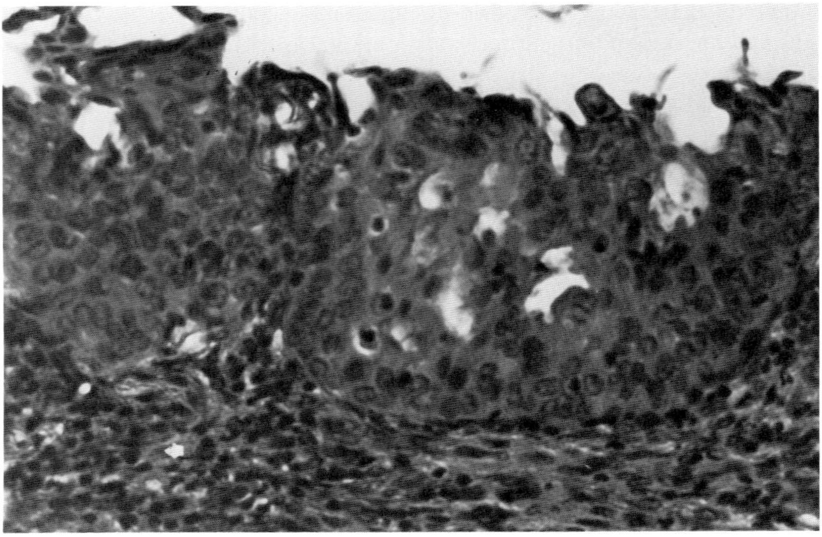

FIGURE 5. Squamous metaplasia. The metaplastic cells may be seen beneath the columnar cells. The metaplastic cells are regular, have well-defined borders and demonstrate no cellular atypia, although there is little epithelial maturation. Hematoxylin and eosin. X 160.

The chromosome number and karyotype of CIN and corresponding DNA measurements of CIN cells differ from those of normal cells (Atkin 1969). Jones et al. (1967) have suggested that these chromosome abnormalities, i.e., aneuploidy, may be used as diagnostic criteria for differentiating early CIN from active squamous metaplasia. There is no characteristic marker chromosome or chromosome number of the preinvasive lesions; instead, there is more of a random increase in total number of chromosomes. DNA measurements have given similar results to those studies using direct chromosome preparations. There is no characeristic DNA amount in the CIN lesions, but a clustering around the pseudo-diploid and pseudo-tetraploid ranges.

3. CLINICAL OBSERVATIONS

Rubin (1910) first described the lesion now called carcinoma in situ in 1910 when he began to examine histologically areas of the cervix other than the gross carcinoma. Thus the original intraepithelial neoplasias were found adjacent to areas of invasive cancers, having all the cellular characteristics of the cancer but lacking invasion. A few patients who had prior cervical biopsies later went on to develop invasive cancer. In retrospect, the changes of CIN were found in these earlier biopsies. A number of earlier "prospective" studies (Richart 1973) indicated that in spite of extensive biopsies that indeed may have removed the lesion to be followed, a high percentage of patients with CIS went on to develop invasive cancer or progress up the spectrum of CIN. The only nonbiopsied or manipulated prospective study is that of Richart and Barron (1969) in which patients with established CIN were followed by cytology, colpomicroscopy, and colposcopy, without biopsy, and only 5 of 557 patients observed up to 3 years did not progress.

The colposcope gives another dimension to clinical observation as well as adding a dimension to the gross "pathology" of the lesions of CIN. Even before this instrument was perfected, Schiller noted a difference in the staining reaction to iodine solution between areas of the cervix now identified as CIN and the normal epithelium. This is the result of the glycogen content of the normal epithelium which takes up the iodine stain. Unfortunately, lesions other than CIN also fail to stain so the "Schiller test" is rather nonspecific when used alone. Paul Younge (1965) however, was able to identify accurately areas of CIN by combining the Schiller stain and the astute observation of the gross characteristics of CIN. Areas of CIN show a peculiar "blush" in color and "roughness" in texture. Kolstad and Stafl (1977) refined these gross observations with the colposcope using vascular and epithelial characteristics as illustrated in Figs. 6 and 7. The changes are characteristic enough to be of use in the practical clinical management of patients with CIN. Many clinics have an accuracy of more than 90% in "diagnosing" the lesion later identified by biopsy (Stafl and Mattingly 1973).

These vascular and epithelial changes have been extensively studied (Kolstad and Stafl 1977). In summary, the normal squamous epithelium has a fine, flat, capillary network between the stroma and the epithelium. There are regular intercapillary distances (Fig. 6). In CIN, the distance between the capillaries can vary within relatively wide margins, but in general this distance is increased. The epithelium has an irregular surface and a change in "color tone." The lesions are sharply demarkated from the normal epithelium (Fig. 7a). Usually, the more irregular the epithelial and vascular pattern, the more severe the histologic changes. Invasive cancer, even microinvasion, is marked by terminal capillaries that are strikingly irregular in shape, caliber, consistency, and spatial configuration. These vessels run parallel and just below the surface of the epithelium (Fig. 7b). Probably as a result of these widely spaced and irregular vessels, the oxygen tension of CIN and invasive cancer is less that that of the normal cervix (Kolstad 1964). Stafl and Mattingly (1975) have followed a few patients

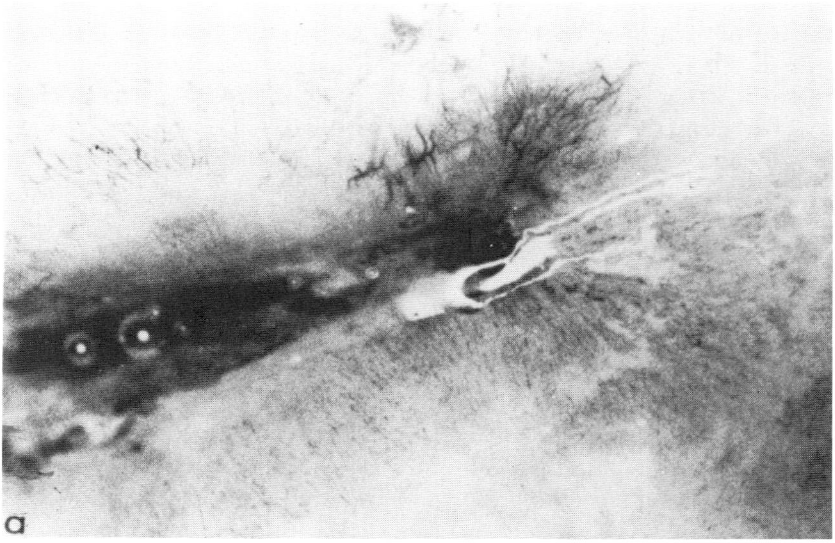

FIGURE 6. a. Colpophotograph of a normal cervix showing the external os (transverse opening). The original squamous epithelium shows fully differentiated multilayered epithelium with normal maturation; note the orderly blood vessel pattern.

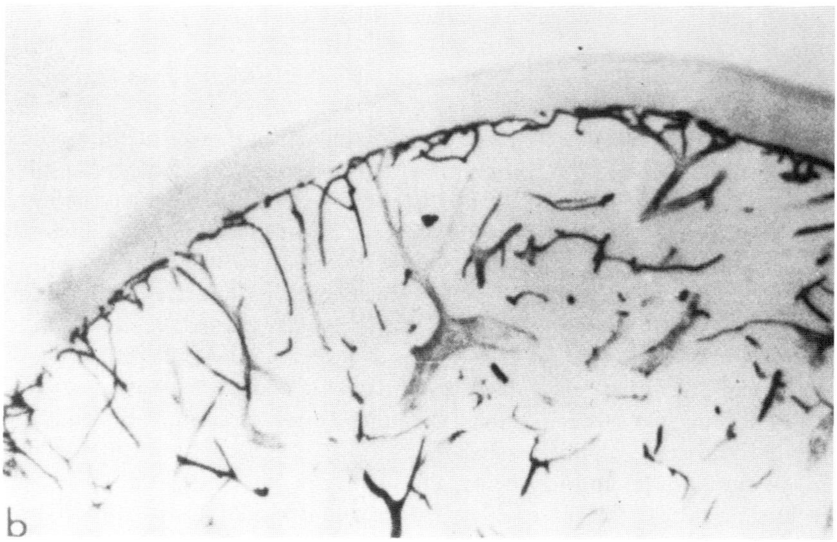

b. Histologic vascular preparation (100 μm thick section incubated with alkaline phosphatase) shows a flat capillary network at the border between the stroma and the epithelium. (Reproduced from Kolstad and Stafl, 1977, by permission.)

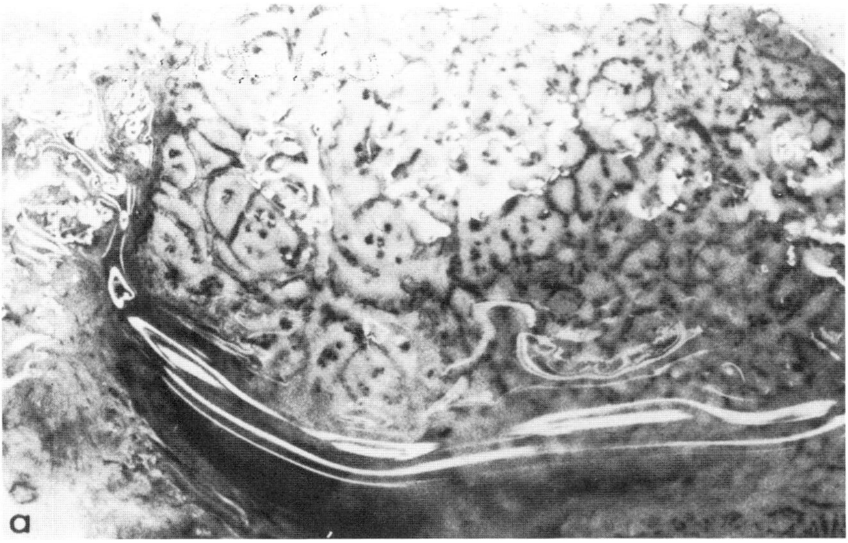

FIGURE 7. a. Colpophotograph of an area of CIN 3 with microinvasion and surrounding CIN 2. The course and irregular mosaic pattern, the extremely large intercapillary distances, and the whiteness of the epithelium all indicate that invasion is present. In the most abnormal area there was invasion of the stroma, although this was less than 5 mm.

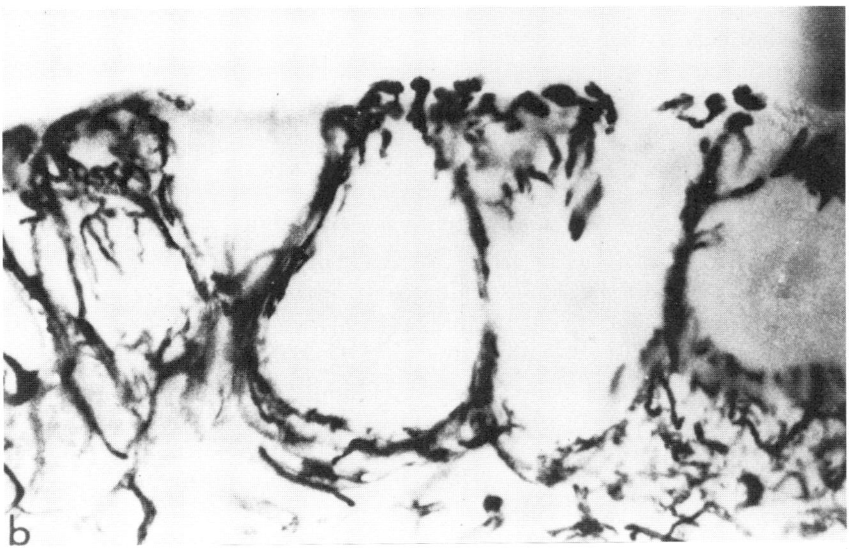

b. The vascular pattern demonstrates a significantly increased intercapillary distance with a completely chaotic arrangement of parallel vessels near the surface. (Reproduced from Kolstad and Stafl 1977, by permission.)

in whom characteristic vascular changes of CIN were seen to precede the histological cellular changes. Initially, the vascular abnormalities were in an area of histologically normal epithelium which later developed into histologically confirmed CIN.

4. ETIOLOGY

Patients with invasive squamous cell of the cervix, CIS, and dysplasia have certain common epidemiological characteristics. These women tend to begin coitus early, have multiple sexual partners, and have the first child before age 20 years (Kessler 1976). In contrast, cervical carcinoma is extremely rare in nuns, and thus behaves like a venereal disease.

One of the agents implicated in cervical carcinoma is the Herpes Simplex Virus, Type II (HSV-2). The possible correlation between cervical carcinoma and its precursors and HSV-2 is a complex one that has been reviewed recently (Herpesvirus and cervical cancer, 1973). Simply, women with cervical carcinoma and CIN have significantly higher titers to serum neutralizing antibodies for HSV-2 than do control women from the same country. Melnick et al. (1974) calculated the relative risk of developing invasive cancer for women with antibodies to HSV-2. If equal weight is given to the relative risk estimated from each area studied, the mean values of relative risk for invasive cancer, CIS, and dysplasia are very similar: 4.4, 4.7, and 4.5, respectively. From these estimates, the authors speculate that women with antibodies to HSV-2 are about 4.5 times more likely to develop cervical cancer than are women without antibodies and that the presence of antibodies to the virus also increases the risk of developing preinvasive lesions by a similar factor.

5. EXPERIMENTAL OBSERVATIONS

5:1 IMMUNOLOGIC STUDIES

Royston and Aurelian (1970) demonstrated the presence of HSV-2 antigens in cervical tumor cells exfoliated from human cervical carcinoma and its precursors, but could not demonstrate specific HSV-2 antigens by similar immunofluorescent techniques in biopsy material of tumors from these same individuals. Nahmias et al. (1975) have demonstrated HSV-2 antigens in biopsies of invasive cervical cancer by means of anticomplement immunofluorescence. Roizman and Frankel (1973) found nucleotide sequences corresponding to a fragment of the HSV-2 genome in a cervical cancer from one patient. They have not reported confirmatory studies on tumors from additional patients. An important requirement of the HSV-2 cervical cancer theory is to be able to isolate the virus from a human cancer or its precursor. Aurealian et al. (1971) have isolated infectious HSV-2 from cells grown in culture from one patient with CIS. They have not been able to repeat the isolation from additional patients and no one has confirmed the experiment. These isolated reports are intriguing, but the consistent isolation of an HSV-2 virus and/or the consistent identification of a portion of the HSV-2 genome in tumor tissue from patients with cervical cancer and its precursors must be the final link in what is thus far a circumstantial association.

Looking for more specific immunologic markers for cervical cancer and CIN, Aurelian (1976) and Hollinshead et al. (1973) have found a more specific antibody in patients with cervical cancer. The data on this antigen are not complete as Sabin (1974) reported he was unable to confirm earlier work reported from his laboratory by Sabin and Tarro (1973). Singer et al. (1975) reported finding cellular immunity to human basic myelin protein (EF) in women with CIN. Unfortunately, other studies have shown up to 31% of patients with nonmalignant conditions may be sensitized to EF. These data are preliminary, but if reproducible may identify a specific immunologic marker for CIN.

5:2 ANIMAL STUDIES

Animal models have been used to illustrate the continuum of early cervical neoplasia and to test various carcinogens. Reagan et al. (1969) produced dysplasia, CIS, and invasive cancer in various rodents using a variety of chemical carcinogens. More recently Wentz et al. have produced dysplasia in the mouse cervix using irradiated and other inactivated HSV-2 virus (personal communication). Palmer et al. (1976) have produced dysplasia in the cervix of the Cebus monkey with HSV-2, but have not produced an invasive carcinoma. The use of animal models tends to support the process of CIN as a continuum, but has not specifically indicated the primary carcinogen involved.

5:3 IN VITRO STUDIES

Several in vitro studies support the theories of this continuum. Richart (1963) applied a short-term tritiated thymidine incubation technique to a large number of cervical biopsies with diagnoses varying from normal through CIN Grades, I, II, and III. The labeling index was found to increase logarithmically almost as a straight line with the severity of the lesion (see also chapter 13). Averette has reported similar findings from in vivo experiments (Averette et al. 1970). These indicate a continuum, rather than two different cell populations, representing dysplasia and CIS.

Tissue culture has been used to study the lesions of CIN with varying degrees of success (Wilbanks 1969). Normal epithelium from the adult human cervix is difficult to grow. It has not been maintained in culture and no cell line has been established. Wilbanks (1969) and Richart (1973) have noted an aggressive behavior of normal epithelium in culture, which they have compared to certain clinical observations of healing of the biopsied lesions. They have had success in growing normal epithelium for short-term experiments.

Most researchers have found CIS to have in vitro characteristics either similar to invasive carcinoma or somewhat in between normal and invasive carcinoma. Dysplasia (including various atypias) usually is reported as having characteristics that differ from the normal in most parameters and is either similar to CIS or in between normal and CIN. Simeckova et al. (1962) found good correlation between growth characteristics in vitro and histopathological correlation, but Richart (1973) did not find such a correlation.

In general, the normal cervical cells grow as a sheet of attached cells, with little overlapping. The cells in culture gradually "differentiate" and lift off the glass. The culture cannot be transferred and does not survive more than 6–8 weeks. In contrast, cells from CIN (varying grades) grow more as individual cells, with some overlapping and can be transferred and maintained in culture up to 20–30 passages (Wilbanks 1969).

The CIN cells have some loss of contact inhibition, but not complete loss as in most invasive cancers. Using the electron microscope, both transmission (Shingleton and Wilbanks 1974) and scanning electron microscopy (Ferenczy and Richart 1974; Roizman and Frenkel 1973), the normal cells and CIN cells in tissue culture have characteristics similar to the same lesions in biopsy specimens.

6. SUMMARY

The human uterine cervix and the oral cavity seem to be similar in that they offer a unique opportunity to study the early lesions of epithelial carcinoma. Data from the uterine cervix suggest that cervical neoplasia is a continuum beginning with mild dysplasia (CIN 1) usually progressing through more severe grades of CIN (CIS) to invasive cancer. The earliest lesion of CIN has chromosomal and/or DNA aneuploidy suggestive of malignancy. Clinical observations and epidemiologic studies suggest a venereal nature to the disease. Immunologic-epidemiologic and some laboratory research data suggest HSV-2 as a possible carcinogen, although so far the majority of the data is circumstantial. Other animal and in vitro studies support these hypotheses. It is hoped that the combining of some of the basic, clinical, and epidemiologic data form the study of early lesions of oral cavity and cervix may speed the answers to many of the questions of these two common human neoplasias.

REFERENCES

Atkin, N. B. 1969. Perimodal variations of DNA values of normal and malignant cells. *Acta Cytol.* **13**, 270–273.

Aurelian, L. 1976. Coitus and cancer. *Bull. N. Y. Acad. Med.* **52**, 910–934.

Aurelian, L., Strandberg, J. D., Melendez, L. V., and Johnson, L. A. 1971. Herpes virus type 2 isolated from cervical tumor cells grown in tissue culture. *Science* **174**, 704–707.

Averette, H. E., Weinstein, G. D., and Frost, P. 1970. Audioradiographic analysis of cell proliferation kinetics in human genital tissues. I. Normal cervix and vagina. *Am. J. Obstet. Gynecol.* **108**, 8–17.

Coppleson, M., and Reid, B. 1975. Origin of premalignant lesions of cervix uteri. In: *Progress in Gynecology.* (Edited by Taymor, M. C., and Green, T. H.), Vol. 6, pp. 517–539. Grune and Stratton, New York.

Ferenczy, A., and Richart, R. M. 1974. *Female Reproductive System: Dynamics of Scan and Transmission Electron Microscopy.* John Wiley, New York.

Fox, C. H., Turner, F. G., Johnson, W. L., and Thornton, W. N. 1962. Endometrial cytology, a new technique. *Am. J. Obstet. Gynecol.* **83**, 1582–1591.

Gall, S. A., and Haines, H. G. 1974. Cervical carcinoma antigen and the relationship to HSV-2. *Gynecol. Oncol.* **2**, 451–459.

Haenszel, W., and Hillhouse, M. 1959. Uterine-cancer morbidity in New York City and its relation to the pattern of regional variation within the United States. *J. Natl. Cancer Inst.* **22**, 1157–1181.

Hollinshead, A. C., Lee, O., Chretien, T. B., Tarpley, J. L., Rawls, W. E., and Adam, E. 1973. Antibodies to herpesvirus nonviron antigens in squamous carcinomas. *Science* **182**, 713–715.

Johnson, L. D. 1969. The histological approach to early cervical neoplasia. *Obstet. Gynecol. Survey* **24**, 735–767.

Jones, H. W., Katayama, K. P., Stafl, A., and Davis, H. J. 1967. Chromosomes of cervical atypia, carcinoma in situ and epidermoid carcinoma of the cervix. *Obstet. Gynecol.* **30**, 790–805.

Kessler, I. I. 1976. Human cervical cancer as a venereal disease. *Cancer Res.* **36**, 783–791.

Kolstad, P. 1964. *Vascularization, Oxygen Tension and Radiocurability in Cancer of the Cervix.* Universitetsforlaget, Oslo.

Kolstad, P., and Stafl, A. 1977. *Atlas of Colposcopy.* 2d. rev. ed. University Park Press, Baltimore.

Melnick, J. L., Adam, E., and Rawls, W. E. 1974. The causative role of herpesvirus type 2 in cervical cancer. *Cancer* **34**, 1375–1385.

Murphy, J. F., Allen, J. M., Jordan, J. A., and Williams, A. E. 1975. Scanning electron microscopy of normal and abnormal exfoliated cervical squamous cells. *Br. J. Obstet. Gynaecol.* **82**, 44–51.

Murphy, J. F., Jordan, J. A., Allen, J. M., and Williams, A. E. 1974. Correlation of scanning electron microscopy, colposcopy and histology in 50 patients presenting with abnormal cervical cytology. *J. Obstet. Gynaecol. Br. Commonw.* **81**, 236–241.

Nahmias, A. J., Del Buono, I., and Ibrahin, J. 1975. Antigenic relationship between herpes simplex viruses, human cervical cancer and HSV-associated hamster tumours. In: *Oncogenesis and Herpesviruses.* (Edited by de-Thé, G., Epstein, M. A., and zur Hausen, H.), Vol. 2, Part 1, pp. 309–313. (IARC Scientific Publications No. 11). International Agency for Research on Cancer, Lyon.

Palmer, A. E., London, W. T., Nahmias, A. J., Naib, Z. M., Tunca, J., Fuccillo, D. A., Ellenberg, J. H., and Sever, J. L. 1976. A preliminary report on investigation of oncogenic potential of herpes simplex virus type 2 in Cebus monkeys. *Cancer Res.* **36**, 807–809.

Reagan, J. W., Ng, A. B. P., and Wentz, W. B. 1969. Concepts of genesis and development in early cervical neoplasia. *Obstet. Gynec. Survey* **24**, 860–873.

Richart, R. M. 1963. A radioautographic analysis of cellular proliferation in dysplasia and carcinoma in situ of the uterine cervix. *Am. J. Obstet. Gynecol.* **86**, 925–930.

Richart, R. M. 1973. Cervical intraepithelial neoplasia. In: *Pathology Annual.* (Edited by Sommers, S. C.), Vol. 8, pp. 301–328. Appleton-Century-Crofts, New York.

Richart, R. M., and Barron, B. A. 1969. A follow-up study of patients with cervical dysplasia. *Am. J. Obstet. Gynecol.* **105**, 386–393.

Roizman, B., and Frenkel, N. 1973. The transcription and state of herpes simplex virus DNA in productive infection and in human cervical cancer tissue. *Cancer Res.* **33**, 1402–1416.

Royston, I., and Aurelian, L. 1970. The association of genital herpesvirus with cervical atypia and carcinoma in situ. *Am. J. Epidemiol.* **91**, 531–538.

Rubin, I. C. 1910. The pathological diagnosis of incipient carcinoma of the uterus. *Am. J. Obstet.* **62**, 668–676.

Sabin, A. 1974. Herpes simplex-genitalis virus nonviron antigens and their implication in certain human cancers: Unconfirmed. *Proc. Natl. Acad. Sci. USA* **71**, 3248–3252.

Sabin, A. B., and Tarrow, G. 1973. Herpes simplex and herpes genitalis viruses in etiology of some human cancers. *Proc. Natl. Acad. Sci. USA* **70**, 3225–3229.

Shingleton, H. M., Richart, R. M., Wiener, J., and Spiro, D. 1968. Human cervical intraepithelial neoplasia: Fine structure of dysplasia and carcinoma in situ. *Cancer Res.* **28**, 695–706.

Shingleton, H. M., and Wilbanks, G. D. 1974. Fine structure of human cervical intraepithelial neoplasia in vivo and in vitro. *Cancer* **33**, 981–989.

Simeckova, M., Nichols, E., and Lonser, E. 1962. Tissue cultures in gynecologic research. *Obstet. Gynecol.* **20**, 251–255.

Singer, A., Shelton, J., Hill, S., and Pottern, C. 1975. Cellular immunity to human basic myelin protein in women with dysplasia and carcinoma in situ of the cervix. *Br. J. Obstet. Gynaecol.* **82**, 820–825.

Stafl, A., and Mattingly, R. F. 1973. Colposcopic diagnosis of cervical neoplasia. *Obstet. Gynecol.* **41**, 168–176.

Stafl, A., and Mattingly, R. F. 1975. Angiogenesis of cervical neoplasia. *Am. J. Obstet. Gynecol.* **121**, 845–852.

Weid, G. L. 1961. *International Congress of Exfoliated Cytology.* Proceedings. 1st. 1961. (Edited by Weid, G. L.), p. 283. Lippincott, Philadelphia.

Wilbanks, G. D. 1969. Tissue culture in early cervical neoplasia. A review and prospectus. *Obstet. Gynecol Survey* **24**, 804–837.

Wilbanks, G. D. 1976. In vivo and in vitro 'markers' of human cervical intraepithelial neoplasia. *Cancer Res.* **36**, 2485–2494.

Williams, A. E., Jordan, J. A., Allen, J. M., and Murphy, J. F. 1973. The surface ultrastructure of normal and metaplastic cervical epithelial and of carcinoma in situ. *Cancer Res.* **33**, 504–513.

Younge, P. A. 1965. The natural history of carcinoma in situ of the cervix uteri. *J. Obstet. Gynaecol. Br. Commonw.* **72**, 9–16.

Discussion

Dr. Solt asked Professor Smith whether a step-wise mechanism of initiation and promotion has been clearly demonstrated in hamster cheekpouch carcinogenesis. Professor Smith replied that a two-step process has been demonstrated by the use of low doses of DMBA followed by croton oil. Dr. Slavkin commented that mice have been widely used in studies of skin carcinogenesis and asked Professor Smith whether the observed resistance to development to oral carcinoma in mice might be related to choice of strains that had been used for examination and whether there has been an exhaustive study of the use of mice for oral carcinogenesis. Professor Smith replied that mice have not been exhaustively studied, perhaps because early in the development of a model of oral cancer, the hamster cheek pouch had proved so successful. Dr. Outzen suggested that the longer retention of carcinogen in the blind-ending pouch might account for a greater effectiveness of a carcinogen which would be washed away more rapidly by saliva from other parts of the oral cavity. Dr. Squier referred to work by Wallenius (1965; 1966) which had shown that skin transplanted to the oral cavity of the rat is similarly resistant to carcinogenesis indicating an effect of saliva. However it appeared that, rather than a washing effect, the role of saliva might be in forming a barrier at the surface which prevents penetration of lipid soluble carcinogens. Dr. Mackenzie commented that he had noticed that agents such as hexadecane, which produce a marked hyperplasia of the epidermis, fail to do so when applied to the oral mucosa unless used in conjunction with dimethylsulfoxide which presumably acts to increase mucosal permeability. Dr. Outzen, referring to Professor Smith's comment that most of the lesions seen in the cheek pouch during experimental carcinogenesis progress quite rapidly to carcinoma, asked whether this might be a dosage effect. Human carcinogenesis appears to be associated with exposure to weak carcinogens over a long period of time. Would a model more closely mimicking the latent period for human carcinogenesis be obtained by using lower doses for longer periods? Professor Smith agreed that this might be possible, but added that the cheek pouch model has been primarily intended to study the carcinoma stage of the lesion. A rapid development has therefore been considered desirable and information that might be relevant to premalignancy has mostly been obtained only coincidentally.

Dr. Wilbanks, replying to a question from Dr. Smith as to whether changes in the properties of contact inhibition of normal cervical cells in culture have been observed as the result of infection with herpes virus, said that he has spent several years attempting to develop a method of examining carcinogenesis of cervical epithelium in vitro. So far, little information is available. Addition of herpes virus to cultures leads to such rapid cell destruction that changes in cell contact properties cannot be examined. Following various modifications of viral action, for example by UV light, heat, or antibodies, cells remained vital, but changes typical of transformation have not been observed. Dr. Wilbanks added that classical concepts of contact inhibition, developed for examination of fibroblasts, do not readily apply to cultures of normal cervical epithelial cells which move as a sheet and not as individual cells. Cultures of carcinomatous cells from the cervix, do, however, grow and move as individual cells and it is interesting that cells from lesions of carcinoma in situ appear to behave in an intermediate fashion.

Dr. Slavkin asked whether assays for the localization of actin might be a way of identifying groups of epithelial cells which were about to metastasize. Dr. Dabelsteen replied that unpublished studies he had undertaken with Dr. Birkedal-Hansen in Copenhagen, using immunofluorescent staining methods, have shown the presence of actin in the cells of advancing edges of sheets of growing epithelial cells in culture. The staining for actin disappeared when the cells reached confluence. An examination of actin in premalignant lesions, carcinoma, and wounds of the oral mucosa has shown actin in fibroblasts associated with healing wounds but not in any of the epithelial cells. Dr. Dabelsteen added, however, that he is aware of differences in the antigenicity of the range of actin and actin-like substances that might be present in the epithelial cells. His work has been limited to human anti-actin antibodies which are of uncertain specificity.

Dr. Johnson stated that work with microphotometry appears to show a correlation between the DNA content of the cells of an overtly malignant lesion and the subsequent behavior of the lesion. By and large, lesions with near-normal diploid cells have the better prognosis except in the cervix where the reverse seems to hold (Atkin 1976). He asked Dr. Wilbanks if there was any explanation for this peculiarity. Dr. Wilbanks said he had no clear explanation for these observations but that, in the cervix, perhaps the more nearly normal cells are less readily recognized by the body as altered and therefore have a better opportunity to metastasize.

Dr. Waldron asked Dr. Wilbanks about the progression of cervical dysplasia and how certain it was that a mild dysplasia would eventually become carcinoma in situ. Dr. Wilbanks felt that this was the normal course of events. This progression was clearly shown by the follow-up studies of Richart (1973). Dr. Dabelsteen asked whether cervical carcinoma in situ shows evidence of a monoclonal origin. Dr. Wilbanks replied that although carcinoma in situ of the cervix has been extensively investigated, there appears to be no consistent chromosomal marker or other change apparent within the group of cells forming the carcinoma in situ. However, some sort of stem cell line appears to become established upon epithelial invasion.

REFERENCES

Atkin, N. B. 1976. Prognostic significance of ploidy level in human tumours. II. Extra-uterine cancers and summary of data on 1171 tumours. *Cytobios* **15**, 233–237.

Richart, R. M. 1973. Cervical intraepithelial neoplasia. In: *Pathology Annual*. (Edited by Sommers, S. C.), Vol. 8, pp. 301–328. Appleton-Century-Crofts, New York.

Wallenius, K. 1965. Effect of 7, 12-dimethylbenz(a)anthracene in the rat's cheek skin transplanted to the buccal cavity. *Odontol. Revy* **16**, 204–215.

Wallenius, K. 1966. Experimental oral cancer in the rat. With special reference to the influence of saliva. *Acta Pathol. Microbiol. Scand.* Suppl. **180**, 1–91.

PART FOUR
PATTERNS OF CELL BEHAVIOR IN NORMAL AND PREMALIGNANT TISSUES

9

Structure of Normal Oral Mucosa

C. A. SQUIER

Dows Institute for Dental Research, College of Dentistry, University of Iowa, Iowa City, Iowa

1. INTRODUCTION

This chapter has two main purposes: to provide a brief account of the normal organization of the human oral mucosa, and to discuss some aspects of its structure and function that may be relevant to a consideration of malignant change.

Although the oral cavity represents the beginning of the digestive tube, most of its lining is derived from the ectoderm that during embryological development gives rise to the skin. The oral mucosa thus shows varied properties, resembling the intestinal mucosa in having a moist surface and an epithelium with a relatively high rate of cell turnover but, on the other hand, having many of the characteristics of the skin including, in some regions, a keratinized surface virtually indistinguishable in its structure from the epidermis.

2. ORGANIZATION OF THE ORAL MUCOSA

The oral mucosa is usually divided on a functional basis into three main types (Stern 1976): (a) a lining mucosa, covering much of the surface of the mouth including the inside of the lips and cheeks, the floor of mouth, underside of tongue and soft palate; (b) a masticatory mucosa which covers the gingivae and hard palate; and (c) the specialized mucosa of the dorsum of the tongue which, although functionally a masticatory mucosa, bears the specialized lingual papillae and taste buds. These mucosae differ in their structure and in their attachment to underlying structures and this reflects the different functional demands of each region. Thus, lining mucosa covers mobile structures and is flexible and distensible, consisting of a nonkeratinized epithelial surface and a loosely fibrous connective tissue flexibly attached to underlying muscle or bone, while masticatory mucosa, which is exposed to the mechanical compression and friction of mastication, usually has a keratinized epithelium overlying a dense fibrous connective tissue and is firmly adherent to underlying structures.

3. THE ORAL EPITHELIUM

The most characteristic histological changes of oral premalignancy are seen in the epithelium, and it is this tissue that will now be considered in more detail. In all regions of the oral cavity the surface epithelium is a stratified squamous epithelium which serves as the primary barrier of the mucosa. In fulfilling this role, the surface cells are constantly lost or desquamated and replaced by divisions in the deeper layers which provide new cells that differentiate or mature as they move to the surface. The rate of proliferation, the number of cell layers, and the type of maturation and the nature of the surface layer are all features of the epithelium which vary in different regions, as does the overall thickness of the epithelium and the contours of the epithelium-connective tissue interface. These latter features have recently been quantified by Klein-Szanto and Schroeder (1977) and some of their data is presented in Table 1. Thus, in the floor of the mouth there is a thin epithelium with a few shallow epithelial ridges whereas the gingiva is a thick tissue with numerous deep ridges. Such variation means that there are considerable differences in the ratio of the area of the epithelium-connective tissue interface to that of the epithelial surface which may allow for different rates of metabolic exchange and different degrees of mechanical attachment between epithelium and connective tissue in various regions (Scapino 1971).

Ultrastructurally, the basal complex or basal lamina between epithelium and connective tissue consists of a lamina lucida and a lamina densa into which are inserted small anchoring fibrils (Fig. 1). The morphology and dimensions of the basal lamina are similar in all oral regions, as they are in most other organs of the body (Kefalides 1975). There has often been some emphasis placed on discontinuities and duplication of the lamina densa as an indicator of incipient malignant change of the epithelium (Tarin 1967). However, breaks may occupy up to 9% of the area of the basal lamina in apparently normal tissue (Franklin, personal communication) and duplication is frequently a consequence of nonspecific inflammation (MacCallum et al. 1975). The significance of these features are further discussed in chapters 11 and 21.

3:1 EPITHELIAL PROLIFERATION

It has already been mentioned that the surface cells are constantly being lost from the surface and replaced by division so that normally the epithelium maintains a constant thickness (see chapter 12). However, as the tissue has a different thickness and a different pattern of maturation in different regions, it is not surprising that the rate of cell proliferation also varies from region to region. As Hill points out in chapter 13, the variety of methods for measuring cell proliferation and the different ways of expressing the results make it difficult to present accurate data, but Table 2 represents comparative data for approximate turnover times in different regions of human oral epithelium. While the range gives some idea of the enormous variation encountered in the literature, a few points emerge. Turnover is generally faster in oral epithelium than in epidermis, with a tendency for the thicker, nonkeratinized epithelium to turn over more rapidly than keratinized regions such as the gingiva. There are factors such as inflammation (Hopps and Johnson 1975), friction (Mackenzie and Miles 1973), and chemical agents (Baird et al. 1971) that may frequently affect turnover rates, and this makes studies of proliferation in pathological situations particularly complex (see chapter 13).

TABLE 1

Regional Variation of Human Oral Epithelium and the Epithelium-Connective Tissue Interface

Site	*Average thickness* (μm)	*Height of connective tissue papillae* (μm)	*Number of connective tissue papillae* (*per* mm^2)
Floor of mouth	86	30	16
Alveolar mucosa	260	165	46
Lip	370	245	76
Cheek	480	340	73
Hard palate	248	190	114
Attached gingiva	255	170	119

Based on Klein-Szanto and Schroeder (1977).

TABLE 2

Turnover Times of Various Epithelia

Skin	52–75 days (1)
Gingiva	41–57 days (2)
Buccal mucosa	25 days (3)

The time given is that required for the total thickness of the epithelium to be replaced. The wide range of values arise by the use of different techniques to evaluate the rate of cell proliferation.

(1) Halprin (1972).
(2) Calculated from Meyer et al. (1956).
(3) Alvares et al. (1972).

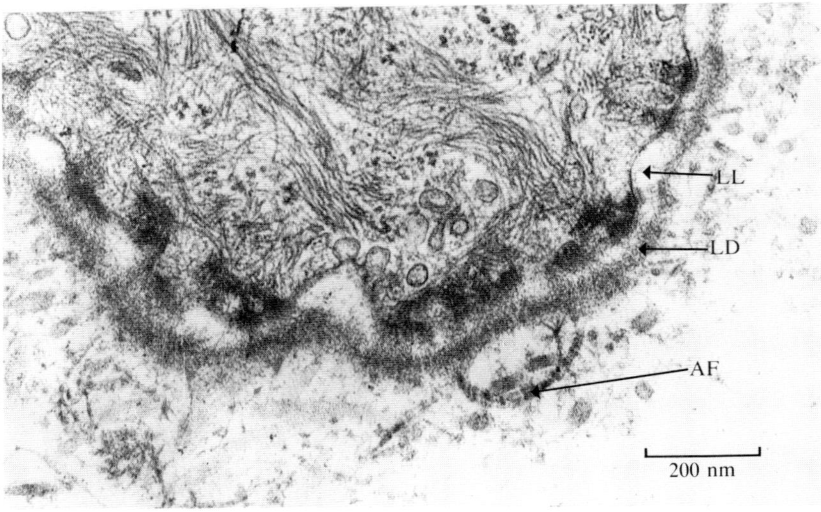

FIGURE 1. Electron micrograph of the basal complex of oral mucosa showing the lamina lucida (LL), lamina densa (LD), and an anchoring fibril (AF). Marker represents 200 nm.

Within any given epithelium there is still some uncertainty as to where divisions take place. Thus, while many authors assume that mitosis only occurs in the basal layer (Cameron 1966; Cutright and Bauer 1967), there have been reports of as many as 40% of the divisions appearing in the spinous layer in some human oral epithelia (Kaidbey and Kurban 1971; Kittler et al. 1969). Generally, it appears that most dividing cells lie on the basement membrane, and all are within three cell layers of it (Löe et al. 1972). A similar confusion has arisen over the distribution of mitosis along the basement membrane. It has often been claimed that division occurs randomly at any point on the basement membrane (Leblond et al. 1964), but there is evidence that there may be clustering of divisions at certain sites. For example, they are seen at the bottom of the epithelial ridges in gingiva (Löe et al. 1972) and palate (Mackenzie, I. C. and Dabelsteen, E., personal communication). This has important implications for the determination and maintenance of patterns of tissue organization (see chapter 14).

3:2 EPITHELIAL MATURATION

In morphological terms, differences such as the rate of cell proliferation and the distribution of mitoses are not as obvious as the patterns of epithelial maturation, and in particular the type of surface layer formed in different regions of the oral mucosa. The human oral epithelium shows a

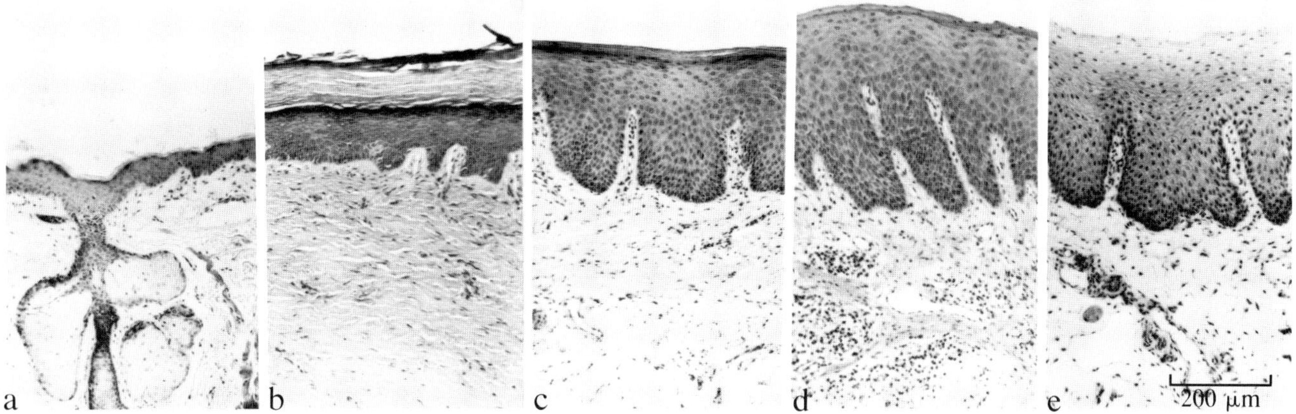

FIGURE 2. The range of appearances of human oral epithelium (b-e) compared with skin (a). Note the difference in thickness and in type of surface layer: (a) skin containing sebaceous gland from the face, (b) hyperkeratotic epithelium from palate of a smoker, (c) normal orthokeratinized palatal epithelium, (d) parakeratinized gingival epithelium, (e) nonkeratinized buccal epithelium. Marker represents 200 μm.

considerable diversity of appearances ranging from a thick orthokeratinized layer to parakeratinization and nonkeratinization (Fig. 2). The events that produce these different patterns of maturation consist of a series of cellular changes taking place in each stratum of the epithelium, the end product in a keratinized (or parakeratinized) epithelium being keratin. In the epidermis, keratin is envisaged as a system of protein microfilaments embedded in a matrix that is rich in sulphur (Fraser et al. 1972) (Fig. 3), and the arrangement is probably similar in keratinized oral epithelium, although there has been very little detailed analysis (Dale et al. 1977). The filaments in keratin seem to be derived from the tonofilaments which are seen at all levels in the keratinizing epithelium (Meyer and Schroeder 1975). These become arranged in bundles called tonofibrils as the epithelial cell migrates from the basal layer and are conspicuous in the prickle cell layer (Fig. 4a). As the cell moves to the granular layer (Fig. 5a), there is a change in its shape and in its content of organelles made particularly evident by the appearance of numbers of irregular dense granules, the keratohyalin granules. These granules are intimately associated with the tonofilaments (Fig. 5a inset), which they are believed to coat so as to form a matrix by the time the cell reaches the keratinized layer (Brody 1959; Chen and Meyer 1971). Between the granular layer and the keratinized layer there is a loss of all the organelles except for the filaments, and the cells become dehydrated and flattened (Fig. 4b). The superficial cells are thus filled entirely with a mass of fibrillar protein that is both mechanically tough and insoluble (Iqbal and Gerson 1971). Parakeratinization, which is common in some regions of the oral cavity such as the palate and gingiva (Fig. 2), represents a pattern of maturation similar to that of orthokeratinization, but without a total loss of organelles in the granular layer so that the nuclei, for example, persist in the surface layer as shrunken, pyknotic structures (Silverman 1971).

By contrast with ortho- and parakeratinized oral epithelium, the morphological changes in nonkeratinized oral epithelium are less striking. Tonofilaments are again present at all levels, but they are arranged as a loose network and not aggregated into bundles (Fig. 4b) (Chen and Meyer 1971; Landay and Schroeder 1977). There is again a change in shape of the cells as they move to the surface, but this is not so marked as in keratinized epithelium. Keratohyalin granules are occasionally seen (Meyer et al. 1967; Rubinstein et al. 1970; Silverman 1971), and glycogen is often present in the superficial part of the epithelium. Some of the organelles, including the nuclei, persist to the surface (Landay and Schroeder 1977) (Fig. 5b). In morphological terms, this picture is very similar to that of the normal nonkeratinized cervical epithelium (Hackemann et al. 1968) (see chapter 8).

3:3 QUANTITATIVE STUDIES OF EPITHELIAL MATURATION

The events taking place during maturation of epidermis and various oral epithelia have recently been quantified by Schroeder and his coworkers

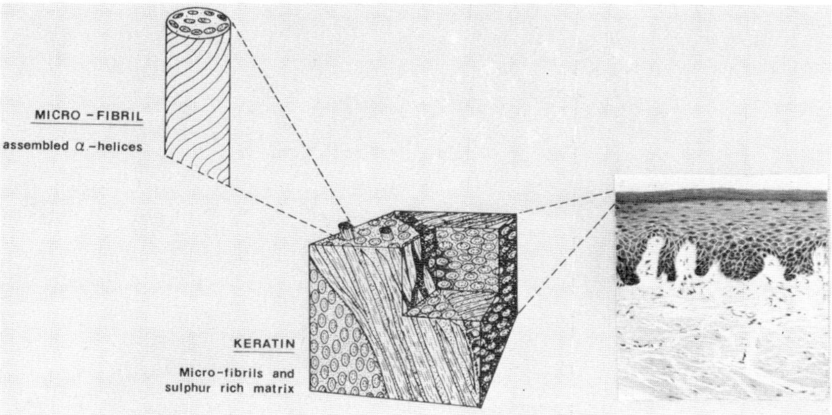

FIGURE 3. Diagram of the macromolecular organization of keratin. (Based on data from Brody, 1959 and Fraser et al., 1972).

(Meyer and Schroeder 1975; Klein-Szanto et al. 1976; Bernimoulin and Schroeder 1977; Landay and Schroeder 1977). The basis for these procedures is described more fully in chapter 15, but the method essentially provides information about the composition of a unit volume of epithelium so that the ultrastructural organization can be compared at different levels in the same epithelium and between the same levels of different epithelia.

Data from an analysis of the nucleated layers of epidermis, keratinized palatal epithelium and nonkeratinized buccal epithelium, is presented in graphical form in Figure 6. The changes in concentration of the various organelles from layer to layer seen in epidermis and keratinized oral epithelium are very similar; there is a gradual increase in filaments and a decrease in organelles except for the relatively rapid increase of keratohyalin granules. The Figure does not include values for the stratum corneum, where there would be no organelles, a high concentration of filaments, and some cytoplasmic ground substance (Schroeder, H. E.,

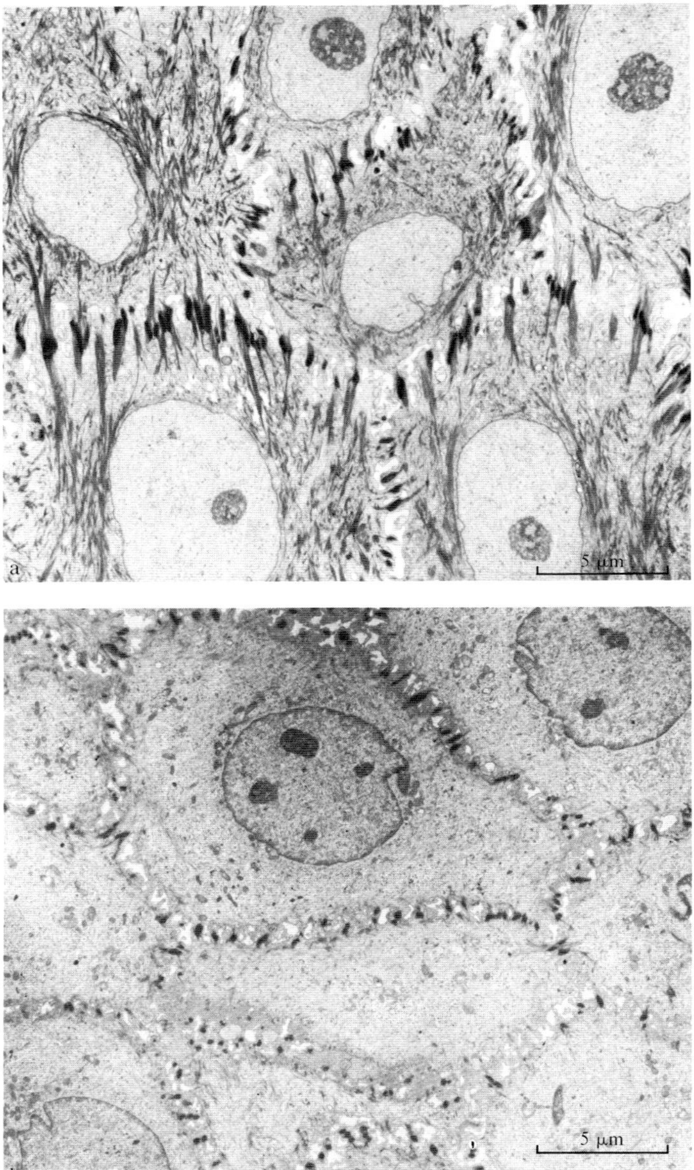

FIGURE 4. Cells from the prickle cell layer of (a) keratinized and (b) nonkeratinized oral epithelium. Note the striking difference in the arrangement of tonofilaments. Marker represents 5 μm.

personal communication). Thus, quantitatively, maturation proceeds steadily through each layer in these keratinized epithelia, with the greatest qualitative change taking place between the granular and keratinized layers.

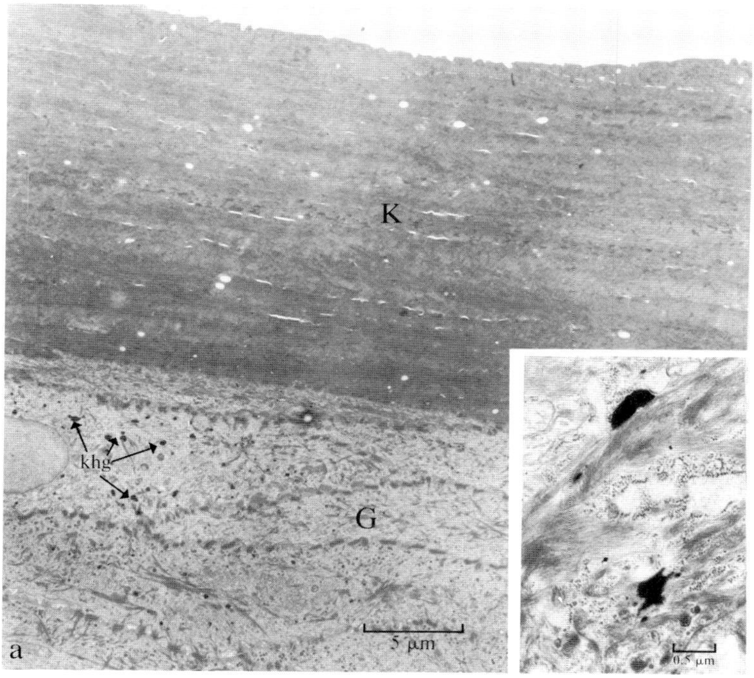

FIGURE 5. a. Keratinized (k) and granular cell layers (G) from gingival epithelium. A number of small dense keratohyalin granules (khg) are evident in the granular layer; their irregular form and intimate association with tonofibrils is shown in the inset. The junction between the two layers is abrupt. Marker represents 5 μm. Inset: marker represents 0-5 μm.

In nonkeratinized oral epithelium, we know from morphological observations (Figs. 4b and 5b) that there is a retention of organelles in the surface layers, and that tonofilaments, but not tonofibril bundles, are present. What has not hitherto been suspected is the extent to which organelles are lost, and the existence of very high concentrations of tonofilaments. In fact, on a unit volume basis, there tend to be more filaments in nonkeratinized than in keratinized oral epithelium (Meyer and

Schroeder 1975), although the grouping of the filaments into bundles (tonofibrils) in keratinized epithelium tends to make them more conspicuous. This finding emphasizes the subjective nature of most morphological descriptions. In contrast to keratinized epithelium, the major events in maturation in nonkeratinized epithelium take place between the basal and spinous layers, and there is subsequently a uniform gradient of maturation to the surface (Landay and Schroeder 1977).

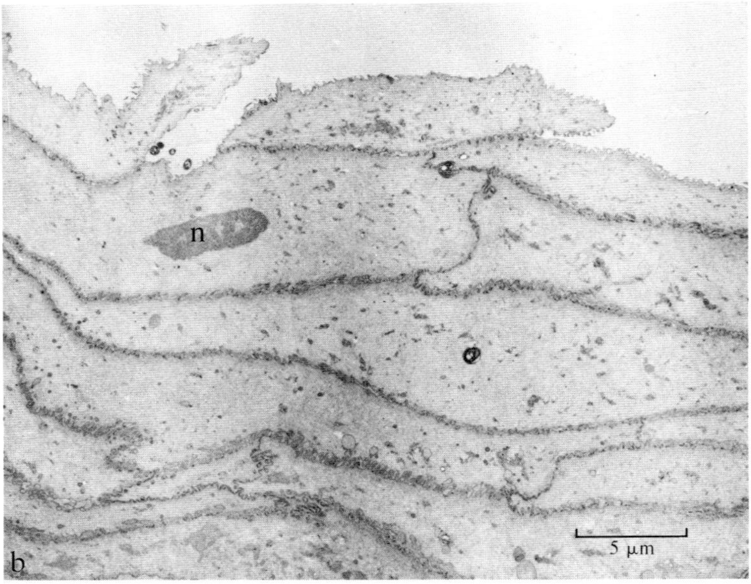

FIGURE 5. b. Superficial cell layer from nonkeratinized alveolar mucosa. The cells show only slight flattening and retain some cell organelles including nuclei (n). Compare with Figure 5a which is reproduced at a similar magnification. Marker represents 5 µm.

4. NONKERATINOCYTES

There are present in the oral epithelium a population of cells that differ from the epithelial cells in not possessing desmosomes or tonofilaments. These cells are the nonkeratinocytes, and can represent up to approximately 10% of the cell population of the epithelium (Meyer et al. 1976); they are represented principally by the melanocyte and the Langerhans cells. These cells have often been called "clear cells," probably because of their tendency to shrink in histological preparations, which gives rise to a clear halo around the nucleus (Cattoni 1953).

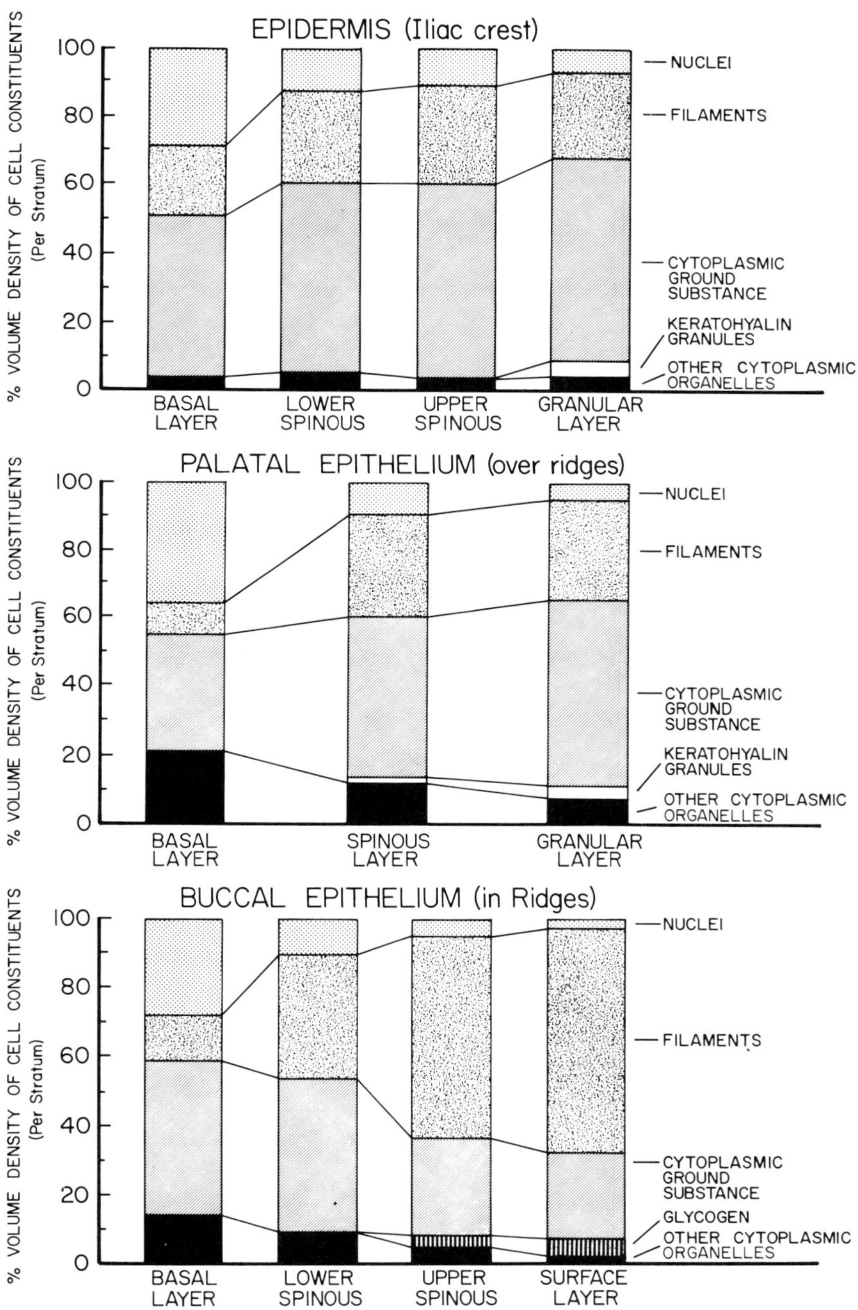

FIGURE 6. Changes in the relative concentrations of various cell organelles in different cell layers of epidermis and keratinized and nonkeratinized oral epithelium. The data is expressed as volume density, i.e., number of structures per unit volume of tissue, and was kindly provided by Dr. H. E. Schroeder.

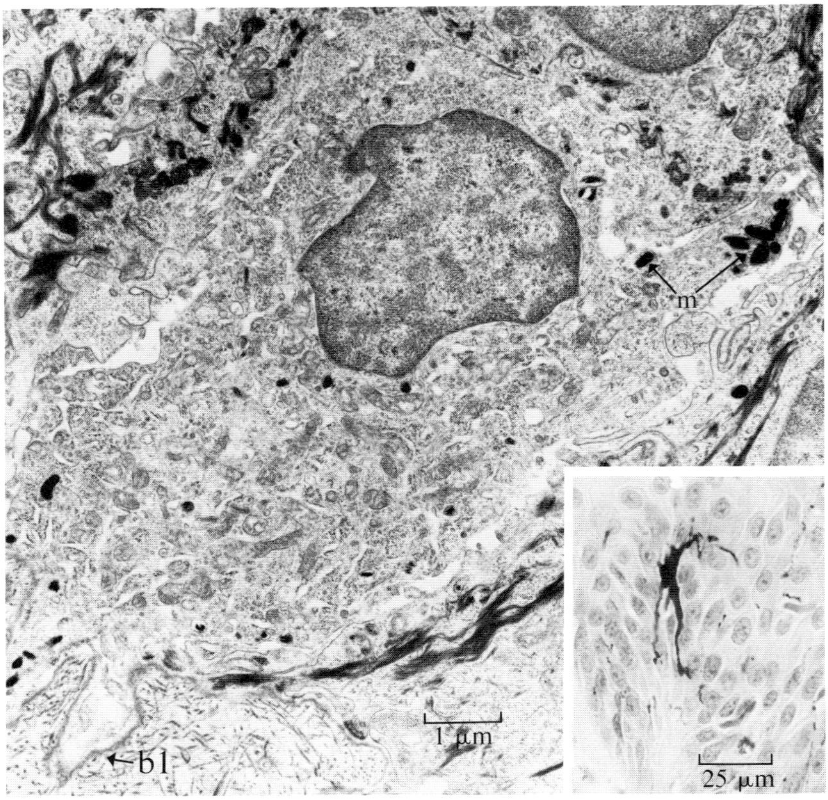

FIGURE 7. Electron micrograph of a melanocyte in the epithelial basal cell layer. The cell lacks tonofilaments and desmosomes but contains numbers of dense melanosomes (m); bl-basal lamina. Marker represents 1 μm. Inset: a histological section of gingival epithelium containing a dendritic melanocyte, demonstrated by the DOPA reaction. Marker represents 25 μm.

4:1 MELANOCYTES

The melanocytes, formerly termed melanoblasts, melanodendrocytes, or melanophores, are the pigment cells of the oral epithelium. These cells originate from neural crest ectoderm and migrate into the oral epithelium and epidermis during embryological development, forming a self-perpetuating population, located in the basal region of the epithelium (Breathnach 1971). Melanocytes are extensively dendritic (Fig. 7) and it is by means of these dendritic processes that the pigment granules (melanosomes) synthesized in the cell are passed into adjacent epithelial cells (Schroeder 1969). When melanosomes are present in groups they form the melanin granules visible in histological sections in the light microscope.

The degree of melanin pigmentation of the oral mucosa tends to mirror the pigmentation of the epidermis (Dummet and Barens 1971), usually being very slight or absent in Caucasians (Fry and Almeyda 1968). However one interesting finding is that, regardless of race, similar areas of the body have similar numbers of melanocytes (Szabo 1954), different degrees of pigmentation resulting from variation in the activity of the melanocyte in synthesizing melanin and distributing it to the epithelial cells (Hori et al. 1968). In heavily pigmented areas it is not unusual to see melanin which has originated from epithelial melanocytes in phagocytes in the connective tissue; these are often termed melanophages (Breathnach 1971).

4:2 LANGERHANS CELLS

The Langerhans cell is a dendritic cell frequently situated at a higher level in the epithelium than the melanocyte, which has often led to it being called a "high level clear cell." Ultrastructurally, the Langerhans cell is recognized by its indented nucleus, the presence of lysosome-like organelles, and a characteristic rod or racquet-shaped granule, the Langerhans granule (Fig. 8) (Sagebiel et al. 1971). The cell enters the epithelium during embryological development (Breathnach 1971) and remains as a self-reproducing population (Mackenzie 1975), but its origin and functions are enigmatic. Although it has been variously described as a neural element (Langerhans 1868), a degenerate melanocyte (Billingham and Medawar 1953), an epithelial regulatory cell (Sagebiel et al. 1971), and an epithelial stem cell (Potten and Allen 1976), there is little evidence for any of these roles. There have been accounts of Langerhans cells in or associated with various neoplasms including ameloblastoma (Lee et al. 1972), extra-mammary Paget's disease (Nagao and Sekiguchi 1973), and melanoma (Szekeres and Orfanos 1978), but the significance of such findings is unknown. Most recently there have been suggestions that the Langerhans cell has a macrophagic function, serving as an antigen trap and processing material that enters the epidermis and presenting it to cells of the lymphoid series (Silberberg 1973; Shelley and Juhlin 1977). Immunological evidence for such a role in skin is accumulating (Shelley and Juhlin 1978; Stingl et al. 1978) and it would not be surprising if this cell has a similar function in oral mucosa.

5. PERMEABILITY OF ORAL EPITHELIUM

The process of maturation in oral epithelia produces surface layers that are appropriate to the function they fulfill—the keratinized surface is tough, rigid, and resists mechanical damage; the nonkeratinized surface is flexible and withstands the distension of the mucosa it covers. These are the mechanical aspects of the barrier function of oral epithelium. There is, in addition, another role that many lining or covering tissues fulfill which is that of a permeability barrier, restricting loss of interstitial fluid from the tissues, and preventing entry of substances from the exterior.

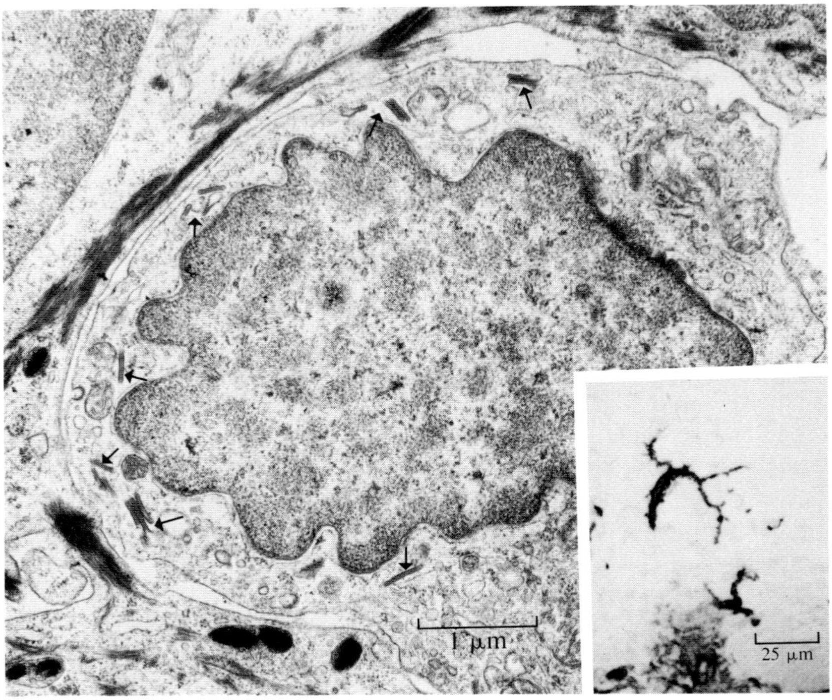

FIGURE 8. Electron micrograph of a Langerhans cell containing numbers of characteristic rod-shaped granules (arrows); no tonofilaments or desmosomes are associated with this cell. Marker represents 1 μm. Inset: the dendritic nature and suprabasal location of the Langerhans cell can be seen in this histological preparation stained for ATPase. Marker represents 25 μm. Section kindly supplied by Dr. I. C. Mackenzie.

From the point of view of the etiology of oral cancer, permeability is an important property, for there are many substances that come into contact with the surface of the oral mucosa which, if they could gain access to the tissue, may have carcinogenic potential. However, one puzzling feature of experimental oral carcinogenesis has been the greater frequency with which the common chemical carcinogens produce tumors in the skin as compared with the oral mucosa (Levy et al. 1951; Kolas 1955). This was originally thought to be a consequence of the absence of appendages from oral mucosa, such as hair follicles and sweat glands (Goldhaber 1958) which offer ready pathways for the entry of substances into the skin (Scheuplein 1976), but Wallenius (1965) showed that when skin with appendages was grafted into the oral cavity it showed no greater capacity for tumor production than the adjacent mucosa. Wallenius suggested that it was the saliva which had a protective role and confirmed this by suppressing salivary secretion and obtaining a far greater tumor yield (Wallenius 1966). Thus, saliva may have a role as a primary barrier against the penetration of certain substances, and Adams (1975) has demonstrated a saliva-derived mucopolysaccharide coating over the surface cells of oral epithelium. On the other hand, many compounds dissolve in saliva and will be maintained in solution at the surface, thus facilitating their penetration. In this regard, it is interesting that tumors have been readily produced in oral mucosa using the water soluble carcinogen, 4-nitro-quinoline N-oxide (4NQo) (see chapter 7).

It is well known that the physical and chemical properties of substances, and particularly solubility, influence their penetration through stratified squamous epithelium (Tregear 1966; Scheuplein 1972). In general, lipid-soluble substances move more rapidly across mucosal epithelium than water-soluble ones, and those with a solubility in both penetrate most rapidly (Siegel et al. 1971; Squier and Johnson 1975). The oral mucosa has often been thought to be more permeable than skin, although many of the workers who have claimed this have been under the misapprehension that the whole of the oral mucosa is nonkeratinized (Malkinson 1964; Winkelman 1969). Kaaber (1974) has studied the movement of certain ions and water across the human oral mucosa in vivo and has shown that there is little penetration across palatal mucosa, the rate approximating that in epidermis. Similarly, studies using an intercellular tracer protein, horseradish peroxidase, have demonstrated an intercellular barrier to this substance in keratinized oral epithelium that is comparable to that existing in the epidermis (Fig. 9) (Squier 1973). In contrast to results from the palate, Kaaber (1974) found that water passed rapidly across buccal mucosa although ions did not, and studies in vitro (Galey et al. 1976), using separated mucosal sheets have demonstrated that this region is more permeable than skin to a range of different substances. Thus, not only are there differences in the penetration due to the nature of the penetrant but also as a consequence of the regional differences in the structure of the oral mucosa.

Penetration through skin or oral mucosa is not an active process, but is governed by the laws of diffusion (Tregear 1966; Siegel et al. 1971), and so the rate of penetration will depend on the thickness of the barrier, the concentration of the penetrant, and the duration of application. The floor of the mouth not only lacks keratin but is an extremely thin tissue (see Table 1), and this seems to correspond with its observed permeability to drugs (Altman et al. 1960). Cawson (1975) has pointed out that there is often widespread keratosis of the palate in pipe smokers, although cancer usually develops in the floor of the mouth, possibly where the saliva containing the carcinogens drains and accumulates (see chapter 18). It must also be remembered that oral mucosa is particularly susceptible to damage that can cause breaks in the epithelial covering or to pathological conditions affecting its cohesion, and these will also increase its permeability (Squier and Johnson 1975).

Finally, there is evidence that the immune system may play a part in restricting entry of foreign material across the oral mucosa membrane. Several workers have suggested that antigenic material which penetrates the surface layers of the epithelium may be trapped by antibodies as immune complexes within or beneath the epithelium (McDougall 1974; Tolo and Jonsen 1975). Recently, Brandtzaeg and Tolo (1977) have quantified this effect and have also claimed that such activity may be at the expense of the barrier function to other molecules. Their explanation is that the structural integrity of the epithelium suffers as a result of the activities of neutrophils entering the tissue to phagocytose immune complexes. Whether this is a significant threat to the integrity of the mucosa remains to be seen.

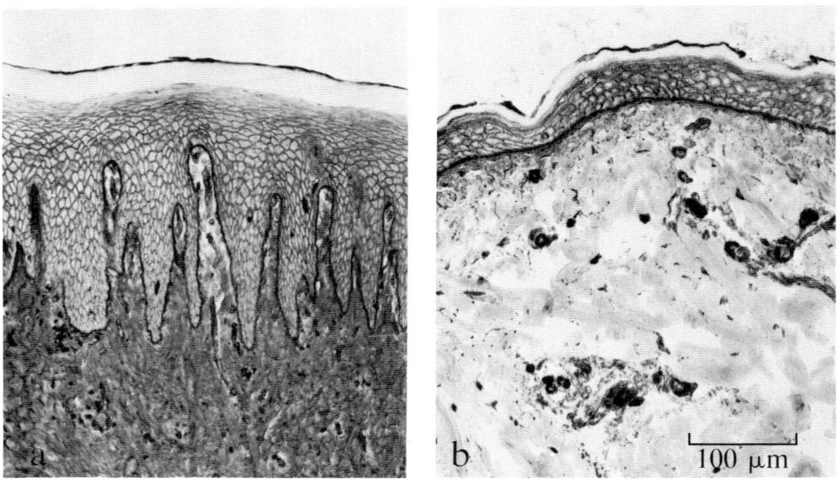

FIGURE 9. Sections of palate (a) and skin (b) that have been treated with the intercellular tracer protein horseradish peroxidase. While the tracer can be seen within the deeper portions of the epithelium and on the surface, it has not entered the keratinized layer, which represents a permeability barrier to this substance. Marker represents 100 μm.

REFERENCES

Adams, D. 1975. The mucus barrier and absorption through the oral mucosa. *J. Dent Res.* **54**, Special Issue B, B19–B26.

Altman, G. E., Riseman, J. E., and Koretsky, S. 1960. Sublingual erythrol tetranitrate in the treatment of angina pectoris. Effect of varying the dose and rate of administration. *Am. J. Med. Sci.* **240**, 100–110.

Alvares, O., Skougaard, M. R., Pindborg, J. J., and Roed-Petersen, B. 1972. In vitro incorporation of tritiated thymidine in oral homogeneous leukoplakias. *Scand. J. Dent. Res.* **80**, 510–514.

Baird, W. M., Sedgwick, J. A., and Boutwell, R. K. 1971. Effects of phorbol and four diesters of phorbol on the incorporation of tritiated precursors into DNA, RNA, and protein in mouse epidermis. *Cancer Res.* **31**, 1434–1439.

Bernimoulin, J. P., and Schroeder, H. E. 1977. Quantitative electron microscopic analysis of the epithelium of normal human alveolar mucosa. *Cell Tissue Res.* **180**, 383–401.

Billingham, R. E., and Medawar, P. B. 1953. A study of the branched cells of the mammalian epidermis with special reference to the fate of their division products. *Philos. Trans. R. Soc. Lond. [Biol.]* **237**, 151–171.

Brandtzaeg, P., and Tolo, K. 1977. Mucosal penetrability enhanced by serum-derived antibodies. *Nature* **266**, 262–263.

Breathnach, A. S. 1971. *An Atlas of Ultrastructure of Human Skin: Development, Differentiation, and Post-natal Features.* J. N. Churchill, London.

Brody, I. 1959. An ultrastructural study on the role of the keratohyalin granules in the keratinization process. *J. Ultrastruct. Res.* **3**, 84–104.

Cameron, I. L. 1966. Cell proliferation, migration, and specialization in the epithelium of the mouse tongue. *J. Exp. Zool.* **163**, 271–283.

Cattoni, M. 1953. Melanoblasts in the inflamed gingiva. *Oral Surg.* **6**, 1095–1110.

Cawson, R. A. 1975. Premalignant lesions in the mouth. *Br. Med. Bull.* **31**, 164–168.

Chen, S. Y., and Meyer, J. 1971. Regional differences in tonofilaments and keratohyaline granules. In: *Current Concepts of the Histology of Oral Mucosa.* (Edited by Squier, C. A., and Meyer, J.), Chap. 6, pp. 114–128. Charles C Thomas, Springfield, Illinois.

Cutright, D. E., and Bauer, H. 1967. Cell renewal in the oral mucosa and skin of the rat. II. DNA conservation and reutilization during the renewal cycle in vivo and in tissue explants. *Oral Surg.* **23**, 260–271.

Dale, B. A., Stern, I. B., and Clagett, J. A. 1977. Initial characterization of the proteins of keratinized epithelium of rat oral mucosa. *Arch. Oral Biol.* **22**, 75–82.

Dummet, C. O., and Barens, G. 1971. Oromucosal pigmentation: An updated literary review. *J. Periodontol.* **42**, 726–736.

Fraser, R. D. B., MacRae, T. P., and Rogers, G. E. 1972. *Keratins, Their Composition, Structure and Biosynthesis,* pp. 83–210. Charles C Thomas, Springfield, Illinois.

Fry, L., and Almeyda, J. R. 1968. The incidence of buccal pigmentation in Caucasoids and Negroids in Britain. *Br. J. Derm.* **80**, 244–247.

Galey, W. R., Lonsdale, H. K., and Nacht, S. 1976. The in vitro permeability of skin and buccal mucosa to selected drugs and tritiated water. *J. Invest Dermatol.* **67**, 713–717.

Goldhaber, P. 1958. Further studies on experimental oral carcinogenesis. *J. Dent. Res.* **37**, 18–19.

Hackemann, M.,,Grubb, C., and Hill, K. R. 1968. The ultrastructure of normal squamous epithelium of the human cervix uteri. *J. Ultrastruct. Res.* **22**, 443–457.

Halprin, K. M. 1972. Epidermal "turnover time"—a reexamination. *Br. J. Dermatol.* **86**, 14–19.

Hopps, R. M., and Johnson, N. W. 1975. Relationship between histological degree of inflammation and epithelial proliferation in macaque gingiva. *J. Periodontol. Res.* **9**, 273–283.

Hori, Y., Toda, K., Pathalk, M. A., Clark, W. H., and Fitzpatrick, T. B. 1968. A fine-structure study of the human epidermal melanosome complex and its acid phosphatase activity. *J. Ultrastruct. Res.* **25**, 109–120.

Iqbal, M., and Gerson, S. 1971. Biochemical features of oral epithelium. In: *Current Concepts of the Histology of Oral Mucosa.* (Edited by Squier, C. A., and Meyer, J.), Chap. 2, pp. 34–60. Charles C Thomas, Springfield, Illinois.

Kaaber, S. 1974. The permeability and barrier functions of the oral mucosa with respect to water and electrolytes. *Acta Odont. Scand.*, Suppl. **66**, 1–47.

Kaidbey, K. H., and Kurban, A. K. 1971. Mitotic behaviour of the buccal mucosal epithelium in psoriasis. *Br. J. Dermatol.* **85**, 162–166.

Kefalides, N. A. 1975. Basement membranes: Current concepts of structure and synthesis. *Dermatologica* **150**, 4–15.

Kittler, G., Lauckner, H., and Mieler, I. 1969. Der Mitosekoeffizient der gesunden und ent zündlich erkrankten. Interdental papillen. I. (Mitosis coefficient of healthy and inflamed interdental papillae.) *Deutsch. Zahn. Mund. Kieferheilk.* **53**, 16–18.

Klein-Szanto, A. J., and Schroeder, H. E. 1977. Architecture and density of the connective tissue papillae of the human oral mucosa. *J. Anat.* **123**, 93–109.

Kolas, S. 1955. Investigation of normal human saliva for possible anticarcinogenic action and chemical carcinogenesis in mucous membranes. *Oral Surg.* **8**, 1192–1203.

Landay, M. A., and Schroeder, H. E. 1977. Quantitative electron microscopic analysis of the stratified epithelium of normal human buccal mucosa. *Cell Tissue Res.* **177**, 383–405.

Langerhans, V. P. 1868. Ueber die Nerven der menschlichen Haut. *Arch. Path. Anat. Physiol.* **44**, 325–337.

Leblond, C. P., Greulich, R. C., and Pereira, J. P. M. 1964. Relationship of cell formation and cell migration in the renewal of stratified squamous epithelia. In: *Wound Healing: Advances in Biology of the Skin*, Vol. 5. (Edited by Montagna, W., and Billingham, R. E.), pp. 39–67. Macmillan, New York.

Lee, K. W., El-Labban, N. G., and Kramer, I. R. 1972. Ultrastructure of a simple ameloblastoma. *J. Pathol.* **108**, 173–176.

Levy, B. M., Gorlin, R., and Gottsegen, R. 1951. Histology of early reactions of skin and mucous membrane of the lip of the mouse to a single application of a carcinogen. *J. Natl. Cancer Inst.* **12**, 275–285.

Löe, H., Karring, T., and Hara, K. 1972. The site of mitotic activity in rat and human oral epithelium. *Scand. J. Dent. Res.* **80**, 111–119.

MacCallum, D. K., Lillie, J. H., and Scaletta, L. J. 1975. Evidence for basal lamina biosynthesis and epithelial-connective tissue remodelling in normal and inflamed human gingivae. (Abstract) *J. Dent. Res.* **54**, L26.

Mackenzie, I. C. 1975. Labelling of murine epidermal Langerhans cells with H^3-thymidine. *Am. J. Anat.* **144**, 127–136

Mackenzie, I. C., and Miles, A. E. 1973. The effect of chronic frictional stimulation on hamster cheek pouch epithelium. *Arch. Oral Biol.* **18**, 1341–1349.

Malkinson, F. D. 1964. Permeability of the stratum corneum. In: *The Epidermis.* (Edited by Montagna, W., and Lobitz, W. C.), Chap. 21, pp. 435–452. Academic Press, New York.

McDougall, W. A. 1974. The effect of topical antigen on the gingiva of sensitized rabbits. *J. Periodont. Res.* **9**, 153–164.

Meyer, J., Marwah, A. S., and Weinmann, J. P. 1956. Mitotic rate of gingival epithelium in two age groups. *J. Invest. Derm.* **27**, 237–247.

Meyer, J., Daftary, D. K., and Pindborg, J. J. 1967. Studies in oral leukoplakias. XI. Histopathology of leukoplakias in Indians chewing "pan" with tobacco. *Acta Odontol. Scand.* **25**, 397–435.

Meyer, J., Alvares, O. F., and Gerson, S. J. 1976. The structure and function of the oral mucosa. In: *Scientific Foundations of Dentistry.* (Edited by Cohen, B., and Kramer, I. R.), pp. 449–458. W. Heinemann Medical Books, London.

Meyer, M., and Schroeder, H. E. 1975. A quantitative electron microscopic analysis of the keratinizing epithelium of normal hard palate. *Cell Tissue Res.* **158**, 177–203.

Nagao, S., and Sekiguchi, T. 1973. Ultrastructural study of a case of extramammary Paget's disease with special reference to cellular changes in melanocytes and a Langerhans cell. *Fukushima J. Med. Sci.* **19**, 41–55.

Potten, C. S., and Allen, T. D. 1976. A model implicating the Langerhans cell in keratinocyte proliferation control. *Differentiation* **5**, 43–47.

Rubinstein, A. S., Medak, H., and Meyer, J. 1970. Early effects of smoking on surface cytology of the oral mucosa. I. Regional differences in surface cytology of smokers and non-smokers. *Oral Surg.* **30**, 131–141.

Sagebiel, R. W., Clarke, M. A., and Hutchens, L. H. 1971. Dendritic cells in oral epithelium. In: *Current Concepts of the Histology of Oral Mucosa.* (Edited by Squier, C. A., and Meyer, J.), Chap. 8, pp. 143–166. Charles C Thomas, Springfield, Illinois.

Scapino, R. P. 1971. Biomechanics of masticatory and lining mucosa. In: *Current Concepts of the Histology of Oral Mucosa.* (Edited by Squier, C. A., and Meyer, J.), Chap. 11, pp. 181–202. Charles C Thomas, Springfield, Illinois.

Scheuplein, R. J. 1972. Properties of the skin as a membrane. In: *Pharmacology and the Skin. Advances in Biology of the Skin,* Vol. 12. (Edited by Montagna, W., Van Scott, E. J., and Stoughton, R. B.), pp. 125–152. Appleton-Century-Crofts, New York.

Scheuplein, R. J. 1976. Permeability of the skin; a review of major concepts and some new developments. *J. Invest. Derm.* **67**, 672–676.

Schroeder, H. E. 1969. Melanin containing organelles in cells of the human gingiva. I. Epithelial melanocytes. *J. Periodontol. Res.* **4**, 1–8. II. Keratinocytes. *J. Periodontol. Res.* **4**, 235–247.

Shelley, W. B., and Juhlin, L. 1976. Langerhans cells for a reticuloepithelial trap for external contact antigens. *Nature* **261**, 46–47.

Shelley, W. B., and Juhlin, L. 1977. Selective uptake of contact allergens by the Langerhans cell. *Arch. Dermatol.* **113**, 187–192.

Shelley, W. B., and Juhlin, L. 1978. The Langerhans cell; its origin, nature and function. *Acta Derm. Venereol. (Stockh.)* **58**, Suppl. **79,** 7–22.

Siegel, I. A., Hall, S. H., and Stambaugh, R. 1971. Permeability of the oral mucosa. In: *Current Concepts of the Histology of Oral Mucosa.* (Edited by Squier, C. A., and Meyer, J.), Chap. 17, pp. 274–286. Charles C Thomas, Springfield, Illinois.

Silberberg, J. 1973. Apposition of mononuclear cells to Langerhans cells in contact allergic reactions. *Acta Derm. Venereol.* **53**, 1–12.

Silverman, S. 1971. Nonkeratinization and kertinization; the extremes of the human range. In: *Current Concepts of the Histology of Oral Mucosa.* (Edited by Squier, C. A., and Meyer, J.), Chap 4, pp. 80–96. Charles C Thomas, Springfield, Illinois.

Squier, C. A. 1973. The permeability of keratinized and non-keratinized oral epithelium to horseradish peroxidase. *J. Ultrastruct. Res.* **43**, 160–177.

Squier, C. A., and Johnson, N. W. 1975. Permeability of oral mucosa. *Br. Med. Bull.* **31**, 169–175.

Squier, C. A., Johnson, N. W., and Hackemann, M. 1975. Structure and function of normal human oral mucosa. In: *Oral Mucosa in Health and Disease.* (Edited by Dolby, A. E.), Chap. 1, pp. 1–112. Blackwell Scientific Publications, Oxford.

Stern, I. B. 1976. Oral mucous membrane. In: *Orban's Oral Histology and Embryology*, 8th ed. (Edited by Bhaskar, S. N.), pp. 253–327. C. V. Mosby, St. Louis, Missouri.

Stingl, G., Katz, S. I., Shevach, E. M., Rosenthal, A. S., and Green, I. 1978. Analogous functions of macrophages and Langerhans cells in the initiation of the immune response. *J. Invest Dermatol.* **71**, 59–64.

Szabo, G. 1954. The number of melanocytes in human epidermis. *Br. Med. J.* **1**, 1016–1017.

Szekeres, L., and Orfanos, C. E. 1978. Alterations of the clinically noninvolved skin in patients with malignant melanoma. An electron microscopic study before and after repeated application of BCG. *Dermatologica* **156**, 142–154.

Tarin, D. 1967. Sequential electron microscopical study of experimental mouse skin carcinogenesis. *Int. J. Cancer* **2**, 195–211.

Tregear, R. T. 1966. *Physical Functions of Skin*, pp. 37–46. Academic Press, London.

Tolo, K., and Jonsen, J. 1975. In vitro penetration of tritiated dextrans through rabbit oral mucosa. *Arch. Oral Biol.* **20**, 419–422.

Wallenius, K. 1965. Effect of 7, 12-dimethylbenz(a)anthracene in the rat's cheek skin transplanted to the buccal cavity. *Odontol. Revy.* **16**, 204–215.

Wallenius, K. 1966. Experimental oral cancer in the rat. With special reference to the influence of saliva. *Acta Path. Microbiol. Scand.* Suppl. **180**, 1–91.

Winkelmann, R. K. 1969. The relationship of the structure of the epidermis to percutaneous absorption. *Br. J. Derm.* **81**, Suppl. 4, 11–22.

10

Epithelial-Mesenchymal Interactions and Normal Epithelial Differentiation

H. C. SLAVKIN

Laboratory for Developmental Biology, Ethel Percy Andrus Gerontology Center
and Department of Biochemistry and Nutrition, School of Dentistry,
University of Southern California, Los Angeles, California

1. INTRODUCTION

The regulatory processes operating during epithelial-mesenchymal interactions are as yet obscure. Whereas the descriptive and experimental embryology of many epithelial-mesenchymal systems has been reported (for example, reviews by Moscona 1964; Grobstein 1963; Slavkin 1974; Slavkin et al. 1977), little information is available related to the actual mechanisms of heterotypic tissue interactions.

The objective of this chapter is to review information regarding possible mechanisms by which close-range intercellular communication affects a specific epithelial phenotype. It is evident that the instructions necessary to initiate and maintain epithelial cell differentiation reside in part within mesenchymal cell surface molecules (see reviews Saxén et al. 1976; Slavkin et al. 1977). Embryonic induction and epithelial-mesenchymal interactions describe those processes related to tissue-specific morphogenetic signaling and the response to those signals. Cytodifferentiation and morphogenesis result from numerous regulatory processes including cell to cell communication between heterotypic cell types. There is no disagreement regarding the importance of these interactions, however, despite more than fifty years of active research in experimental embryology and developmental biology, many fundamental questions remain unanswered.

2. EPITHELIAL-MESENCHYMAL INTERACTIONS

In 1953, Grobstein introduced a novel tissue culture approach to investigate cell to cell communication related to epithelial-mesenchymal interactions during salivary gland morphogenesis. This approach focused upon the role of the extracellular matrix to mediate information transfer between heterotypic tissue. Using an experimental design which allows separation of the tissues by various filters, Grobstein designed experiments to test the effect of various types of mesenchyme upon epithelial cytodifferentiation in vitro. He interpreted his findings (Grobstein 1953, 1963, 1967, 1975) to indicate that there were at least three types of mechanisms which affected epithelial-mesenchymal interactions: (1) direct cell to cell interactions, (2) long-range interactions, and (3) extracellular matrix interactions (Fig. 1).

Several very important ideas have emerged since Grobstein's original observations. In genetics and molecular biology the term "induction" is used to describe activation of repressed structural genes and the *de novo* transcription of messenger ribonucleic acid (mRNA) from the DNA. If the structural gene or genes are activated, epigenetic factors (i.e., extra-chromosomal factors) may function to repress or amplify gene expression. Grobstein and others in contrast have used "induction" to describe the state of tissue in which developmental events were already determined (protodifferentiated) *before* they began their experiments.

If one is seeking to demonstrate the *induction* of differentiation experimentally in salivary gland acinar cells, in terms of amylase production (a gene product reflecting this unique phenotype), one must first isolate cells which are not synthesizing amylase mRNA and/or the gene product. If this lack of synthesis can be established, then one can assay for the effects of various factors associated with control of differentiation such as NGF (Nerve Growth Factor) on the induction of amylase. However, if amylase mRNA and/or amylase are present in the cells at low levels at the start of the experiment, then one can assess important physiological processes such as amplification (see section 3) in this experimental system.

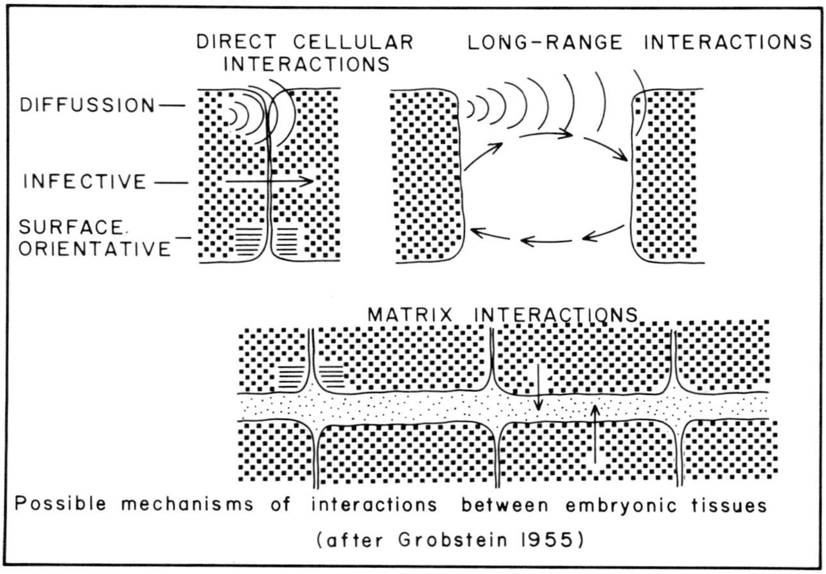

FIGURE 1. Cell-cell-matrix interactions (after Grobstein 1955).

This is important in evaluating secondary embryonic inductions during embryogenesis (Fig. 2).

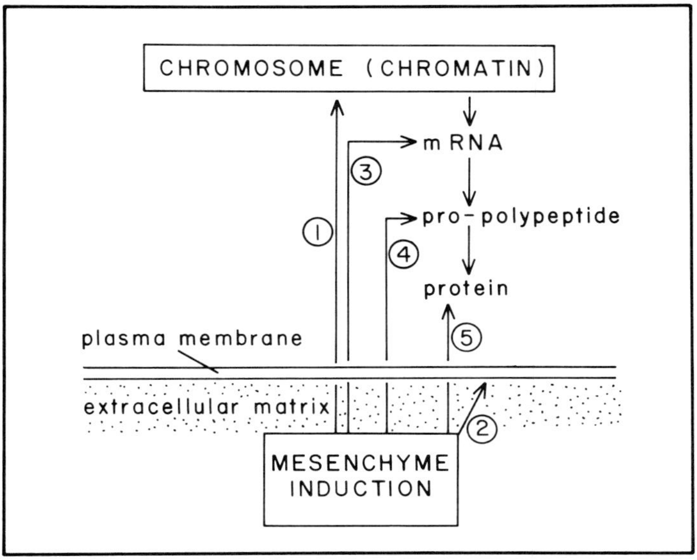

FIGURE 2. Five levels of mesenchyme induction upon a responding epithelium are described: (1) direct gene activation; (2) mesenchyme inducing factors binding to cell surface receptors; (3) amplification of preexisting mRNAs reflecting a unique epithelial phenotype; (4) translational control of protein synthesis; and (5) post-translational modifications of existing gene products.

3. MESENCHYMAL SPECIFICITY: A MODEL TO STUDY EPITHELIAL-MESENCHYMAL INTERACTIONS

An understanding of some of the principles associated with tissue interactions has been acquired primarily through experimental intervention during embryonic organ development: thus the developmental capabilities of tissues have been tested in vitro and in tissue recombination experiments using various heterotypic tissues. By these methods it has been repeatedly shown that, in general, epithelium depends upon the influence of an underlying mesenchyme in order to undergo histological differentiation and morphogenesis (see review by Saxén et al. 1976). Numerous embryonic organ rudiments, such as the pancreas, salivary gland, tooth organs, kidney, thyroid, skin, lung, and mammary gland, can be isolated and continue to differentiate and express their phenotypic characteristics when cultured in vitro. The epithelium and mesenchyme of an organ can be dissociated and when recombined in vitro will continue to express the developmental characteristics of the organ. However, isolated tissue will not differentiate when cultured without its interactant. In general, the organ specificity of the mesenchyme will influence a "responsive" epithelium to differentiate into complementary epithelium even across different vertebrate species (Grobstein 1975; Slavkin 1974). For example, embryonic rabbit mammary gland mesenchyme has been shown to induce avian flank epithelium to differentiate into mammary gland-like epithelium complete with branching tubule formation.

Evidence from other studies indicates that mesenchyme produces a specific set of molecular instructions which determine the cytodifferentiation of the associated epithelium. For example, mouse embryonic lung mesenchyme can elicit branching morphogenesis in tracheal epithelium, a tissue which does not normally branch. Tooth organ mesenchyme from embryonic mouse molar has been shown to induce mouse foot pad epithelium to differentate into ameloblasts and form a tooth complete with dentine and enamel matrices (see the extensive review by Slavkin 1974). The results obtained from a number of studies indicate that mesenchyme also produces permissive and/or growth rate-limiting factors which accomodate the phenotypic expression of previously determined or protodifferentiated epithelia in tissue recombinants. Mesenchymal specificity in this sense is analogous to an "amplification phenomenon" in which previously determined developmental events are provided with a stimulus conducive to the expression of a particular phenotype (Fig. 3).

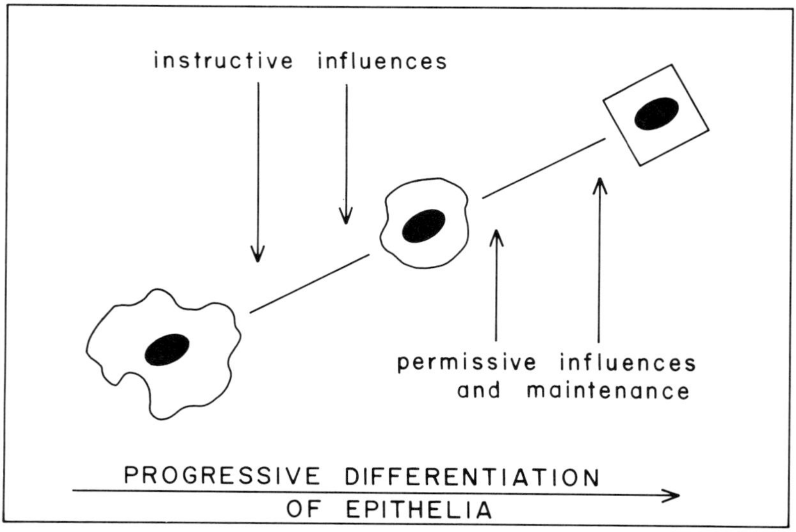

FIGURE 3. Mesenchymal influences upon adjacent epithelial cells can be instructive and/or permissive (see reviews by Bell 1964; Grobstein 1975; Hay 1977; and Slavkin et al. 1977).

In almost all published studies of epithelial-mesenchymal interactions, morphogenesis (e.g., branching tubule formation, metachromatic extracellular matrix deposition, cessation of mitosis, etc.) has been used as the criterion to assess mesenchyme specificity. In a defined system, no evidence as yet has been reported which unequivocally demonstrates mesenchymal induction of *new* gene transcription, translation, posttranslational modifications or secretion of unique macromolecules by a responding epithelium. Therefore, one of the central issues is to design experiments which might provide evidence which could discriminate between (1) developmental instructions derived from the mesenchyme, and (2) permissive and/or growth rate-limiting factors which might amplify or retard the synthesis and secretion of epithelial gene products.

4. REGULATION OF EPITHELIAL CELL DIFFERENTIATION

A major part of cellular differentiation is protein synthesis. The control of protein synthesis is a complex mechanism involving many cellular and biochemical events. Evidence is now available describing some of the cellular and biochemical changes during epidermal cell differentiation (see reviews by Bernstein et al. 1977; Freedberg 1976; Mercer 1964; and Moscona 1964), including substantial advances in our understanding of the chemistry and synthesis of keratin (Fraser et al. 1972). The morphogenesis of several structures derived from skin has been extensively studied including teeth (see review by Slavkin 1974) and feathers (see review by Sengel 1976). During embryonic chick feather morphogenesis, the synthesis of keratin proteins has been described (Kemp et al. 1974a). Further, chick feather keratin mRNA has been isolated and translated in both rabbit reticulocyte and wheat germ cell-free systems (Partington et al. 1973; and Kemp et al. 1974b). In experiments where the feather keratin mRNA was translated (i.e., used as a template for protein synthesis) using the cell free systems, a homogeneous group of polypeptides was synthesized having a similar molecular weight and chemical composition to that reported for the polypeptides for chick embryo feather keratin (Fig. 4).

Many stratified squamous epithelia are keratinized; some epithelial cells in the oral mucosa are known to keratinize given the proper conditions and are capable of expressing those genes responsible for transcription of the mRNAs required for keratin synthesis. The phenotypic expression of nonkeratinized epithelium may either involve repression of the transcription of the keratinization genes or of the translation of the mRNA involved in keratinization. An epithelial cell in which all the genes involved in keratinization (i.e., the cistron for keratinization) would be freely transcribing mRNA's for keratin synthesis can be considered as a "wild" genotype. Conversely, a "wild" genotype repressed may indicate an epithelial cell in which keratin synthesis is repressed at either the transcriptional or the translational level. In order for a keratinizing epithelium to become a nonkeratinizing type, a repressor molecule may serve to prevent keratin synthesis, and each epithelial cell derived from the dividing progenitor basal cell may receive this repressor molecule prior to leaving the basal cell layer. If this regulation is not exercised the cell will become a keratinizing epithelia. This hypothesis suggests that a nonkeratinizing epithelium could become "derepressed" and synthesize keratin.

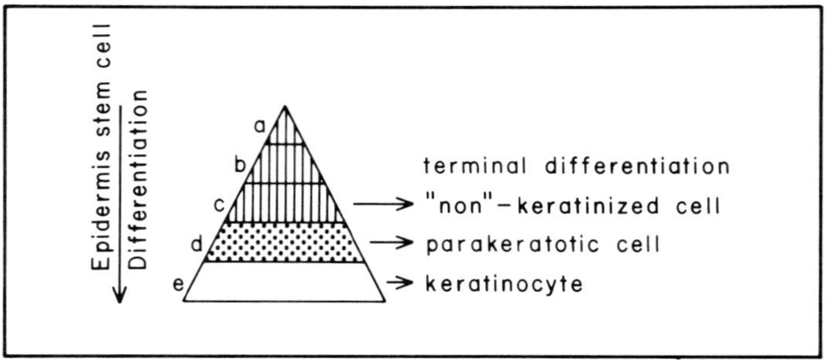

FIGURE 4. A model for stem cell differentiation-dependent regulation of keratin synthesis. The triangle corresponds to the epidermal stem cell compartment and postulated stages of epithelial cell differentiation, a to e. Commitment to keratin synthesis is considered to be inversely related to degree of epithelial stem cells (basal cells). Differentiation stages a, b, and c are associated with the ability of cells to produce large amounts of keratin in terminally differentiated cells derived from these stages. Commitment to keratin is decided in a stochastic fashion in the progeny of burst-forming units of the differentiation stage (d, stippled area). Stage 3 (white area) is associated with only keratin production in the terminally differentiated progeny. The determination of various types of epithelial cytodifferentiation is exquisitely regulated by the immediately adjacent mesenchyme.

If repression is involved, it is possible that the suggested repressor molecule could be present in serum. Evidence exists that the development of embryonic chick skin is initiated by a "humoral factor" which permits it to differentiate even when cultured in partly defined media (Sengel and Mauger 1976), or completely defined media (Bell 1964). Repressor influence on the epithelium could therefore be mediated either directly or indirectly through the underlying connective tissue.

5. FUTURE POSSIBILITIES FOR EXPERIMENTAL INVESTIGATION

Immunochemistry can be used to localize antigens in tissue and cell preparations, and antisera is now available to various types of keratin.

Immunofluorescence microscopy can therefore be used to detect small concentrations of keratin proteins within cells. It is now possible to isolate mRNAs which may code for keratin. A complementary DNA (cDNA) probe can be synthesized from the mRNA, using an enzyme such as reverse transcriptase and thereby producing in vitro the structural gene for keratin. These methods and reagents can be used to assay the results of epithelial-mesenchymal interactions and to evaluate the effect of mesenchyme upon epithelial cell differentiation in the oral mucosa.

SUMMARY

Oral mucosa develops as a consequence of epithelial-mesenchymal interactions. The mesenchyme instructs and maintains the phenotype of the adjacent epithelium. The epithelial phenotype can be studied using keratin biosynthesis as a phenotypic marker. *De novo* gene activation, transcription to form mRNA, translation to form polypeptides, and subsequent posttranslational modifications are levels of cell function available to study neoplasia in normal and abnormal epithelium.

ACKNOWLEDGMENTS

The original concepts discussed in this manuscript were contributed by Drs. Spemann (1938), Needham (1942), Weiss (1968), and Grobstein (1953, 1963, 1967, 1975). An understanding of these concepts and the pursuit of experimentation designed towards acquiring an understanding of epithelial-mesenchymal interactions was made possible, in part, by research and training supported by DE-02848-07, DE-03513-06, DE-03569-05, DE-00094-05, from the National Institute for Dental Research, U.S. Public Health Service. I also wish to acknowledge the efforts of Barbara Klein and Cecelia Keaton for preparing this manuscript. I wish to also acknowledge the drawings prepared by Pablo Bringas, Jr.

REFERENCES

Bell, E. 1964. Protein synthesis in differentiating chick skin. In: *Metabolic Control Mechanisms in Animal Cells.* (Edited by Rutter, W. J.) *Natl. Cancer Inst. Monogr.* **13**, 1–11.

Bernstein, I. A., Sachs, L., Ball, R., and Walker, G. 1977. Regulation in epidermal differentiation. In: *Biochemistry of Cutaneous Epidermal Differentiation.* (Edited by Seiji, M., and Bernstein, I. A.), pp. 243–250. University Park Press, Baltimore.

Cunha, G. R. 1976. Alterations in the developmental properties of stroma during the development of the urogenital ridge into ductus deferens and uterus in embryonic and neonatal mice. *J. Exp. Zool.* **197**, 375–388.

Foulds, L. 1969. *Neoplastic Development*, Vol. 1, pp. 41–89. Academic Press, New York.

Fraser, R. D. B., MacRae, T. P., and Rogers, G. E. 1972. *Keratins: Their Composition, Structure and Biosynthesis.* Charles C Thomas, Springfield, Illinois.

Freedberg, I. M. 1976. Biochemistry of keratinization in hair: Protein synthesis, pathways and controls. In: *Biology and Disease of the Hair.* International Symposium on Biology and Disease of the Hair, Proceedings, 1st, Tokyo, 1975. (Edited by Kobori, T., Montagna, W., and Toda, K.), pp. 105–124. University Park Press, Baltimore.

Grobstein, C. 1953. Morphogenetic interaction between embryonic mouse tissues separated by membrane filter. *Nature* **172**, 869–871.

Grobstein, C. 1963. Cytodifferentiation and macromolecular synthesis. In: *Society for Developmental Biology, Symposium, 21st. Cytodifferentiation and Macromolecular Synthesis.* (Edited by Locke, M.), pp. 1–14. Academic Press, New York.

Grobstein, C. 1967. Mechanisms of organogenetic tissue interaction. *Natl. Cancer Inst. Monogr.* **26**, 279–299.

Grobstein, C. 1975. Developmental role of intercellular matrix. In: *Extracellular Matrix Influences on Gene Expression.* Santa Catalina Island Colloquium, 2d, 1974. (Edited by Slavkin, H. C., and Greulich, R. C.), pp. 9–16. Academic Press, New York.

Hay, E. D. 1973. Origin and role of collagen in the embryo. *Am. Zool.* **13**, 1085–1107.

Hay, E. D. 1977. Cell-matrix interaction in embryonic induction. In: *International Cell Biology 1976–1977.* (Edited by Brinkley, B. R., and Porter, K. R.), pp. 50–57. Rockefeller University Press, New York.

Hay, E. D., and Dodson, J. W. 1973. Secretion of collagen by corneal epithelium. I. Morphology of the collagenous products produced by isolated epithelia grown on frozen-killed lens. *J. Cell Biol.* **57**, 190–213.

Holtzer, H., Dienstman, S., Biehl, J., and Holtzer, S. 1975. Generation of cell diversity. In: *Extracellular Matrix Influences on Gene Expression. Proceedings.* (Edited by Slavkin, H. C., and Greulich, R. C.), pp. 253–257. Academic Press, New York.

Kemp, D. J., Dyer, P. Y., and Rogers, G. E. 1974a. Keratin synthesis during development of the embryonic chick feather. *J. Cell Biol.* **62**, 114–131.

Kemp, D. J., Schwinghamer, M. W., and Rogers, G. E. 1974b. Translation of pure feather keratin mRNA in a wheat embryo cell-free system. *Mol. Biol. Rep.* **1**, 441–446.

Main, J. H. P. 1972. Developmental considerations: Carcinogenesis and oncology. In: *Developmental Aspects of Oral Biology.* (Edited by Slavkin, H. C., and Bavetta, L. A.), pp. 385–405. Academic Press, New York.

Masters, J. R. 1976. Epithelial-mesenchymal interaction during lung development: The effect of mesenchymal mass. *Dev. Biol.* **51**, 98–108.

Mercer, E. H. 1964. Protein synthesis and epidermal differentiation. In.: *The Epidermis.* (Edited by Montagna, W., and Lobitz, W. C.), Chap. 10, pp. 161–178. Academic Press, New York.

Moscona, A. A. 1964. Studies on stability of phenotypic traits in embryonic integumental tissues and cells. In: *The Epidermis.* (Edited by Montagna, W., and Lobitz, W. C.), Chap. 5, pp. 83–96. Academic Press, New York.

Needham, J. 1942. *Biochemistry and Morphogenesis*, pp. 165–188. Cambridge University Press, London.

Partington, G. A., Kemp, D. J., and Rogers, G. E. 1973. Isolation of feather keratin mRNA and its translation in a rabbit reticulocyte cell-free system. *Nature (New Biol.)* **246**, 33–36.

Saxén, L., Karkinen-Jääskeläinen, M., Lehtonen, E., Nordling, S., and Wartiovara, J. 1976. Inductive tissue interactions. In: *The Cell Surface in Animal Embryogenesis and Development.* (Edited by Poste, G., and Nicolson, G. L.), pp. 331–407. Elsevier/North Holland, Amsterdam.

Sengel, Philippe. 1976. *Morphogenesis of Skin.* Cambridge University Press, Cambridge.

Sengel, P., and Mauger, A. 1976. Peridermal cell patterning in the feather-forming skin of the chick embryo. *Dev. Biol.* **51**, 166–171.

Slavkin, H. C. 1974. *Embryonic Tooth Formation: A Tool for Developmental Biology.* Oral Sciences Review Series, Vol. 4. (Edited by Melcher, A. H., and Zarb, G. A.) Munksgaard, Copenhagen.

Slavkin, H. C., Matosian, P., Wilson, P., Bringas, P., Mino, W., Croissant, R. D., and Guenther, H. 1975. Epithelial-specific extracellular matrix influences on mesenchyme collagen biosynthesis in vitro. In: *Extracellular Matrix Influences on Gene Expression.* (Edited by Slavkin, H. C., and Greulich, R. C.), pp. 237–251. Academic Press, New York.

Slavkin, H. C., Trump, G. N., Brownell, A., and Sorgente, N. 1977. Epithelial-mesenchymal interactions: Mesenchymal specificity. In: *Cell and Tissue Interactions.* (Edited by Lash, J. W., and Burger, M. N.), pp. 29–46. Raven Press, New York.

Spemann, H. 1938. *Embryonic Development and Induction*, pp. 141–169. Yale University Press, New Haven.

Trelstad, R. L., and Slavkin, H. C. 1974. Collagen synthesis by the epithelial enamel organ of the embryonic rabbit tooth. *Biochem. Biophys. Res. Commun.* **59**, 443–449.

Weiss, P. A. 1968. *Dynamics of Development: Experiments and Inferences.* Academic Press, New York.

11

Connective Tissue Influences on Epithelial Malignancy or Premalignancy

C. J. SMITH

Department of Oral Pathology, University of Sheffield, Sheffield, England

Circumstantial evidence from human pathology suggests a role for the connective tissue in the development and behavior of carcinomas. Pointers include the variable appearance of the stroma in certain tumors (e.g. scirrhus carcinomas), alterations that can be demonstrated in the subepithelial connective tissue of sun-damaged skin (which is more susceptible to the development of carcinomas than normal skin), and the preferential distribution of metastases to certain organs (Tarin 1976). In addition, during experiments with chemical carcinogens in animals, changes can be observed taking place not only in the exposed epithelium but also in the underlying connective tissue.

It is axiomatic that any premalignant epithelium, whether or not it manifests overt signs of epithelial dysplasia or carcinoma in situ, must be supported by connective tissue. The ways in which these two tissues interact could be of significance in several respects:

(a) Connective tissue influences on normal epithelium (see chapter 10) might be disturbed in such a way as to cause the epithelium it supports to develop premalignant or malignant characteristics; for example, chemical carcinogens might exert their primary effect on the connective tissue. This may be difficult to prove, however, as it would be hard to eliminate the possibility that the epithelium had been directly affected by the same substance that caused the alterations in the connective tissue.

(b) Once premalignant characteristics have developed in an epithelium, progression to malignant invasion may be determined by effects that the epithelium is able to exert on the adjacent connective tissue. If the connective tissue resists such influences, then invasion will not occur.

(c) The eventual fate of premalignant epithelium may be determined by effects that the underlying connective tissue is able to exert on the epithelium. Regression, stabilization or invasion may result.

To complicate matters, more than one of these possibilities may exist either simultaneously or sequentially. Thus a premalignant epithelial lesion such as carcinoma in situ may have developed to that state because of connective tissue influences or may be maintained in that state, and perhaps even regress from it, because the connective tissue is not susceptible to epithelial attempts at invasion. There are also important implications for the various forms of therapy provided for premalignant lesions that arise from consideration of the possible interactions between epithelium and connective tissue; these include skin or mucosal grafting procedures, cryosurgery, and chemotherapy. Work that has been carried out on the various influences that might be exerted by epithelium and connective tissue on each other during experimental carcinogenesis, or during the development of human malignant lesions, covers a wide variety of disciplines and laboratory techniques. These can be broadly divided into studies directed at finding out more about (1) the junctional zone between epithelium and connective tissue, (2) the collagenous component of the connective tissue, (3) the noncollagenous components of the connective tissue, (4) the vascular supply, and (5) the inflammatory cell component. As far as the latter is concerned, the reasons for its presence are probably mainly immunological and therefore will be dealt with largely elsewhere (see chapter 16). Consideration has also to be given to information that can be obtained on the interactions between epithelium and connective tissue from experiments involving transplantation and recombination of grafts. Although it is convenient for descriptive purposes to subdivide an approach to the problem in this way, it is necessary to repeat that probably many of the changes that are seen to occur, or influences that seem to have an effect, are acting simultaneously and in variable combinations. How these various factors may be of particular relevance to the problems of human oral premalignancy are considered in the final section of this chapter.

1. THE JUNCTIONAL ZONE BETWEEN EPITHELIUM AND CONNECTIVE TISSUE

1:1 STRUCTURAL CHANGES

Several studies have described the sequential alterations that occur at the boundary between epithelium and connective tissue in experimental chemical carcinogenesis of skin (reviewed by Tarin 1972) and of oral mucosa (reviewed by Smith 1972a). As recognizable premalignant lesions develop, electron microscopy reveals small interruptions in the lamina densa which increase in frequency and extent as carcinogenesis progresses. In addition, fragments of the laminar material accumulate irregularly beneath the basal epithelial cells so that a duplicated or multilayered structure can be seen. At this early stage there are few obvious changes in the connective tissue, though collagen fibers may be smaller than normal (Tarin 1976). When, in both skin and oral mucosal carcinogenesis, small papillomatous surface outgrowths appear, then subepithelial patches of connective tissue destruction may also be seen electron-microscopically. These are often associated with extrusions of pseudopodia without organelles that arise from the basal plasma membrane of the basal epithelial cells and project into the damaged areas of connective tissue (Fig. 1). The collagen fibers in these areas are now less distinct and blood vessels are found close to the epithelium. As carcinogenesis progresses the loss of lamina densa becomes more pronounced and the pseudopodia increase in size, possessing irregular margins and containing occasional organelles, until in invasive carcinomas the loss of lamina densa is almost complete and the pseudopodia fuse to form a fimbriated cell border. What is not known about this sequence of changes is the degree to which they are of significance in the process of invasion and whether the connective tissue damage is a prerequisite for pseudopodia formation or vice versa.

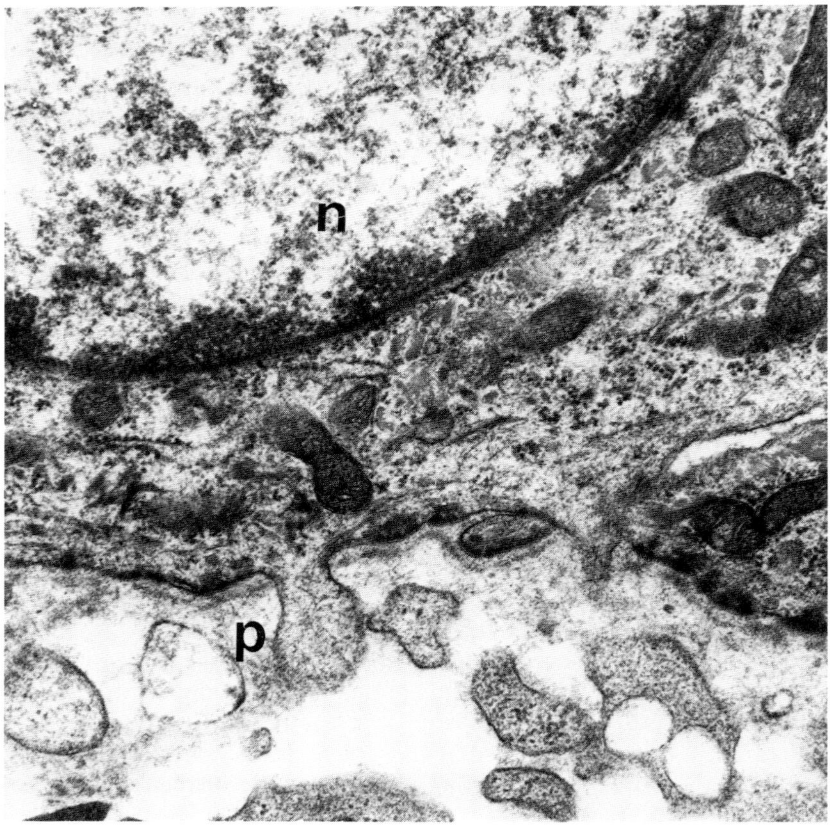

FIGURE 1. Electron micrograph of junction between epithelium and connective tissue in hamster cheek pouch mucosa treated with DMBA and exhibiting epithelial hyperplasia but no obvious dysplasia. An organelle-free pseudopodium extends from the basal epithelial cell through a break in the lamina densa into altered connective tissue. n-nucleus of basal epithelial cell; p-pseudopodium. X 32,000. (Reproduced by permission of F. H. White.)

Similar changes have been described in various human tissues with early malignant or premalignant characteristics (Sugár 1972; Frithiof 1972; Smith 1972a; McNutt 1976) and, conversely, also in several other conditions that are not malignant or premalignant, such as wound healing (Ross and Odland 1968; Odland and Ross 1968; Croft and Tarin 1970; Tarin and Croft 1970), psoriasis (Cox 1969), mucous membrane pemphigoid (Susi and Shklar 1971), epidermolysis bullosa (Briggaman and Wheeler 1975), after trypsinisation (Jensen and Mottet 1970), and as a result of the action of collagenase (Kahl and Pearson 1967). It is thought, therefore, that breakdown of the lamina densa and pseudopodia formation are generally nonspecific indicators of tissue damage (see chapter 21). However, in the nonneoplastic conditions, damage to basal lamina appears to be reversible, whereas in carcinogenesis it is progressive and does not appear to be dependent upon continued application of the carcinogen (Woods and Smith 1969; Tarin 1976). Conceivably there may be as yet undiscovered differences between the damage that occurs prior to the development of carcinomas and that observed in nonneoplastic states. Nonetheless, the gaps that appear in the basal lamina during carcinogenesis may be important in allowing connective tissue influences to have greater access to the basal epithelial cells than usual, or allowing epithelial influences to reach the connective tissue more readily. Histological reduction in connective tissue staining may be related to the above ultrastructural observations (Fig. 2).

1:2 HISTOCHEMICAL OBSERVATIONS

Acid phosphatase and other hydrolytic enzymes, in all probability of lysosomal localization, have been shown to undergo changes in intracellular histochemical staining during chemical carcinogenesis in hamster cheek pouch mucosa (Smith 1972a, 1972b). The most striking alterations occur in some of the basal cells of hyperplastic epithelium where there may be a pronounced increase in reaction product before any evidence of epithelial dysplasia can be found. These focal changes become more widespread and gradually involve other cell layers as carcinogenesis progresses and malignant invasion ensues. At the same time, there is evidence of focal damage to the subepithelial connective tissue (Smith, 1972a, 1972b), though it is still a matter of surmise whether the enzymatic changes in the basal cells are directly related to the altered connective tissue or to ultrastructural damage at the junction between epithelium and connective tissue described in section 1:1 above. A similar distribution of lysosome-like bodies containing napthylamide-splitting enzymes has been described by Sylvén and Bois-Svensson (1964) in tumors transplanted to experimental animals. More recently, detailed quantitative cytochemical and morphological studies at the electron microscope level have confirmed that there are real increases in lysosomal size and number in hamster cheek pouch epithelial cells during carcinogenesis (Gohari 1977).

As well as the changes detected by these enzyme histochemical techniques in epithelial cells, they also serve to demonstrate the influx of macrophages to the subepithelial region during carcinogenesis. Again, the function of these cells in connection with premalignancy is by no means understood, though conceivably they could be participating in removal of damaged cells and tissues or be primarily involved in causing such damage.

Similar histochemical techniques applied to sections from human oral white lesions have revealed that some of these, and it is not known whether these were the premalignant ones or not, demonstrated lysosomal enzyme patterns identical to those in the carcinogen-painted hamster cheek pouch mucosa (Smith, 1972a, 1972b).

2. THE COLLAGENOUS COMPONENT OF THE CONNECTIVE TISSUE

During experimental skin carcinogenesis it has been shown that, in addition to the subjective impression of collagen destruction, biochemical measurements always show a marked decline in collagen content a long time before any morphological changes can be observed; also, application of a potentially carcinogenic agent does not lead to tumor production if the collagen content does not fall below a critical level (Mazzucco 1972). A decrease in collagen content, however, does not inevitably result in tumor development in the skin; when noncarcinogens produce such a decrease there is a rapid recovery of collagen content, unlike the irreversible loss of collagen observed in prolonged carcinogenesis. From carcinogenesis experiments carried out in sites where the collagen content is variable from time to time (e.g. newt skin) or from area to area (e.g. mouse tail and back skin), it appears that there is an increased susceptibility to tumor development when collagen content is reduced (see Mazzucco 1972; Tarin 1976). Should such a relationship between collagen content and susceptibility to carcinogens be borne out by further experimental work, it might provide at least part of an explanation for the variability in behavior of otherwise apparently similar premalignant lesions and may help to explain variations between sites and individuals in their experience of cancer.

As Mazzucco (1972) has pointed out, there may be several reasons why collagen appears to be lost during carcinogenesis; it may be produced in smaller quantities, its breakdown may be accelerated, or it may simply be diluted by the inflammatory component inevitably found in these areas. Probably all three mechanisms operate to some extent.

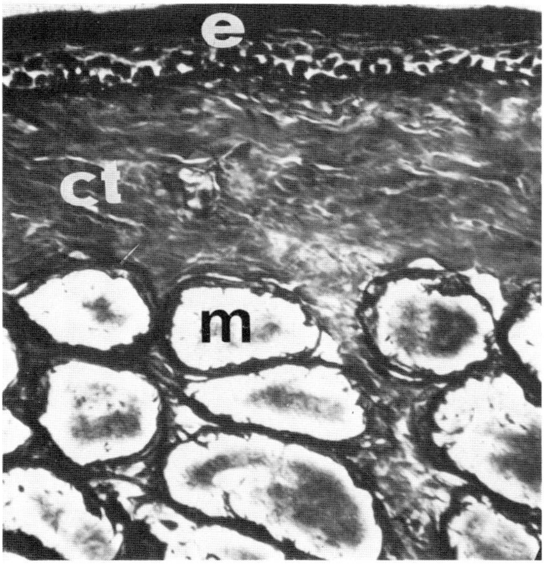

FIGURE 2. a. Normal hamster cheek pouch mucosa. Gomori silver impregnation. e-epithelium; ct-subepithelial connective tissue; m-muscle. X 175.

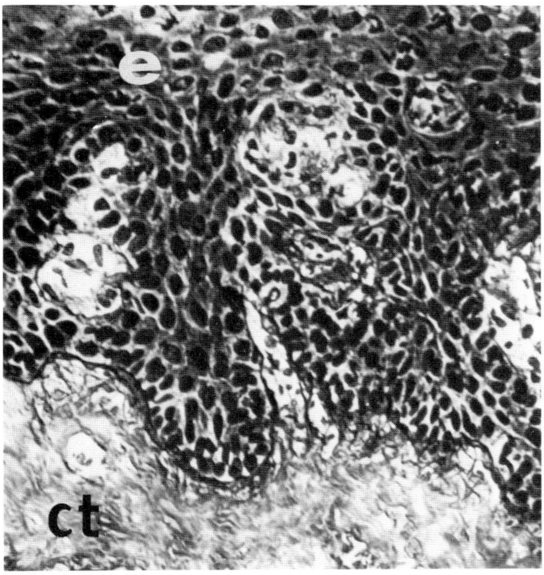

FIGURE 2. b. Hamster cheek pouch mucosa treated for 16 weeks with DMBA and exhibiting epithelial hyperplasia. Subepithelial connective tissue stains less densely than normal. Gomori silver impregnation. e-epithelium; ct-subepithelial connective tissue. X 175.

3. THE NONCOLLAGENOUS COMPONENT OF CONNECTIVE TISSUE

The collection of tumor interstitial fluid, which occupies part of the space between stromal blood vessel walls and tumor cells, can be achieved by two methods that have been reviewed and discussed by Gullino (1975). In one method, fluid is sampled from small pouches created in the tumor by blunt dissection (Sylvén and Bois 1960), though it carries the inherent problem of incorporating fluid from disrupted cells. In the other technique, a Millipore chamber containing small pieces of transplantable tumor is implanted into subcutaneous tissue and the fluid that collects in the chamber is later retrieved; this method suffers from the disadvantage that the influence of the filter may be significant. Several workers have described high levels of proteolytic and lysosomal enzymes in tissue interstitial fluid obtained by these techniques, but their results have not always been confirmed by others (see review by Gullino 1975). The relationship of these enzymes to tumor cell necrosis or invasion is subject to doubt largely on account of the limitations of the sampling procedures.

Connective tissue destruction at the advancing edges of invasive tumors is associated with a much higher content of collagenolytic enzymes than is found in benign tumors or normal tissues, and the most invasive zones have more enzyme activity than central regions of the same tumor (Strauch 1972). Collagenolytic activity has also been described in basal cell carcinomas (Hashimoto et al. 1972; Yamanishi et al. 1972), in squamous cell carcinomas of skin (Hashimoto et al. 1973), and in malignant melanomas (Yaminishi et al. 1973). There is apparently an increase in collagenolytic activity during chemical carcinogenesis of mouse skin, the extent of which is closely correlated with both ultrastructural changes and the development of papillomas and invasive carcinomas (Rohrbach et al. 1970).

Although most workers seem to assume that the collagenases at the tumor periphery emanate from neoplastic epithelial cells (Strauch 1972), the possibility of a contribution from stromal fibroblasts or inflammatory cells has not been entirely excluded.

4. THE VASCULAR SUPPLY

Tumors seem to be capable of releasing a substance, with a molecular weight of about 100,000, that has been dubbed the "tumor angiogenesis factor" (TAF) (Folkman 1974). This factor stimulates the growth of capillary blood vessels towards viable implanted tumor cells, which can be demonstrated to exert their angiogenic effect across a Millipore membrane. The growth of new capillaries affects the growth of the tumor implants

(Gimbrone et al. 1972, 1973, 1974) and continuation of tumor growth would appear to be dependent upon the continuing capacity of the tumor to induce new blood vessel development at its periphery. It has been suggested, therefore, that if such angiogenesis could be inhibited, this might provide an alternative approach to the control of tumors (Folkman et al. 1971).

There is as yet no clear indication of the way in which the presence of the newly-induced blood vessels around a tumor may exert their influence; presumably, tumor growth may be affected through their capacity to provide a nutritional lifeline, allow the dissemination of waste products, or act as a pathway for spread of tumor cells.

Gimbrone and Gullino (1976), using an experimental system whereby mouse mammary tissue could be transplanted to rabbit iris, were able to demonstrate that preneoplastic mammary tissue could be recognized by its ability to elicit angiogenesis before any morphological signs of neoplasia became evident. The transparent chamber technique devised by Sanders and Shubik (1964) has been used extensively for the study of tumor transplants in hamster cheek pouch. It has proved possible to distinguish between different tumors by careful examination of the pattern of their new blood supply (Goodall et al. 1965). More recent applications of this model for the study of TAF have been described by Shubik et al. (1976). Other studies related to the influences exerted by the blood supply of tumors, such as their vascular volume and the blood flow through them, have been extensively reviewed by Gullino (1975).

The supply of oxygen to tumors, among other essential factors, must be determined at least in part by the efficiency of their blood supply. Lack of oxygen in parts of the tumor that outstrip the blood supply will lead to necrosis. This relationship has been found to be remarkably constant (Thomlinson and Gray 1955), intact tumor cells never being found more than 180 μm from supporting stroma. In cancer therapy, oxygen supply is also of importance as anoxic cells may be capable of escaping the otherwise lethal effect of a prescribed radiation dose (Thomlinson 1973).

Colposcopy allied with exfoliative cytology was used by Rubinstein (1968) for the examination of lesions of the uterine cervix; he found that the condition of "hypemia," in which the capillaries are dilated, coarse, and variable in pattern, whilst the epithelium has a gray or grayish-white color, was associated with a high proportion of dysplastic lesions and carcinomas in situ. As it was also found in inflammatory conditions, "hypemia" could not be considered an absolute diagnostic marker; however, it may be indicative of an altered vascular bed that is of importance in the development of premalignant lesions. Although it is known that in carcinogenesis the vascularity of the dermis increases (Tarin 1972), the part played by angiogenic factors and the overall contribution of vascular supply to the development and outcome of premalignant epithelial lesions has been subjected to little scientific enquiry. In view of the potential therapeutic implications, however, there would seem to be some merit in extending investigations into this area.

5. CELLULAR INFILTRATES

The stroma around human carcinomas, beneath premalignant lesions and beneath epithelial surfaces painted experimentally with carcinogenic solutions is commonly seen to contain a varyingly dense infiltrate of "inflammatory" cells. Sometimes this observation is complicated by the presence of ulceration or trauma to the tissues, but in many instances the infiltrate appears to be predominantly of immunological origin and composed of cells of the lymphoid series. Ioachim (1976) has recently reviewed this topic in relation to human cancers, pointing out why such an infiltrate is believed to represent a favorable host reaction to the neoplasm and indicating its potential for studies on prognosis. The fundamental immunological changes associated with malignant neoplasia that may help to explain the presence of such infiltrates are discussed by Outzen (see chapter 16). There is scope for further work on this subject, particularly by well-controlled in vitro tests of cell function and in vivo analysis of the different cell types through the use of more sophisticated immunological staining reactions.

In experimental carcinogenesis of hamster cheek pouch mucosa, it is evident that macrophages are particularly prominent in the stroma from an early stage (Smith 1972b; Gohari and Johnson 1974); their role, however, remains enigmatic. Attention has also been focused on the presence of mast cells in this experimental system, but with conflicting results (Smith 1967; Homburger 1969) and no satisfactory explanation for their possible significance.

6. TRANSPLANTATION AND RECOMBINATION EXPERIMENTS

The work of Orr and his coworkers (Billingham, et al. 1951; Marchant and Orr 1953; Orr and Spencer 1972) has been one of the main sources of the belief that connective tissue influences are responsible for the development of malignant epithelial neoplasms. In essence, they found that if the epithelium is removed from a skin site painted with a chemical carcinogen and is replaced by an epithelial graft from an area not exposed to carcinogen, then tumors will develop in the epithelial graft. Transplantation of the original carcinogen-treated epithelium to a dermal site not previously exposed to carcinogen, however, does not result in the development of tumors. Objections to these conclusions have been raised, some substantiated by experimental results, on the grounds that remnants of original epithelium were left behind in the graft site, or grew in from its edges; more important, perhaps, is the possibility that carcinogen may have become pooled in the connective tissue beneath painted sites and was from there able to exert its effect on the newly-grafted unpainted donor epithelium. Through the use of skin grafting experiments similar to those originally described by Billingham et al. (1951), but this time employing grafts from a purebred strain transplanted to carcinogen-painted sites in F_1 hybrid mice, Steinmuller (1971) was able to show that tumors developing in the treated and denuded areas were derived from host epithelial cells and not from those of donor epithelium.

Of further relevance to this question are the results of experiments described by Dawe (1972) in which tumors were produced in embryonic salivary gland tissues by infecting them with polyoma virus. When epithelial and connective tissue components of the susceptible embryonic glands were separated prior to infection and then reimplanted individually into living animals, no tumors were produced in either tissue. However, if the epithelial and connective tissue portions were recombined after infection with the virus and then implanted into host animals, tumors did develop. Apparently the epithelium and connective tissue must be provided with the opportunity to interact before tumors can be formed. Moreover, this process is apparently specific, for salivary gland epithelium combined with connective tissue from another organ that is also susceptible to the tumor-promoting properties of the polyoma virus does not give rise to tumors following infection and reimplantation. The earlier interpretations of this work have recently been called into question, however, by further work in which the mesenchymal component does not appear to be necessary for the induction of neoplasms in embryonic salivary gland epithelium by polyoma virus (Dawe et al. 1976).

A new method for looking at stromal-epithelial interactions in tumor induction has been devised by Hodges et al. (1977). This work relies upon the characteristic alterations that can be observed by scanning electron microscopy in the process of differentiation and early neoplasia in rat bladder epithelium. The carcinogen N-methyl-N-nitrosourea was used as a direct-acting bladder carcinogen and the adult tissues were studied not only in vivo but also in an in vitro organ culture system. Structural changes in the cell surface pattern of normal and carcinogen-treated bladder epithelium were observed and those characteristic of neoplastic change were identified. Similar modifications to the surface epithelial features were then sought in recombinant cultures prepared from normal and MNU-treated adult rat bladders. Hodges et al. (1977) conclude from their experiments that the carcinogen may have an effect on the epithelium by causing a disturbance to the function of supporting stromal tissues.

7. IMPLICATIONS FOR HUMAN ORAL PRECANCER

Much of the evidence described above concerning the interaction of epithelium and mesenchyme in the development of carcinomas is inconclusive or at an early stage of comprehension. That such interactions exist would appear to be beyond doubt but their precise role and significance has yet to be ascertained. Nevertheless, it is pertinent to consider some of the possible implications of such interactions for our understanding of the different appearances and behavior patterns that may be observed in human oral precancerous lesions.

Although much of the intraoral regional variation in distribution of premalignant lesions is probably attributable to differences in the influence of extrinsic etiological factors (see chapters 2 and 18), it is not unreasonable to suppose that some sites may be more prone to develop such lesions because their connective tissue is different from that found in other sites (see chapter 9). Not only might variations in susceptibility be influenced by etiological and connective tissue factors but so also might the eventual outcome of the lesion; it is known that oral leukoplakia in certain sites has a greater tendency to develop into carcinoma than in other sites (Kramer et al. 1978). One could further speculate that some of the otherwise unexplained racial or individual variations in occurrence of oral premalignancy could be due to genetic or nutritional influences being exerted on the oral subepithelial connective tissues.

At the histological level, some oral leukoplakias have a noticeably thickened "basement membrane" region; this could possibly be of some significance with regard to the reduplicated basal lamina observed both in these human lesions and during experimental oral carcinogenesis. Whether this phenomenon and that of basal cell pseudopodia extending into underlying connective tissue through interruptions in the basal lamina prove to be "precancer associated," as they now seem, rather than "precancer specific," is deserving of further investigation.

Increased vascularity of connective tissues beneath carcinogen-treated hamster cheek pouch epithelium would appear to follow the pattern described in other experimental sites; there may therefore be advantages to be gained from looking more closely at the distribution of blood vessels in human oral mucosal lesions of possible malignant potential.

The most likely candidate for a human oral premalignant lesion being strongly influenced by stromal interaction is the condition of submucous fibrosis (see chapter 1). Although the evidence for this being premalignant is not conclusive, there is apparently a close association between oral cancer and submucous fibrosis in India (Pindborg 1972). Furthermore, it has been demonstrated that submucous fibrosis is characterised at the light microscope level by amorphous connective tissue lacking fiber bundles (Hamner et al. 1971) and by irregularly dispersed, thin collagen fibers of variable diameter at the electron microscopical level (Binnie and Cawson 1972).

The author has compared the nature and extent of the inflammatory cell infiltrate beneath oral epithelium in a variety of conditions (unpublished data). These included oral leukoplakias which were known to have become malignant later, as well as those that had not; leukoplakias from Indian patients were compared with those from Danes and other lesions included in the study were oral submucous fibrosis, oral candidosis, and oral lichen planus. Although differences were detected in the predominant types of cells and their distribution between the various conditions, none was distinctive enough to distinguish known premalignant lesions from the other groups. One observation from a different study that may be important in this respect, however, is that Russell bodies, which are believed to represent immunoglobulin aggregates derived from plasma cells, appeared to be more often found in the infiltrate beneath oral leukoplakias that became malignant than beneath a control group of oral keratoses that did not develop carcinomas (Kramer et al. 1970 and chapter 19).

Should connective tissue influences be at all important in determining the outcome of oral premalignant lesions, then clearly any attempts at treatment would have to take these into account. The procedures for which such influences would appear to be most relevant are those where an attempt is made to obliterate the superficial part of the lesion, usually the entire epithelial layer at least, but not to destroy much of the supporting tissues because of anatomical or functional considerations. Thus the technique of stripping affected mucosa from its underlying connective tissue bed and replacing the surface by a skin graft is to an extent comparable to some of the experimental work with grafts described above. Close surveillance of such sites is clearly warranted and the long-term results of these procedures are awaited with interest. Similarly, the effect of cryosurgery is to destroy superficial tissues and allow healing to occur from adjacent normal areas; what effect this has, however, on the capacity of underlying connective tissue to continue to exert any influence on the new epithelial covering also awaits the outcome of appropriate studies.

CONCLUSIONS

From the diverse pieces of information derived from a variety of observations on different aspects of this topic, there would seem to be little reason to doubt that interactions between the epithelial and connective tissue components of oral mucosa have considerable significance for the development and outcome of oral premalignant lesions. The exact nature of these influences is far from being accurately determined and the methods by which they might be revealed are only in an early stage of development. However, it is important that the concept of the potential role of the connective tissue starts to take a more prominent place in our approach to problems of the etiology, diagnosis, prognosis and control of human oral premalignant lesions.

REFERENCES

Billingham, R. E., Orr, J. W., and Woodhouse, D. L. 1951. Transplantation of skin components during chemical carcinogenesis with 20-methylcholanthrene. *Br. J. Cancer* **5**, 417–432.

Binnie, W. H., and Cawson, R. A. 1972. A new ultrastructural finding in oral submucous fibrosis. *Br. J. Dermatol.* **86**, 286–290.

Briggaman, R. A., and Wheeler, C. E., Jr. 1975. Epidermolysis bullosa dystrophica-recessive: A possible role of anchoring fibrils in the pathogenesis. *J. Invest Dermatol.* **65**, 203–211.

Cox, A. J. 1969. The dermal-epidermal junction in psoriasis. *J. Invest. Dermatol.* **53**, 428–435.

Croft, C. B., and Tarin, D. 1970. Ultrastructural studies of wound healing in mouse skin. I. Epithelial behaviour. *J. Anat.* **106**, 63–77.

Dawe, C. J. 1972. Epithelial-mesenchymal interactions in relation to the genesis of polyoma virus-induced tumours of mouse salivary gland. In: *Tissue Interactions in Carcinogenesis.* (Edited by Tarin, D.), Chap. 10, pp. 305–358. Academic Press, London.

Dawe, C. J., Morgan, W. D., Williams, J. E., and Summerow. J. P. 1976. Inductive epithelio-mesenchymal interaction: Is it involved in the development of epithelial neoplasms? In: *Progress in Differentiation Research.* (Edited by Muller-Berat, N.), pp. 305–318. International Conference on Differentiation, 2d., Copenhagen, 1975. Elsevier/North Holland, Amsterdam.

Folkman, J. 1974. Proceedings: Tumor angiogenesis factor. *Cancer Res.* **34**, 2109–2113.

Folkman, J., Merler, E., Abernathy, C., and Williams, G. 1971. Isolation of a tumor factor responsible for angiogenesis. *J. Exp. Med.* **133**, 275–288.

Frithiof, L. 1972. Ultrastructural changes at the epithelial-stromal junction in human oral preinvasive and invasive carcinoma. In: *Tissue Interactions in Carcinogenesis.* (Edited by Tarin, D.), Chap. 6, pp. 161–189. Academic Press, London.

Gimbrone, M. A., Jr., and Gullino, P. M. 1976. Neovascularization induced by intraocular xenografts of normal, preneoplastic, and neoplastic mouse mammary tissues. *J. Natl. Cancer Inst.* **56**, 305–318.

Gimbrone, M. A., Jr., Cotran, R. S., Leapman, S. B., and Folkman, J. 1974. Tumor growth and neovascularization: An experimental model using the rabbit cornea. *J. Natl. Cancer Inst.* **52**, 413–428.

Gimbrone, M. A., Jr., Leapman, S. B., Cotran, R. S., and Folkman, J. 1972. Tumor dormancy in vivo by prevention of neovascularization. *J. Exp. Med.* **136**, 261–276.

Gimbrone, M. A., Jr., Leapman, S. B., Cotran, R. S., and Folkman, J. 1973. Tumor angiogenesis: Iris neovascularization at a distance from experimental intraocular tumors. *J. Natl. Cancer Inst.* **50**, 219–228.

Gohari, K. 1977. A quantitative morphological and cytochemical study of the synthetic and metabolic apparatus in hamster cheek pouch epithelium during chemical carcinogenesis. Ph.D. dissertation, University of Sheffield.

Gohari, K., and Johnson, N. W. 1974. A quantitative study of the inflammatory response to chemically-induced carcinoma in hamster cheek pouch. Abstract. *J. Dent. Res.* **53**, 1062.

Goodall, C. M., Sanders, A. G., and Shubik, P. 1965. Studies of vascular patterns in living tumors with a transparent chamber inserted in hamster cheek pouch. *J. Natl. Cancer Inst.* **35**, 497–521.

Gullino, P. A. 1975. Extracellular compartments of solid tumors. In: *Cancer: A Comprehensive Treatise. Vol. III. Biology of Tumors: Cellular Biology and Tumor Growth.* (Edited by Becker, F. F.), Chap. 12, pp. 327–354. Plenum Press, New York.

Hamner, J. E., Mehta, F. S., Pindborg, J. J., and Daftary, D. K. 1971. Altered staining reaction of connective tissues in 53 submucous fibrosis patients. *J. Dent. Res.* **50**, 388–392.

Hashimoto, K., Yamanishi, Y., and Dabbous, M. K. 1972. Electron microscopic observations of collagenolytic activity of basal cell epithelioma of the skin in vivo and in vitro. *Cancer Res.* **32**, 2561–2567.

Hashimoto, K., Yamanishi, Y., Maeyens, E., Dabbous, M. K., and Kanzaki, T. 1973. Collagenolytic activities of squamous cell carcinoma of the skin. *Cancer Res.* **33**, 2790–2801.

Hodges, G. M., Hicks, R. M., and Spacey, G. D. 1977. Epithelialstromal interactions in normal and chemical carcinogen-treated adult bladder. *Cancer Res.* **37**, 3720–3730.

Homburger, F. 1969. Chemical carcinogenesis in the Syrian golden hamster: A review. *Cancer* **23**, 313–338.

Ioachim, H. L. 1976. The stromal reaction of tumors: An expression of immune surveillance. *J. Natl. Cancer Inst.* **57**, 465–475.

Jensen, H. M., and Mottet, N. K. 1970. Ultrastructural changes in keratinizing epithelium following trypsinization, epidermal detachment and apposition to mesenchymes. *J. Cell Sci.* **6**, 511–535.

Kahl, F. R., and Pearson, R. W. 1967. Ultrastructural studies of experimental vesiculation. II. Collagenase. *J. Invest. Dermatol.* **49**, 616–631.

Kramer, I. R. H., El-Labban, N., and Lee, K. W. 1978. The clinical features and risk of malignant transformation in sublingual keratosis. *Brit. Dent. J.* **144**, 171–180.

Kramer, I. R. H., Lucas, R. B., El-Labban, N., and Lister, L. 1970. The use of discriminant analysis for examining the histological features of oral keratoses and lichen planus. *Br. J. Cancer* **24**, 673–683.

Marchant, J., and Orr, J. W. 1953. Further attempts to analyse the roles of epidermis and deeper tissues in experimental chemical carcinogenesis by transplantation and other methods. *Br. J. Cancer* **7**, 329–341.

Mazzucco, K. 1972. The role of collagen in tissue interactions during carcinogenesis in mouse skin. In: *Tissue Interactions in Carcinogenesis.* (Edited by Tarin, D.), Chap. 12, pp. 377–398. Academic Press, London.

McNutt, N. S. 1976. Ultrastructural comparison of the interface between epithelium and stroma in basal cell carcinoma and control human skin. *Lab. Invest.* **35**, 132–142.

Odland, G., and Ross, R. 1968. Human wound repair. I. Epidermal regeneration. *J. Cell Biol.* **39**, 135–151.

Orr, J. W., and Spencer, A. T. 1972. Transplantation studies of the role of the stroma in epidermal carcinogenesis. In: *Tissue Interactions in Carcinogenesis.* (Edited by Tarin, D.), Chap. 9, pp. 291–303. Academic Press, London.

Pindborg, J. J. 1972. Is submucous fibrosis a precancerous condition in the oral cavity? *Int. Dent. J.* **22**, 474–480.

Rohrbach, R., Thomas, C., Rümpler, R., and Lau, M. 1970. Die Kollagenasen aktivität und der kollagengehalt der Haut während der Carcinogenese. *Verh. Dtsch. Ges. Pathol.* **54**, 442–450. (Cited by L. Strauch, 1972.)

Ross, R., and Odland, G. 1968. Human wound repair: II. Inflammatory cells, epithelial-mesenchymal interrelations, and fibrogenesis. *J. Cell Biol.* **39**, 152–168.

Rubinstein, E. 1968. Vascular insufficiency in premalignant and pre-invasive squamous epithelium. *Acta Radiol.* **7**, 289–296.

Sanders, A. G., and Shubik, P. 1964. A transparent window for use in the Syrian hamster. Abstract. *Isr. J. Exp. Med.* **11**, 118.

Shubik, P., Feldman, R., Garcia, H., and Warren, B. A. 1976. Vascularization induced in the cheek pouch of the Syrian hamster by tumor and non-tumor substances. *J. Natl. Cancer Inst.* **57**, 769–774.

Smith, C. J. 1967. Effects of carcinogen and cortisone on mast cells in the hamster cheek pouch. *Br. J. Cancer* **21**, 190–197.

Smith, C. J. 1972a. The epithelial-connective tissue junction in the pathogenesis of human and experimental oral cancer. In: *Tissue Interactions in Carcinogenesis.* (Edited by Tarin, D.), Chap. 7, pp. 191–225. Academic Press, London.

Smith, C. J. 1972b. Variations in histochemical properties of hydrolytic enzymes in oral precancerous conditions. *J. Dent. Res.* **51**, 308–318.

Steinmuller, D. 1971. A reinvestigation of epidermal transplantation during chemical carcinogenesis. *Cancer Res.* **31**, 2080–2084.

Strauch, L. 1972. The role of collagenases in tumour invasion. In: *Tissue Interactions in Carcinogenesis.* (Edited by Tarin, D.), Chap. 13, pp. 399–433. Academic Press, London.

Sugár, J. 1972. Ultrastructural and histochemical changes during the development of cancer in various human organs. In: *Tissue Interactions in Carcinogenesis.* (Edited by Tarin, D.), Chap. 5, pp. 127–159. Academic Press, London.

Susi, F. R., and Shklar, G. 1971. Histochemistry and fine structure of oral lesions of mucous membrane pemphigoid: Preliminary observations. *Arch. Dermatol.* **104**, 244–253.

Sylvén, B., and Bois, I. 1960. Protein content and enzymatic assays of intersitital fluid from some normal tissues and transplanted mouse tumors. *Cancer Res.* **20**, 831–836.

Sylvén, B., and Bois-Svensson, I. 1964. Studies on the histochemical "leucine aminopeptidase" reaction: IV. Chemical and histochemical characterization of the intracellular and stromal LNA reactions in solid tumor transplants. *Histochemie* **4**, 135–149.

Tarin, D., and Croft, C. B. 1970. Ultrastructural studies of wound healing in mouse skin. II. Dermo-epidermal interrelationships. *J. Anat.* **106**, 71–91.

Tarin, D. 1972. Morphological studies on the mechanism of carcinogenesis. In: *Tissue Interactions in Carcinogenesis.* (Edited by Tarin, D.), Chap. 8, pp. 227–289. Academic Press, London.

Tarin, D. 1976. Cellular interactions in neoplasia. In: *Fundamental Aspects of Metastasis.* (Edited by Weiss, L.), pp. 151–187. Elsevier/North Holland, Amsterdam.

Thomlinson, R. H. 1973. Radiation and the vascularity of tumours. *Br. Med. Bull.* **29**, 29–32.

Thomlinson, R. H., and Gray, L. H. 1955. The histological structure of some human lung cancers and the possible implications for radiotherapy. *Br. J. Cancer* **9**, 539–549.

Woods, D. A., and Smith, C. J. 1969. The effects of 4-hydroxyanisole on hamster cheek pouch. *Exp. Molec. Path.* **10**, 107–114.

Yamanishi, Y., Dabbous, M. K., and Hashimoto, K. 1972. Effect of collagenolytic activity in basal cell epitheliomas of the skin on reconstituted collagen and physical properties and kinetics of crude enzyme. *Cancer Res.* **32**, 2551–2560.

Yamanishi, Y., Maeyens, E., Dabbous, M. K., Ohyama, H., and Hashimoto, K. 1973. Collagenolytic activity in malignant melanoma: Physicochemical studies. *Cancer Res.* **33**, 2507–2512.

12

The Regulation of Cell Proliferation in Normal Epithelia

E. B. LAURENCE

Mitosis Research Laboratory, Birkbeck College, London, England

1. INTRODUCTION

The basic function common to all epithelia is protection of the underlying tissues from the surrounding external environment, but the variation found in the functional epithelial architecture tends to obscure a basic common pattern of tissue regulation. As in the life cycle of the organism itself, this pattern is one of birth, followed by maturation and death so that any normal tissue is in steady state where cell death is equal to cell birth. Cell proliferation is a process common to all tissues and many techniques have been developed for its study, whereas cell death is specific to each tissue, for it is linked to and consequently obscured by functional processes such as the keratinization and desquamation seen in the epidermal cells. Thus, far more is known about cell proliferation than cell death. Cancer is a state where cell death is exceeded by cell proliferation and so both are of equal importance and may be accomplished by either an increase in cell production or a decrease in the death rate of the cells.

Epithelia are a group of tissues in which regional variations in structure and function are accompanied by differences in rate of cell proliferation, which in the normal state are apparently under the tissues' own homeostatic control. These patterns change abruptly at the boundary of each epithelium (see chapter 14). Thus, it is important to determine the basic mechanisms regulating cell proliferation in various epithelia and to determine the specific epithelial regulating factors which maintain the homeostatic state of each epithelium.

To consider all epithelia is beyond the scope of this article and the theme of this volume and the selection of illustrative examples has been deliberately restricted.

2. STEM CELLS AND EPITHELIAL CELL REPLACEMENT

A typical epithelium is composed of a layer of replicating cells which are situated on a basement membrane separating it from the underlying connective tissue. These cells, after division, move outwards towards the surface as they mature and ultimately are desquamated at the surface. Only in pathological conditions do these epithelial cells pass inwards through the basement membrane and retain their capacity for division.

Regional and functional variations in this basic pattern of epithelial organization occur so that the adult epithelium may be one cell thick, as in the alveolar region of the lung, columnar and ciliated as in the trachea (Fig. 1A), multilayered and nonkeratinizing as in the cornea (Fig. 2A) and many regions of the mouth, keratinizing as in the skin (Figs. 2B and C) and some regions of the mouth, or parakeratotic as in other oral epithelia (Fig. 1F), esophagus (Fig. 1E), and forestomach.

The epithelium lining the vagina may be squamous keratinizing (Fig. 1C) or nonkeratinizing mucous secreting (Fig. 1D), depending on the stage of the estrus cycle of the animal. As different again is the single layered epithelium covering the lens of the eye (Fig. 1B), where in mammals the proliferating region is equatorial and the maturing cells elongate as they develop into the fibers which are constantly being added to the lens throughout the life of the animal (Harding et al. 1971). Thus, this is one organ which never loses cells but is constantly producing them in a very well regulated manner (see Figs. 1 and 2).

The rate of cell production varies for each epithelium (Cameron 1971). For example, there are very few new cells produced in the trachea of the adult mammal, whereas there is a very high rate of cell proliferation in the esophagus. In general, it has been shown that the greater the rate of new cell production, the thicker the epithelium and the shorter the cell life cycle, so that the transit of the cells through the epithelium is faster and the cells are desquamated at a younger stage (Christophers and Laurence 1976). This is true for different regions of skin epidermis, of oral epithelium (see chapter 9), and for some pathological conditions (Christophers and Laurence 1973, 1976; Laurence 1973b; Potten 1975 a and b). For example, in normal skin the very thick keratinizing epithelium of the sole of foot of the mouse has almost three times as many proliferating cells as does the pinna epidermis, and the thickness is almost three times as great (Christophers and Laurence 1973).

In the pinna epidermis the differentiating cells are found amongst the proliferating cells of the basal layer (Christophers 1971a and b; Iversen et al. 1968), and movement of cells from the basement membrane takes place in an ordered fashion so that vertical columns of cells are formed (Mackenzie 1969; Christophers 1971a and b; Allen and Potten 1974). It has been considered that this architecture is the result of an ordered pattern of low cell death and cell production rates resulting in the cells being organized into vertical columns (Christophers et al. 1974) called Epidermal Proliferative Units (EPU) by Potten (1974).

As this thin epidermis, with its horizontal and vertical architecture, is easier to study than the apparently disorganized thicker epithelium, it has been the subject of much speculation concerning the factors controlling its

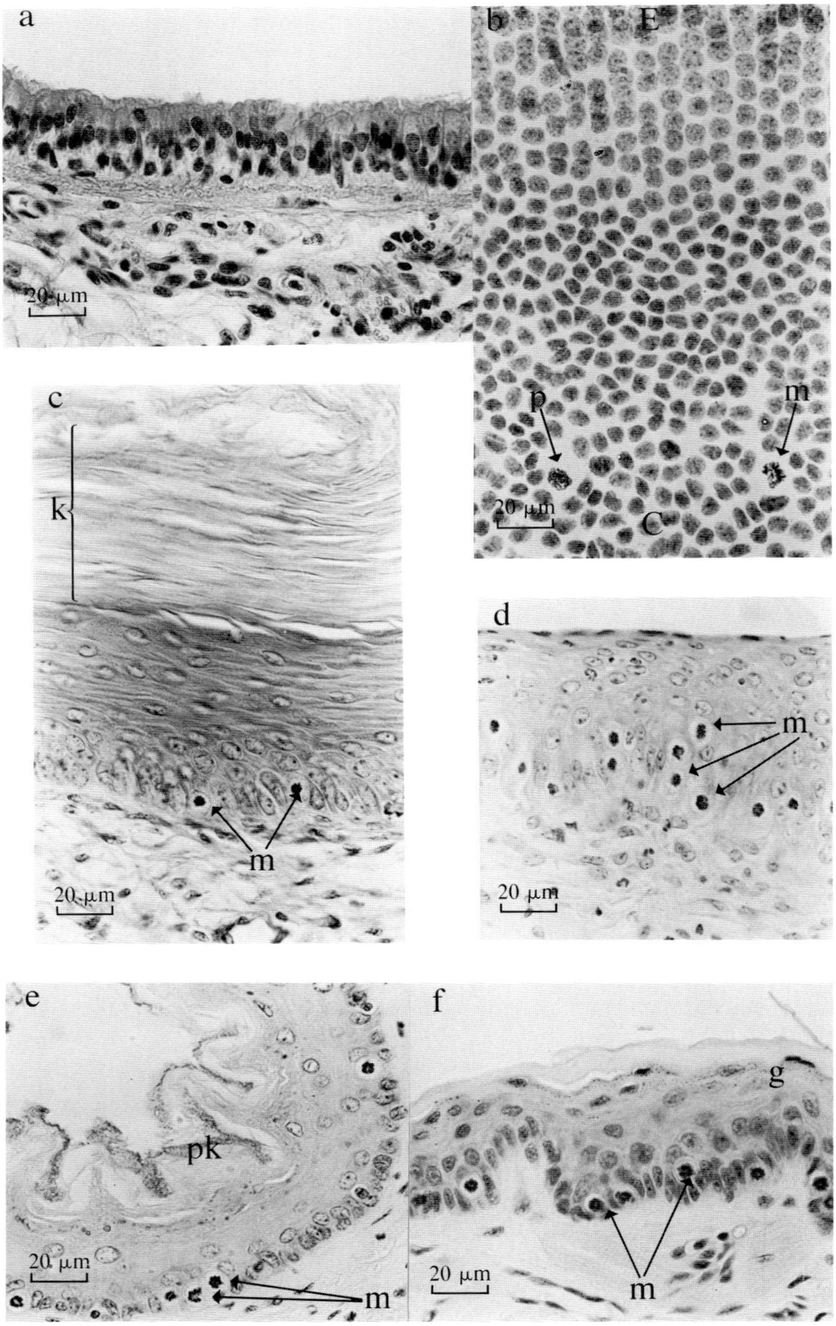

a
20 μm
b
E
p
m
20 μm
C
c
k
m
20 μm
d
m
20 μm
e
pk
20 μm
m
f
g
20 μm
m

FIGURE 1. a. Transverse section of ciliated, columnar epithelium of mouse trachea. Mitoses are seldom found but they can be stimulated by wounding (Gordon and Lane 1977). Hematoxylin and eosin.

b. Single layered flat sheet of epithelial cells stripped from the anterior surface of the lens of the mouse eye. Two dividing cells are seen; one in prophase (p) and the other in metaphase (m). The cells as they mature form into columns at the equator of the lens (E). Towards the center of the epithelial sheet of cells (C) only few mitoses are found although all cells can be stimulated to divide. Feulgen.

c. Transverse section of mouse vagina at estrus phase of the estrus cycle to show considerable cell proliferation (m) and keratinization (k). Hematoxylin and eosin.

d. Transverse section of mouse vagina at diestrus phase of the estrus cycle to show cell proliferation (m) but no keratinization. Hematoxylin and eosin.

e. Transverse section of mouse esophagus to show colcemid arrested metaphases (m) in basal layer, parakeratosis (pk), and absence of granular layer. Hematoxylin and eosin.

f. Transverse section of the lower surface of the mouse tongue to show the parakeratotic epithelium with pronounced granular layer (g) and mitoses, which have been arrested by colcemid at the metaphase (m). Hematoxylin and eosin.

proliferation. The presence of columns may be correlated with a low rate of cell proliferation and slow maturation rate (Christophers 1972a), the cell proliferation occurring in the outer basal cells demarcating the outer limits of each column (Mackenzie 1975; Mackenzie et al. 1975). Christophers et al. (1974) showed that the keratinization process and the ultimate formation of the cornified layer contributed to the column structure as much as the slow rate of cell proliferation in the basal layer.

Potten (1976) likened the epidermal columns to crypts of the intestinal epithelium and considered that there was a central cell which acted as a stem cell, the immediate daughter cells of which never leave the basement membrane and are destined for division only (see Cairnie et al. 1976). He went on to presume an identification of these as Langerhans cells (which are known to have a very low rate of cell production) since, in mouse ear epidermis, one Langerhans cell is found at the central position of each column (Potten and Allen 1976). Mackenzie et al. (1975) severely

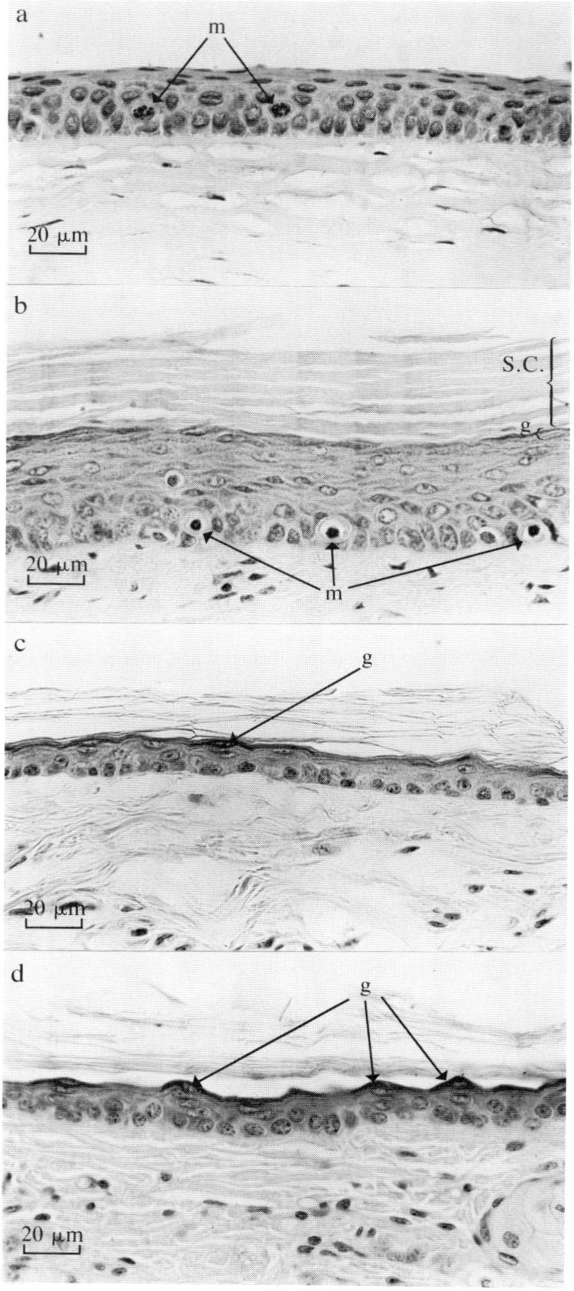
a
m
20 μm
b
S.C.
g
20 μm
m
c
g
20 μm
d
g
20 μm

FIGURE 2. a. Transverse section of mouse cornea to show nonkeratinizing epithelium and mitoses in suprabasal layer (m). Hematoxylin and eosin.

b. Transverse section of epidermis from mouse sole of foot to show well developed granular layer (g), stratum corneum (s.c.) and colcemid arrested mitoses. Hematoxylin and eosin.

c. Transverse section of thin epidermis of the mouse pinna. The vertical columns of cells can be seen although no special procedures have been used. The granular layer (g) can be seen occasionally as a single cell in some columns only. Hematoxylin and eosin.

d. Transverse section of epidermis of mouse ear 7 days after immersion for one minute in water 45° C. There are more cells in the vertical columns than normal and the granular layer is more pronounced (g). Hematoxylin and eosin.

contested this finding as Potten had chosen one of the few examples where this occurred. Mackenzie et al. (1975) showed that in hamster epidermis, where the columns are very pronounced, the population of Langerhans cells is very sparse and there are very many columns without these cells. It is therefore most unlikely that the Langerhans cells, which are found in various positions in a number of epithelia, act as stem cells.

There is little doubt that stem cells exist in other tissues, e.g., various regions of the alimentary canal, the blood forming cells, spermatogonia, etc. (see Cairnie et al. 1976), and so Potten (1976) has constructed a similar model for epidermis, based on the Epidermal Proliferative Unit which acts as a distinct clone of cells. He is of the firm opinion that stem cells exist which have different kinetic values from the other dividing daughter cells, but his evidence is at the limits of statistical significance and further studies using other species with similarly organized epithelia are needed for confirmation of his hypothesis.

If stem cells do exist in epithelia then the problems of control become more complicated since the stem cell apparently has different cell kinetics and is therefore under the control of different regulating substances from those of its more mature and neighboring daughter cells. To make a comparison with the blood forming cells, it is necessary to identify an "epidermopoietin," which can act as an inducer of epidermal stem cells.

3. THE CELL CYCLE IN EPITHELIA

The production of a new cell is accomplished by the same process in all tissues (Padilla et al. 1974; Prescott 1976). The nuclear changes during this process act as convenient markers for studying the procedure. The fact that a cell need not divide more than once does not alter the concept of the cell proliferation cycle. For convenience, the beginning of the cycle is marked by the onset of DNA synthesis in the nucleus, a process which continues for 7–18 hours depending on the epithelial site (Cameron 1971; Blenkinsopp 1968). A cell in this state is said to be in S-phase and can be identified using radioisotope techniques (see chapter 13). At the end of the S-phase a gap of indeterminate biochemical activity exists (G_2), the nucleus remaining for a few minutes to some hours before the histologically identifiable process known as mitosis (M-phase) occurs in which the nucleus divides in two. Production of cytoplasmic proteins result in the formation of two daughter cells and the nuclei pass into a "resting" phase known as G_1. The length of this phase is debatable as the cells may pass out of cycle to begin their maturation process or into a quiescent period known as G_0. G_1 is a much neglected stage in the cell life cycle when the subsequent fate of the cell may be determined or even modulated (dichophase, Bullough 1965, 1975; Gelfant 1976; Epifanova 1977). Subsequently, the cells may either progress through their life cycle to mature, function, and die, or undergo division.

In epidermis it may be said that the longer a cell is prevented from dividing, the greater its chances of never doing so, especially if it has begun to mature and function. The least mature cells of an epithelium can be stimulated to divide by insults such as ultraviolet light and x-irradiation damage, chemical carcinogens, surgical incision, or extirpation of an area of the epithelial cells. The resulting cell proliferation is greatly above normal and the cell cycle phases are shortened (Christophers 1972b; Mackenzie and Ettinger 1975; Bullough and Mitrani 1976; Fowler and Denekamp 1976). Cell cycle phases have been studied in various tissues and summarized accordingly (see Cameron 1971). Generally, it may be said that the internal lining epithelia, e.g., tongue, esophagus, etc., have a short cell cycle, whereas in the epidermis of the extremities (such as epidermis of pinna and sole of foot) the phases are longer. There is no correlation between the number of proliferative cells and the length of cell cycle (Laurence, 1973b). Whether the normal rate of cell proliferation is high or low (Gordon and Lane 1977), every epithelium is capable of responding to mechanical injury by increasing the number of proliferating cells and decreasing the duration of the cell cycle. This increase in mitotic rate follows a similar pattern whether there is a gentle short stimulus such as massage (Bullough and Laurence 1960), as shown in Figure 1, or prolonged friction or abrasion (Mackenzie 1973; 1974a and b). The cell proliferation reaches a peak after 1 or 2 days, decreasing to normal subsequently in short term wounding or when the stimulus is stopped as in long term friction. When there is extirpation of the epithelium, the wound is healed by migration from the wound edges where for a distance of 1 mm a high rate of cell proliferation occurs after 24 hours (Bullough and Laurence 1960; Iversen et al. 1974). If the cornified layers are removed by adhesive tape stripping, a similar response occurs, but if the damage is inflicted by applied heat at e.g. 60°C there is a delay of several days before there is a response by increased cell proliferation (Winter 1972). A similar situation arises when the damage is done by x-irradiation (see Fowler and Denekamp, 1976) where no cells are removed. Christophers and Laurence (unpublished results) have attempted to perform a physiological experiment with mouse pinna by not removing any tissue but increasing the blood flow by immersing the ears of mice for only one minute in hand-hot water (45°C) (Fig. 3). Immediately on immersion there was an increase in blood flow through the ears followed by slight edema which lasted a day. The ears then appeared normal macroscopically, although increased cellularity followed the mitotic wave, and the epidermis returned to normal in due course (Figs. 2C and D). Figure 4 shows the same pattern of response with light friction.

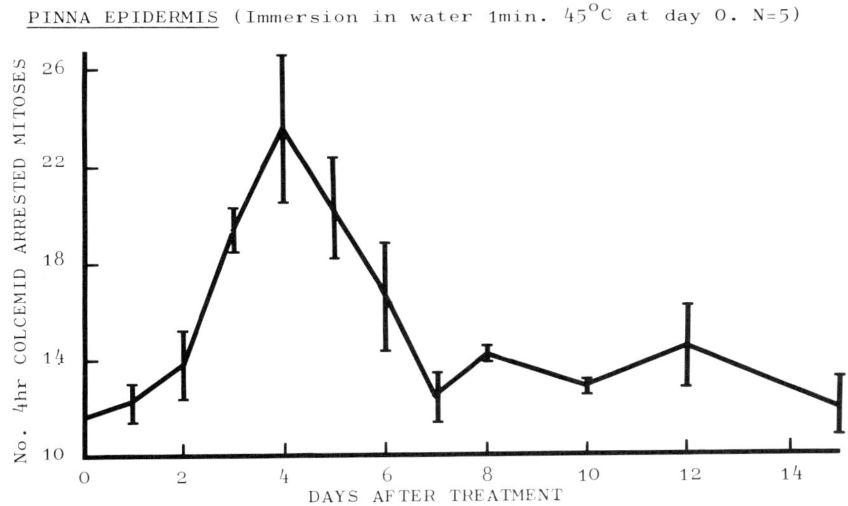

FIGURE 3. Graph of the number of 4 hour colcemid arrested mitoses in 10 mm length of epidermis sectioned at 7 μm. The ears had been immersed for 1 min. in water at 45°C. A group of 5 mice were killed at daily intervals. Each point represents the mean and standard error.

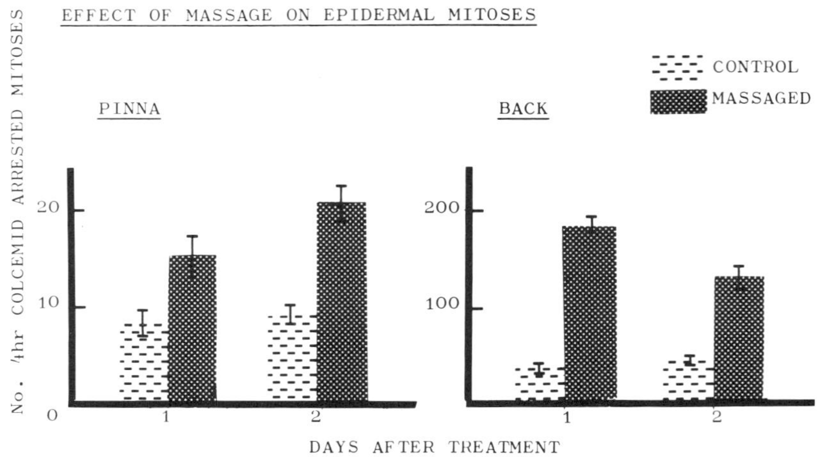

after Bullough & Laurence Proc Roy Soc B 1960. 151, 517-536

FIGURE 4. The number of 4 hour colcemid arrested mitoses in 10 mm length of mouse ear and back skin epidermis one and two days after twenty light massage strokes with the forefinger. As found for incision wounds, the back epidermal mitoses reach a maximum number one day earlier than those of the ear. Results given in detail in Bullough and Laurence (1960).

Thus, it has been shown that normal epithelia can be found in the body with very high mitotic rates or very low. All can be stimulated to increased cell proliferation by various means and, if the underlying dermis is not damaged, (see Laurence 1977) all return to their normal homeostatic state for that particular body site.

4. ENDOGENOUS REGULATING MECHANISMS

4:1 EVIDENCE FOR THE PRESENCE OF SPECIFIC ENDOGENOUS MITOTIC INHIBITORS (CHALONES)

In 1960 Bullough and Laurence, using mouse pinna and body epidermis, presented experimental evidence for the regulation of cell proliferation being effected by an inhibitor which is produced by the epidermis itself. This was later confirmed by Finegold, 1965, and Iversen et al., 1974. By using the very thin mouse pinna Bullough and Laurence showed that when epidermal cells were removed from one side of the ear, there was an increase in cell proliferation in the epidermis immediately opposite the removed area. This increase was not due to mechanical pressure during wounding, for adhesive tape stripping had no effect on the epidermis of the opposite side, unless the epidermis was denuded—a phenomenon also demonstrated by Mackenzie and Ettinger (1975) using friction. "Sham" wounds were also made in an ear of a dead mouse placed over the pinna and no stimulation of cell proliferation resulted in the underlying intact epidermis of the live mouse (Bullough and Laurence 1960). Finegold (1965), using guinea pig ear, and Iversen et al. (1974), using the web of the fruit bat, grafted skin on to the wound and found no increased mitotic rate in the opposite epidermis.

Bullough and Laurence concluded that epidermis was producing a diffusible substance which inhibited the cell proliferation in that tissue. Thus the inhibitor from one side of the ear affected the cell proliferation of the opposite side. The subsequent study using tissue extracts (see Laurence 1973a, and Marks 1976a) resulted in the establishment of a theory of negative feedback control which was effected by tissue-specific, species nonspecific endogenous inhibitors of cell proliferation which Bullough called "chalones" (Bullough 1962). The evidence for chalones as a general concept of tissue regulation has been critically reviewed by Rytömaa (1976) and Thornley (1976). Although there is overwhelming evidence for the existence of chalones, as yet they exist only in impure forms (Thornley and Laurence 1975); their receptor sites or site of origin within the cell have not been established, but there is now a voluminous literature covering all tissues on these chemically elusive substances (Houck and Forscher 1973; Houck 1976).

4.2 EPIDERMAL G_2 CHALONE AND THE STRESS HORMONES

The first epidermal chalone (subsequently known as the Epidermal G_2 Chalone) was isolated in almost pure form by ethanol precipitation, electrophoresis, and dialysis of powdered pig skin (Hondius Boldingh and Laurence 1968). The observation that chalone requires the presence of adrenalin to exert its effect formed the basis of the discriminative "adrenalin-wash" technique in short-term organ culture of mouse pinna devised by Bullough and Laurence (1964). This test showed that when epidermal chalone was present, there was an inhibition of mitoses as determined by colcemide arrest in the first 5 hours of culture. By 9 hours this inhibition was no longer present due to exhaustion of adrenalin. If, after 5 hours of culture with skin extract, the ear pieces were washed in a very dilute solution of adrenalin (0.25 μg/ml) for 30 mins. and subsequently returned to the extract, the inhibition was restored. Table 1 shows the presence of the epidermal G_2 chalone in various tissues from different species which were tested in this way. Extracts of liver and thigh muscle contained no epidermal chalone, while the crystallins of the lens produced a toxic effect which may have been masking the chalone (Table 2). Subsequently, it was found that extracts of tumors of epidermal origin (Table 3) also contained epidermal chalone (Bullough and Laurence 1968b; Laurence and Elgjo 1971; Bullough and Deol 1971), whereas extracts of tumors of nonepidermal origin such as melanomas and lymphomas (Table 4) did not, although they did contain the chalone of their tissue of origin (Bullough and Laurence 1968c, 1970).

The significance of the adrenalin wash was not appreciated at that time, since work on the cAMP system was not well enough advanced. Hormones such as adrenalin apparently do not penetrate the cell membrane but exert their effect through a "second messenger," which in the case of adrenaline is 3'5' cyclic adenosine monophosphoric acid (cAMP) (Robison et al. 1968). Cyclic AMP is produced by adenylate cyclase, which is bound to the cell membrane and becomes activated upon the binding of adrenalin or other such compounds to specific receptors or binding sites on the cell membrane. In the epidermis there may be as many as four specific binding sites on the regulatory subunit to adenylate cyclase. These sites include areas for β adrenergic agents such as adrenalin, adenosine, prostaglandins, and histamine. It was already known that the adrenalin was implicated in the circadian rhythm of mitotic activity in epidermis (Bullough and Laurence 1966) and, furthermore, that the glucocorticoid hormones enhanced and prolonged the effects of adrenalin and chalone (Bullough and Laurence 1968a). In addition the subsequent work by Bullough and Laurence on 2- and 3-day wounds showed the importance of adrenalin and hydrocortisone, rather than epidermal chalone, on the inhibition of mitosis at the edges of the wounds where peak mitosis is usually seen (Bullough 1969). In contrast the work on tumors showed that chalone as well as hydrocortisone and adrenalin were necessary to inhibit mitosis (Bullough and Laurence 1968b and c, 1970; Bullough and Deol 1971). Thus, the proliferating cells at the edge of the wound could not be compared to the proliferating cells of the transplanted carcinomas, and could not be used as a model for cancer cells.

Voorhees et al. (1972) were the first to implicate the cAMP system and chalone in the control of cell proliferation in skin. The evidence on cell proliferation in wounds suggests that the chalone is still being produced by the dividing cells and, therefore, is not the limiting factor. Although this is true for a wound edge, it is not true for carcinomas, nor should it be true for the hyperplasia found in epidermis opposite the wound in the original experiments by Bullough and Laurence (1960). In this context, it is interesting to note here that Rohrbach et al. (1972), Rohrbach and Laerum (1974), and Iversen et al. (1977) have shown that less chalone than normal could be extracted from hyperplastic tissue resulting from carcinogen applications.

As the basal cells of normal epidermis, the migrating edges of incised wounds, and some epidermal cancer cells are not strikingly different in morphological terms, it is necessary to determine whether there are

TABLE 1 Distribution of Epidermal G_2 Chalone

Using the Discriminative "Adrenalin-wash" In Vitro Technique on Mouse Ear Epidermis (N = 10)

Tissue extracts	*Change in Mitotic Count* 5 hours	9 hours	9 hours with "wash" at 5 hours
*Pig palate. 66–80% ethanol ppt.	–49%	0	–52%
*Pig gingiva 66–80% ethanol ppt.	–45%	0	–49%
†Man gingiva crude water extract.	–60%	0	–53%
*Pig esophagus crude water extract.	–41%	0	–44%
*Pig lung 50–70% ethanol ppt.	–43%	0	–44%
‡Rabbit lens α and βS (?) crystallin	–55%	0	–55%
*Man urine preparation	–61%	0	–57%

Prepared by: *Dr. W. Hondius Boldingh, †Dr. E. Randers Hansen, ‡Dr. M. Voaden.

TABLE 2 Extracts From Various Tissues

Using the Discriminative "Adrenalin-wash" In Vitro Technique on Mouse Ear Epidermis (N = 10)

Tissue extracts	*Change in Mitotic Count* 5 hours	9 hours	9 hours with "wash" at 5 hours
*Pig liver crude water extract	0%	0%	—
*Pig thigh muscle water extract	0%	0%	—
‡Rabbit lens α and β crystallins	–54%	–39%	–40%

Prepared by: *Dr. W. Hondius Boldingh, ‡Dr. M. Voaden.

TABLE 3 Extracts from Epidermal Tumors

Using the Discriminative "Adrenalin-wash" In Vitro Technique on Mouse Ear Epidermis (N = 10)

Tumors extracted	*Change in Mitotic Count* 5 hours	9 hours	9 hours with "wash" at 5 hours
*Rabbit Vx2 epidermal tumor	–47%	0%	–50%
†Hamster Chernozemski epid. tumor	–67%	0%	–61%
‡Mouse Hewitt epidermal tumor	–44%	0%	–48%

Prepared by: *Bullough and Laurence 1968, †Laurence and Elgjo 1971, ‡Bullough and Deol 1971.

TABLE 4 Extracts of Tumors Using the Discriminative "Adrenalin-wash" In Vitro Technique on Mouse Ear Epidermis (N = 5)

	Change in Mitotic Count 5 hours	9 hours	9 hours with "wash" at 5 hours
*Mouse Harding Passey melanoma	0%	0%	—
*Hamster Amelanotic melanoma	0%	0%	—
†Mouse lymphoma	0%	0%	—

Prepared by: *Bullough and Laurence 1968, †Bullough and Laurence 1970.

differences in the chalone/β adrenergic receptor/cAMP mechanism which underlie their differing mitotic behavior. Laurence and Thornley (1976a and b) hypothesized that chalones are cell line specific and therefore should regulate according to their embryological origin. In this way, ectodermally derived epidermis should respond to epidermal chalone, while the endodermal esophagus should show no response. All the epithelial tissues tested contained epidermal G_2 chalone, according to the discriminative "adrenalin-wash" technique using mouse ear epidermis (Table 1). Laurence and Randers Hansen (1972) showed that the undersurface of tongue does not respond so much to skin extract as to palatal extract and vice versa, but the tongue was more susceptible to adrenalin than the ear epidermis (Laurence and Randers Hansen 1971). Table 5 shows results of 72–81% ethanol precipitate of pig skin on various epithelia. The esophagus (endodermal in origin) apparently has not been inhibited at all. Later results obtained with the purified epidermal G_2 chalone by Laurence and Brown (unpublished observations) shown here (Table 6) are similar, but, in addition, the ectodermally derived lens epithelium remained unaffected also although the corneal mitoses were inhibited. Now that there is confirmation of the fact that various forms of epithelia produce G_2 chalone, but need not respond to it, and the β adrenergic receptor/cAMP system has been implicated, it also is apparent that changes in the availability of cell receptors may be involved.

It is interesting to note here that Tutton and Barkla (1977) have shown that colon cell proliferation is under the influence of the sympathetic nervous system via the α adrenergic receptors (such as the noradrenalin receptors), which when stimulated resulted in accelerated mitotic activity in colonic crypts but not in colonic tumors, whereas β receptor stimulation by adrenalin inhibited cell proliferation in tumors but not in crypts. This might suggest a changed state of the cancer cell. Rat jejunum resembles colon in being controlled by the autonomic nervous system (Tutton 1973; Tutton and Barkla 1977): however, here α and β adrenergic sites could be stimulated, noradrenalin speeding up mitotic activity while adrenalin slowed it down (Tutton and Helme 1974). Hunt and Tutton (1976) report that buccal epithelial cell proliferation is under β adrenergic control only. There is no reason to suppose that other epithelia, especially those of the eye, should not respond similarly. Whereas noradrenalin (Laurence, unpublished) has been shown to have no effect on epidermal mitosis, which correlates with the work of Uzuka et al. (1977), noradrenalin and cervical ganglionic sympathectomy has been shown to affect lens epithelial mitosis as well as adrenalin (Leeson and Voaden 1970; Voaden 1971).

TABLE 5 72–81% Ethanol Precipitate of Pig Skin

Numbers of colcemid-arrested mitoses after 4 hours treatment (10 mm length of 7μ section of epithelium)

	Change	*Control*	*Ethanol ppt*
Pinna	–67%	10.1 ± 0.28	3.3 ± 0.36
Sole of foot	–39%	36.1 ± 2.35	22.2 ± 1.10
Tongue	–24%	137.8 ± 4.09	105.0 ± 9.12
Esophagus	+3%	126.0 ± 5.18	130.4 ± 9.01
N = number of animals		15	10

TABLE 6 Epidermal G_2 Chalone

Numbers of colcemid-arrested mitoses after 3½ hours treatment (N = 10)

	Change	*Control*	*G_2 Chalone*
*Pinna	–54%	10.8 ± 0.29	5.0 ± 0.29
*Sole of foot	–48%	33.0 ± 2.00	17.0 ± 1.08
*Cornea	–36%	53.2 ± 3.40	33.9 ± 1.32
*Esophagus	–6%	73.7 ± 1.28	69.3 ± 3.01
†Lens	+3%	44.3 ± 3.10	45.7 ± 2.25

*10 mm length of 7μ section of epithelium †10 peripheral fields

The regulation of cell proliferation in the various epithelia considered here seem to be mediated via the β adrenoreceptor/cAMP system.

4:3 EPIDERMAL G_1 CHALONE AND THE cAMP SYSTEM

Using crude water extracts and an in vivo test system with back skin of hairless mice (hr/hr), Elgjo and his coworkers (1971, 1972) gave evidence for the existence of two epidermal chalones, one acting at G_2 phase of the cell cycle (thus confirming the work of Bullough and Laurence) and the other acting at the G_1 phase of the cell cycle. They considered that the former was produced by the basal cells and the latter by the differentiating cells (Elgjo et al. 1971, 1972). Marks (1973, 1975) subsequently isolated the G_1 chalone from pig skin.

Thus, there is very little doubt that there are two epidermal chalones, and both in their most purified form have been extensively tested by Thornley and Laurence (1976). They have shown that the epidermal G_1 chalone expresses its activity at the point of entry into S-phase (Thornley et al. 1977) and the G_2 chalone at entry into M-phase. These chalones are cell-line specific since they do not act on sebaceous glands, a tissue closely related to epidermis both evolutionarily and embryologically (Laurence and Thornley 1976a; Laurence 1977; Laurence et al. 1978).

Normal epidermis and massaged epidermis responds immediately to G_1 chalone treatment, but the stripped epidermis does not respond in the first two days after wounding, and hyperplastic epidermis (treated with phorbol esters) hardly responds at all (Bertsch et al. 1976; Kreig et al. 1976). These results have been explained in terms of the cAMP system, which is affected via the α and β receptor system (Marks 1976b). The nonresponsiveness of newborn epidermis (Bertsch and Marks 1974) to attempts to get a reaction with stimulants and chalones has led Bertsch and Marks (1974) to invoke the epidermal stem cell theory and adopt an old form of terminology for a cancer cell, i.e., that the cancer cell is a dedifferentiated or a potentially embryonic cell. This is discussed later.

4:4 CYCLIC AMP SYSTEM AND ITS ROLE IN THE REGULATION OF CELL PROLIFERATION

There has been much controversy concerning the role of cAMP in the regulation of cell proliferation (Chlapowski et al. 1975). Some indicate it is increased in cell proliferation, others that it is decreased. This is ably reviewed by Halprin (1976) and seems to depend on the assay methods used.

In epidermis grown in culture (either as an explant or as isolated cells), there seems to be general agreement that by raising the cAMP level (Birnbaum et al. 1976), there is an inhibition in mitotic activity, i.e., G_2/M phase block (Chopra 1977a and b; Delescluse et al. 1974). This was shown by Elgjo (1975) using epidermal G_2 chalone in vivo. In epidermis, G_1 chalone did inhibit when the β receptors were blocked, indicating that it perhaps acts at some other point in the cAMP system (Elgjo 1975). As glucocorticoids are regarded as substances which potentiate the effect of adrenalin on the β receptors, the results are consistent with the idea that the cAMP system is implicated with both chalones in the regulation of cell proliferation.

5. SOME OTHER FACTORS EFFECTING CELL PROLIFERATION IN EPITHELIA

5:1 PROSTAGLANDINS

The cAMP system cannot be considered without mentioning the group of substances known as prostaglandins. Prostaglandins (PG) are fatty acid derivatives which can act either in situ or through the circulatory system on their target tissues. There are various classes of these compounds which differ in their chemical composition and are designated by a letter and a number such as PGE_2 or PGF_1. The various classes apparently have different effects. Like the substances involved in the cyclic AMP system, prostaglandins are found in all cells (Mathur and Gandhi 1972). The older work has been confused by the specific prostaglandins not being identified and skin not being separated into its component units so that although certain prostaglandins are known to be released from capillary walls in the dermis, it is not known which they are, nor whether they are involved in the epithelium itself. It is considered that prostaglandins E and F are involved in the stimulation of mitotic activity of epithelium and that corticosteroids suppress their biosynthesis and release from the blood vessels when they are used as antiinflammatory agents (Kantrowitz et al. 1975; Lewis and Piper 1975).

5:2 ESTROGENS

It has been known for many years that some hormones affect cell proliferation in epidermis (Bullough 1943), reaching a maximum as estrus commences, dropping sharply around ovulation, and rising again to peak at metestrus. The pattern is similar for uterus and vagina (Fig. 5) (D. P. Taylor, unpublished), which are particularly responsive to sex hormones, not only changing their cell proliferation rate but also undergoing metaplasia. By spaying the animals, the mitotic rate drops to minimum and can be stimulated by estrogen treatment (Controls Fig. 6). Showing experimentally the effect of chalone becomes a complicated project as dose response to hormones and timing after hormone therapy may play a part in potentiating a chalone effect. The preliminary work of Taylor shown here (Fig. 6) indicates that there may be some epidermal G_2 chalone activity in these tissues. It is not definitely known if chalones and the sex hormones directly interact, but the literature concerning epithelial response to sex hormones is so large that it is only possible to include it here briefly, and variations found during the estrus cycle should be taken into account when work is performed on epithelia in female animals. In addition, circadian rhythms are superimposed on the estrogen effect (Krueger et al. 1975), further complicating the study. These factors are, erroneously, rarely considered of importance.

5:3 EPIDERMAL GROWTH FACTOR

Epidermal growth factor has been isolated and characterized by Cohen using the precocious opening of the eyelid and the eruption of incisors of newborn mice as a test system (Cohen 1972; Cohen and Carpenter 1975). In this context, it has been found to stimulate both cell proliferation and keratinization. Since it is concentrated in the submaxillary gland of the male mouse, it would seem it could be particularly involved in the reported higher rate of cell proliferation in buccal mucosae. Although the chemical structure is known, its true specificity has not been adequately reported. Blosse et al. 1975 reported its ubiquitous action on various epithelia of neonate mice but none whatsoever in the adult animal. It is a strangely reticent substance, which seems only to be active on embryos or on immature cells (Bertsch and Marks 1974).

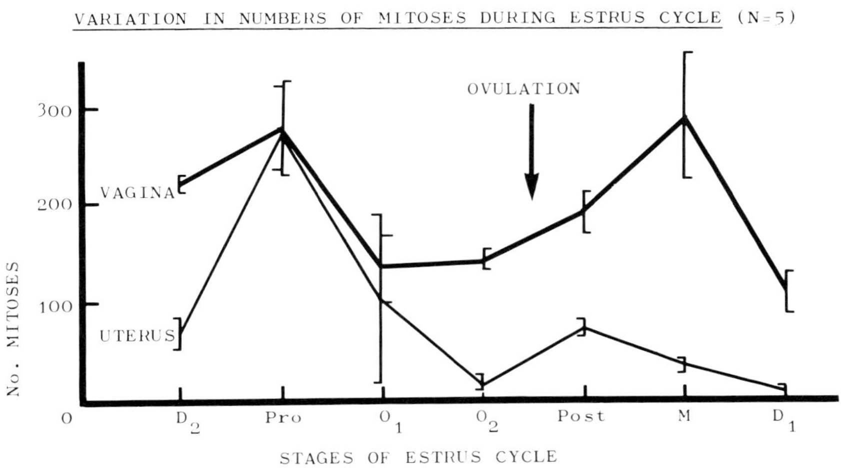

FIGURE 5. Variation of number of mitoses in mouse uterus and vagina at different stages of the estrus cycle. Pro=proestrus; 0_1 and 0_2=the two stages of estrus; Post.=postestrus; M=metestrus, and D_1 and D_2=the two stages of diestrus (Bullough 1943).

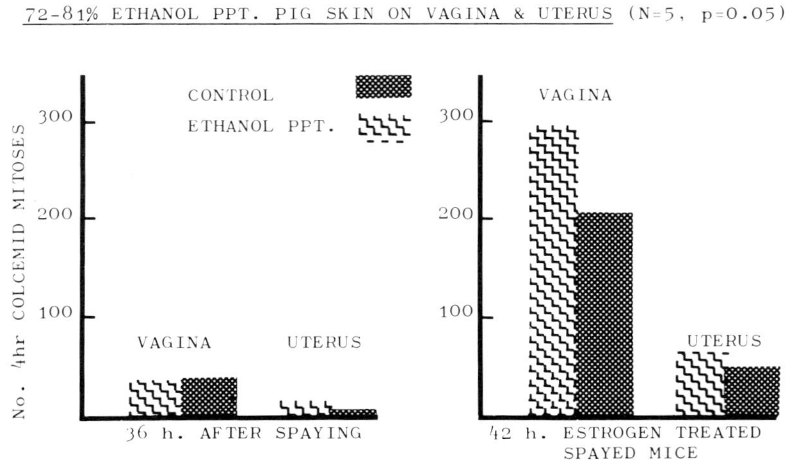

FIGURE 6. The effect of one injection of 72–81% ethanol precipitate of pig skin on uterus and vagina 36 hours after spaying and 42 hours after being given one injection of etriol.

5:4 VITAMIN A

Vitamin A and Vitamin A acid (retinoic acid) have been considered to be epithelial specific in their action as metaplasiagens after increased cell proliferation (Christophers and Wolff 1975). Their role in normal cell proliferation remains obscure and Vitamin A deficient diet may cause keratinization in nonkeratinizing cornea and ciliated tracheal epithelium; hyperkeratinization occurs in gingival epithelium, but hyperplasia and increased cell proliferation occurs in the junctional epithelia (quoted by Schluger et al. 1977). Brown (1975) suggested that the diet of animals and the extent of the level of degradation of Vitamin A accounts for the evolution of mucoid or keratinized epithelia of various animals, although it is difficult to account for the variety of forms found within an adult animal. Although retinoic acid appears to affect maturation or functional differentiation of epithelial cells in culture (Chopra and Flaxman 1975; Christophers and Wolff 1975), its precise mode of action is obscure.

5:5 MESENCHYMAL FACTORS/ANTI-CHALONES

For many years it has been known that epidermal architecture may be dictated by underlying mesenchymal tissues (see chapter 10; Billingham and Silvers 1968), which must reflect some cell kinetic changes although these have not been studied. It may be seen from the examples given here that site variations in epithelial cell proliferation cannot be explained by negative feedback of the inhibitor (chalone). This was pointed out by Laurence et al. (1972), further substantiated by Argyris (1972) using tumor implants, and Bjerknes and Iversen (1974) in a theoretical consideration. Bullough and Mitrani (1976) have indicated that for every tissue that has been studied for mesenchymal factor effects, evidence has been found for its action. The analysis produced here that proliferating cells may have different effector systems, which are all visualized similarly by the process of cell division, suggests that "mesenchymal factors" may cover antichalones, selective β blockers, phosphodiesterase inhibitors, etc. There is considerable evidence for fibroblasts being concerned in this respect (see Sun and Green 1977).

6. CONCLUSIONS

An attempt has been made to review the agents concerned with the regulation of cell proliferation in various epithelia. It has been shown that the literature contains considerable evidence that cells which look morphologically alike, when proliferating, may have different effector mechanisms. Thus, it appears that the cell at the edge of the wound, or in hyperplasia produced by stripping off the stratum corneum, apparently has an altered β receptor/cAMP complex and a normal chalone concentration, whereas there is a low intracellular chalone concentration as well as impaired β receptor/cAMP activity after application of chemical carcinogen or in the implanted tumor. In continuous massage, the chalone mechanism itself is apparently affected. As yet there is no histological method available for recognizing these different cell types. This is also the problem in the identification of premalignant cancer cells.

In no way can carcinomas be regarded as being composed of dedifferentiated or potentially embryonic cells responding only to the G_1 chalone (Marks 1976b). The fact that tumors still produce the chalone of the tissue from which they originate is evidence alone that they cannot be regarded as pluripotential embryonic cells. Although Marrs and Voorhees (1971a and b) extracted their epidermal chalone from epidermis of newborn mice, Bertsch and Marks (1974) found that the G_1 chalone did not inhibit in newborn mouse epidermis, whereas it did contain the chalone, and that this epidermis did not repond to tumor promoting phorbol esters in the same way as adults. Elgjo and Cromarty (1977) showed great variation in cell proliferation between the mice at different ages, and in their response to the epidermal G_1 and G_2 chalone, but this was due to the in vivo state as, in vitro, these cells are still responsive to phorbol esters and respond to G_1 chalone in a manner similar to the adult. Kariniemi and Rytömaa (1976) have shown that the implanted Hewitt epidermal carcinoma causes a depression of cell proliferation similar to that reported here in Table 5, but DNA synthesis was measured instead of mitoses. Korsgaard et al. (1978) have suggested that by recognizing the particular chalones, the tissue of origin may be identified when examining histologically undifferentiated tumors or metastasis as pathological specimens. This negates the claim of Marks (1976b) that G_1 chalone is concerned with regulation of epidermal stem cells only. Because a cell has changed its biochemical architecture so that it no longer shows functional differentiation, it may be said to be functionally undifferentiated. To regard it as dedifferentiated and to even suggest a concept of dedifferentiation as a driving force for tumor promotion is misleading in the light of the evidence presented here.

It is shown here that various tissues contain epidermal G_2 chalone but need not respond to it. The reason is not known, but it need no longer be considered a series of anomalous results. There are indications that this may not be due solely to the different embryological origin of the tissues as similar results have been obtained with epidermis that has been subjected to insult. An altered β-receptor/cAMP system, chalone mechanism, or an excess of mitotic stimulant are also factors to be considered. The actual role that chalones play is not fully understood yet. Laurence and Thornley (1976a) have shown that, depending on the author, chalones have been considered as either primarily cell proliferation inhibitors so that cells remain in the dormant state (G_0), or alternatively chalones may primarily promote cell maturation so that proliferation is inhibited. Their importance is in the tissue specificity of their action.

ACKNOWLEDGEMENTS

I wish to thank the organizers for their invitation to this symposium. Only a stimulus such as this would have made me coordinate the results of over 20 years. I am particularly indebted to my colleagues: Donald Spargo, who has given so much in the preliminary discussion of the ideas presented here; Gillian Brown for her work on lens and corneal epithelium; Paul Taylor for his work on vagina and uterus; and Shirley Knibb for her excellent technical skills. I wish to thank Richard Parker for Figures 1 and 2.

The research is supported by generous grants from the Cancer Research Campaign, the Central Research Fund, University of London, the Medical Research Council, and the Wellcome Trust.

REFERENCES

Allen, T. D, and Potten, C. S. 1974. Fine-structural identification and organization of the epidermal proliferative unit. *J. Cell. Sci.* **15**, 291–319.

Argyris, T. S. 1972. Chalones and the control of normal, regenerative, and neoplastic growth of the skin. *Am. Zool.* **12**, 137–149.

Bertsch, S., and Marks, F. 1974. Proceedings: Lack of an effect of tumor-promoting phorbol esters and of epidermal G1 chalone on DNA synthesis in the epidermis of newborn mice. *Cancer Res.* **34**, 3283–3288.

Bertsch, S., Csontos, K., Schweizer, J. and Marks, F. 1976. Effect of mechanical stimulation on cell proliferation in mouse epidermis and on growth regulation by endogenous factors (chalones). *Cell Tiss. Kinet.* **9**, 445–457.

Birnbaum, J. E., Sapp, T. M., Tolman, E. L. 1976. Cyclic AMP-phosphodiesterase and epidermal mitosis. *J. Invest. Dermatol.* **67**, 235–239.

Bjerknes, R., and Iversen, O. H. 1974. "Antichalone": A theoretical treatment of the possible role of antichalone in the growth control system. *Acta Pathol. Microbiol. Scand. [A]* Suppl. **248**, 33–42.

Blenkinsopp, W. K. 1968. Cell proliferation in striated squamous epithelium in mice. *Exp. Cell Res.* **50**, 265–276.

Blosse, P. T., Edwards, D. C., Fenton, E. L., Mercier-Parot, L., and Tuchmann-Duplessis, H. 1975. The biologic action of epidermal growth factor in mice. Abstract. *J. Invest. Dermatol.* **64**, 282–283.

Billingham, R. E., and Silvers, W. K. 1968. Dermoepidermal interactions and epithelial specificity. In: *Epithelial-Mesenchymal Interactions.* (Edited by Fleischmajer, R., and Billingham, R. E.), Chap. 17, pp. 252–266. Williams and Wilkins, Baltimore.

Brown, C. H. 1975. *Structural Materials in Animals*, pp. 302–304. John Wiley, New York.

Bullough, H. F. 1943. Cyclical changes in the skin of the mouse during the oestrous cycle. *J. Endocrinol.* **3**, 280–287.

Bullough, W. S. 1962. The control of mitotic activity in adult mammalian tissues. *Biol. Rev.* **37**, 307–342.

Bullough, W. S. 1965. Mitotic and functional homeostatis: A speculative review. *Cancer Res.* **25**, 1683–1727.

Bullough, W. S. 1969. Epithelial repair. In: *Repair and Regeneration: The Scientific Basis for Surgical Practice.* (Edited by Dunphy, J. E., and Van Winkle, W.), Chap. 4, pp. 35–46. McGraw-Hill, New York.

Bullough, W. S. 1975. Mitotic control in adult mammalian tissues. *Biol. Rev.* **50**, 99–127.

Bullough, W. S., and Deol, J. U. 1971. Chalone-induced mitotic inhibition in the Hewitt keratinising epidermal carcinoma of the mouse. *Eur. J. Cancer* **7**, 425–431.

Bullough, W. S., and Laurence, E. B. 1960. The control of epidermal mitotic activity in the mouse. *Proc. Roy. Soc.* **151**, 517–536.

Bullough, W. S., and Laurence, E. B. 1964. Mitotic control by internal secretion: The role of the chalone-adrenalin complex. *Exp. Cell Res.* **33**, 176–194.

Bullough, W. S., and Laurence, E. B. 1966. The diurnal cycle in epidermal mitotic duration and its relation to chalone and adrenalin. *Exp. Cell Res.* **43**, 343–350.

Bullough, W. S., and Laurence, E. B. 1968a. The role of glucocorticoid hormones in the control of epidermal mitosis. *Cell Tiss. Kinet.* **1**, 5–10.

Bullough, W. S., and Laurence, E. B. 1968b. Control of mitosis in rabbit Vx2 epidermal tumors by means of the epidermal chalone. *Eur. J. Cancer* **4**, 587–594.

Bullough, W. S., and Laurence, E. B. 1968c. Control of mitosis in mouse and hamster melanomata by means of the melanocyte chalone. *Eur. J. Cancer* **4**, 607–615.

Bullough, W. S., and Laurence, E. B. 1970. The lymphocytic chalone and its antimitotic action on a mouse lymphoma in vitro. *Eur. J. Cancer* **6**, 525–531.

Bullough, W. S., and Mitrani, E. 1976. An analysis of the epidermal chalone control mechanism. In: *Chalones*. (Edited by Houck, J. C.), pp. 7–36. Elsevier/North Holland, Amsterdam.

Cairnie, A. B., Lala, P. K., and Osmond, D. G. 1976. *Stem Cells of Renewing Cell Populations*. Academic Press, New York.

Cameron, I. C. 1971. Cell proliferation and renewal in the mammalian body. In: *Cellular and Molecular Renewal in the Mammalian Body*. (Cell Biology: A Series of Monographs). (Edited by Cameron, I. C., and Thrasher, J. D.), pp. 45–85. Academic Press, New York.

Chlapowski, F. J., Kelly, L. A., and Butcher, R. W. 1975. Cyclic nucleotides in cultured cells. *Adv. Cyclic Nucleotide Res.* **6**, 245–338.

Chopra, D. P., and Flaxman, B. A. 1975. The effect of vitamin A on growth and differentiation of human keratinocytes in vitro. *J. Invest. Dermatol.* **64**, 19–22.

Chopra, D. P. 1977a. Effects of theophylline and dibutyryl cyclic AMP on proliferation and keratinization of human keratinocytes in vitro. *Br. J. Dermatol.* **96**, 255–262.

Chopra, D. P. 1977b. Effects of theophylline, epidermal chalone, or X-Irradiation on human keratinocytes in vitro. *Br. J. Dermatol.* In press.

Christophers, E. 1971a. Die epidermale Columnarstruktur. Vorauss et Zungen und Moglicher Entstehungs mechanisms. *Z. Zell. forsch. Mikrosk. Anat.* **114**, 441–450.

Christophers, E. 1971b. Cellular architecture of the stratum corneum. *J. Invest. Dermatol.* **56**, 165–169.

Christophers, E. 1972a. Correlation between column formation, thickness and rate of new cell production in guinea pig epidermis. *Virchows Arch. Zellpathol.* **10**, 286–292.

Christophers, E. 1972b. Kinetic aspects of epidermal wound healing. In: *Epidermal Wound Healing*. (Edited by Maibach, H. I., and Rovee, D. T.), pp. 53–69. Year Book Medical Publishers, Chicago.

Christophers, E., and Laurence, E. B. 1973. Regional variatons in mouse skin: Quantitation of epidermal compartments in two different body sites. *Virchows Arch. Zellpathol.* **12**, 212–222.

Christophers, E., and Laurence, E. B. 1976. Kinetics and structural organization of the epidermis. *Curr. Probl. Dermatol.* **6**, 87–106.

Christophers, E., and Wolff, H. H. 1975. Effects of vitamin A acid in skin: In vivo and in vitro studies. *Acta Derm. Venereol.* **74**, 42–49.

Christophers, E., Wolff, H. H., and Laurence, E. B. 1974. The formation of epidermal cell columns. *J. Invest. Dermatol.* **62**, 555–559.

Cohen, S. 1972. Epidermal growth factor. *J. Invest. Dermatol.* **59**, 13–16.

Cohen, S., and Carpenter, G. 1975. Human epidermal growth factor: Isolation and chemical and biological properties. *Proc. Nat. Acad. Sci. USA* **72**, 1317–1321.

Delescluse, C., Colburn, N. H., Duell, E. A., and Voorhees, J. J. 1974. Cyclic AMP-evaluating agents inhibit proliferation of keratinizing guinea pig epidermal cells. *Differentiation* **2**, 343–350.

Elgjo, K. 1975. Epidermal chalone and cyclic AMP: An in vivo study. *J. Invest. Dermatol.* **64**, 14–18.

Elgjo, K., and Comarty, A. 1977. Growth kinetics in newborn mouse epidermis: response to epidermal chalone. *Virchows Arch. B. Cell Path.* **24**, 101–108.

Elgjo, K., Laerum, O. D., and Edgehill, W. 1971. Growth regulation in mouse epidermis. I. G_2-inhibitor present in the basal cell layer. *Virchows Arch. Zellpathol.* **8**, 277–283.

Elgjo, K., Laerum, O. D., and Edgehill, W. 1972. Growth regulation in mouse epidermis. II. G_1 inhibitor present in the differentiating cell layer. *Virchows Arch. B. Zellpathol.* **10**, 229–236.

Epifanova, O. I. 1977. Mechanisms underlying the differential sensitivity of proliferating and resting cells to external factors. *Int. Rev. Cytol.* (Suppl.) **5**, 303–335.

Finegold, M. J. 1965. Control of cell multiplicaton in epidermis. *Proc. Soc. Exp. Biol. Med.* **119**, 96–100.

Forscher, B. K., and Houck, J. C. 1973. *Chalones: Concepts and Current Researches.* Natl. Cancer Inst. Mongr. 38. U.S. Dept. of Health, Education, and Welfare, Bethesda, Md.

Fowler, J., and Denekamp, J. 1976. Regulation of epidermal stem cells. In: *Stem Cells of Renewing Cell Populations.* Edited by Cairnie, A. B., Lala, P. F., and Osmond, D. G.), pp. 117–134. Academic Press, New York.

Gelfant, S. 1976. The cell cycle in psoriasis: a reappraisal. *Br. J. Dermatol.* **95**, 577–590.

Gordon, R. E., and Lane, B. P. 1977. Cytokinetics of rat tracheal epithelium stimulated by mechanical trauma. *Cell Tissue Kinet.* **10**, 171–181.

Halprin, K. M. 1976. William Montagna lecture. Cyclic nucleotides and epidermal cell proliferation. *J. Invest. Dermatol.* **66**, 339–343.

Harding, C. V., Reddan, J. R., Unakar, N. J., and Bagchi, M. 1971. The control of cell division in the ocular lens. *Int. Rev. Cytol.* **31**, 215–300.

Hondius Boldingh, W., and Laurence, E. B. 1968. Extraction, purification and preliminary characterization of epidermal chalone. *Eur. J. Biochem.* **5**, 191–198.

Houck, J. C. (ed.) 1976. *Chalones.* Elsevier/North Holland, Amsterdam.

Hunt, H., and Tutton, P. J. 1976. Adrenergic factors influencing the mitotic rate in stratified squamous epithelium of the buccal mucosa of the rat. *Clin. Exp. Pharmacol. Physiol.* **3**, 207–215.

Iversen, O. H., Bhangoo, K. S., and Hansen, K. 1974. Control of epidermal cell renewal in the bat web. A study of the cell number, cell size, and mitotic rate in the epidermis on both sides of the web after the removal of the epidermis on the ventral side only with special emphasis on growth control theories. *Virchows Arch. Zellpathol.* **16**, 157–179.

Iversen, O. H., Bjerknes, R., and Devik, F. 1968. Kinetics of cell renewal, cell migration and cell loss in the hairless mouse dorsal epidermis. *Cell Tissue Kinet.* **1**, 351–367.

Iversen, O. H., Clausen, O. P., Elgjo, K., Iversen, U. M., and Rohrbach, R. 1977. Effects of bleomycin on the epidermal content of growth-regulatory substances (chalones). *Cell Tissue Kinet.* **10**, 71–79.

Kantrowitz, F., Robinson, D. R., Maquire, M. B., and Levine, L. 1975. Corticosteroids inhibit prostaglandin production by rheumatoid synovia. *Nature* **258**, 737–739.

Kariniemi, A. L., and Rytömaa, T. 1976. Effect of the Hewitt keratinizing epidermal carcinoma on cell proliferation in different organs of the host mouse and in human psoriatic skin cultured in diffusion chambers. *Br. J. Dermatol.* **94**, 512–522.

Korsgaard, R., Iversen, O. H., Isaksson-Forsen, G., and Burton, D. 1978. Specificity of epidermal chalone extracts for human epidermoid tumor cells in vitro: A preliminary report. *Cell Tissue Kinet.* **11**, 441–443.

Krieg, L., Kühlmann, I., and Marks, F. 1974. Effect of tumor-promoting phorbol esters and of acetic acid on mechanisms controlling DNA synthesis and mitosis (chalones) and on the biosynthesis of histidine-rich protein of mouse epidermis. *Cancer Res.* **34**, 3135–3146.

Krueger, W. A., Bo, W. J., and Hoopes, P. C. 1975. A circadian rhythm of mitotic activity in the uterine luminal epithelium of the rat: Effect of oestrogen. *Anat. Rec.* **183**, 563–566.

Laurence, E. B. 1973a. Experimental approach to the epidermal chalone. In: *Chalones: Concepts and Current Researches.* Natl. Cancer Inst. Monogr. 38. (Edited by Houck, J. C., and Forscher, B. K.), pp. 37–45. U.S. Dept. of Health, Education and Welfare, Bethesda, Md.

Laurence, E. B. 1973b. The epidermal chalones and keratinizing epithelia. In: *Chalones: Concepts and Current Researches.* Natl. Cancer Inst. Monogr. 38. (Edited by Forscher, B. K., and Houck, J. C.), pp. 37–45. U.S. Dept. of Health, Education and Welfare, Bethesda, Md.

Laurence, E. B. 1977. Factors affecting the organization and renewal of epidermis. In: *Cholesteatoma.* First International Conference. (Edited by McCabe, B. F., Sadé, J., and Abramson, M.), pp. 23–37. Aesculapius, Birmingham, Alabama.

Laurence, E. B., and Elgjo, K. 1971. Epidermal chalone and cell proliferation in a transplantable squamous cell carcinoma in hamsters. II. In vitro results. *Virchows Arch. Zellpathol.* **7**, 8–15.

Laurence, E. B., and Randers Hansen, E. 1971. An in vivo study of epidermal chalone and stress hormones on mitosis in tongue epithelium and ear epidermis of the mouse. *Virchows Arch. Zellpathol.* **9**, 271–279.

Laurence, E. B., and Randers Hansen, E. 1972. Regional specificity of the epidermal chalone extracted from two different body sites. *Virchows Arch. Zellpathol.* **11**, 34–42.

Laurence, E. B., Randers Hansen, E., Christophers, E., and Rytömaa, T. 1972. Systemic factors influencing epidermal mitosis. *Rev. Eur. Etud. Clin. Biol.* **17**, 133–139.

Laurence, E. B., Spargo, D. J., Christophers, E., and Thornley, A. L. 1978. Cell proliferation kinetics of epidermis and sebaceous glands: two compatible tissues for demonstrating tissue specificity of the G_1 chalone. Submitted for publication.

Laurence, E. B., and Thornley, A. L. 1976a. Chalone tissue specificity and the embryonic derivation of organs. An appraisal of the problems. In: *Chalones.* (Edited by Houck, J. C.), pp. 273–288. Elsevier/North Holland, Amsterdam.

Laurence, E. B., and Thornley, A. L. 1976b. The influence of epidermal chalone on cell proliferation. In: *Stem Cells of Renewing Cell Populations.* (Edited by Cairnie, A. B., Lala, P. K., Osmond, D. G.), pp. 103–116. Academic Press, New York.

Leeson, S. J., and Voaden, M. J. 1970. A chalone in the mammalian lens. II. Relative effects of adrenaline and noradrenaline on cell division in the rabbit lens. *Exp. Eye Res.* **9**, 67–72.

Lewis, G. P., and Piper, P. J. 1975. Inhibition of release of prostaglandins as an explanation of some of the actions of anti-inflammatory corticosteroids. *Nature* **254**, 308–311.

Mackenzie, I. C. 1969. Ordered structure of the stratum corneum of mammalian skin. *Nature* **222**, 881–882.

Mackenzie, I. C. 1973. The effect of friction on the keratinising epithelia of the oral mucosa and skin of rodents. *Br. Dent. J.* **134**, 231–236.

Mackenzie, I. C. 1974a. The effects of frictional stimulation on mouse ear epidermis. I. Cell proliferation. *J. Invest. Dermatol.* **62**, 80–85.

Mackenzie, I. C. 1974b. The effects of frictional stimulation on mouse ear epidermis. II. Histologic appearance and cell counts. *J. Invest. Dermatol.* **63**, 194–198.

Mackenzie, I. C. 1975. Spatial distribution of mitosis in mouse epidermis. *Anat. Rec.* **181**, 705–710.

Mackenzie, I. C., and Ettinger, R. L. 1975. Differences in the response of rodent oral mucosa and skin to repeated surface trauma. *J. Prosthet. Dent.* **34**, 666–674.

Mackenzie, I. C., Zimmerman, K. L., and Wheelock, D. A. 1975. Patterns of mitosis in hamster epidermis. *Am. J. Anat.* **144**, 461–466.

Marks, F. 1973. A tissue-specific factor inhibiting DNA synthesis in mouse epidermis. In: *Chalones: Concept and Current Researches.* Natl. Cancer Inst. Monogr. 38. (Edited by Forscher, B. K., and Houck, J. C.), pp. 79–90. U.S. Department of Health, Education and Welfare, Bethesda, Md.

Marks, F. 1975. Isolation of an endogenous inhibitor of epidermal DNA synthesis (G_1 chalone) from pig skin. *Hoppe Seyler Z. Physiol. Chem.* **356**, 1989–1992.

Marks, F. 1976a. The epidermal chalones. In: *Chalones.* (Edited by Houck, J. C.), pp. 173–227. Elsevier/North Holland, Amsterdam.

Marks, F. 1976b. Epidermal growth control mechanisms, hyperplasia, and tumor promotion in the skin. *Cancer Res.* **36**, 2636–2643.

Marrs, J. M., and Voorhees, J. J. 1971a. A method for bioassay of an epidermal chalone-like inhibitor. *J. Invest. Dermatol.* **56**, 174–181.

Marrs, J. M., and Voorhees, J. J. 1971b. Preliminary characterization of an epidermal chalone-like inhibitor. *J. Invest. Dermatol.* **56**, 353–358.

Mathur, G. P., and Gandhi, V. M. 1972. Prostaglandin in human and albino rat skin. *J. Invest. Dermatol.* **48**, 291–295.

Nome, O. 1975. Tissue specificity of the epidermal chalones. *Virchows Arch. (Cell Pathol.)* **19**, 1–25.

Okulov, V. B., and Ketlinski, S. A. 1975. Use of immunochemical methods for the characterization and purification of tissue specific inhibitors of mitotic activity (chalones). English Abstract. *Tsitilogia* **17**, 1294–1299.

Padilla, G. M., Cameron, I. L., and Zimmerman, A., eds. 1974. *Cell Cycle Controls.* Academic Press, New York.

Potten, C. S. 1974. The epidermal proliferative unit: The possible role of the central basal cell. *Cell Tissue Kinet.* **7**, 77–88.

Potten, C. S. 1975a. Epidermal transit times. *Br. J. Dermatol.* **93**, 649–658.

Potten, C. S. 1975b. Epidermal cell production rates. *J. Invest. Dermatol.* **65**, 488–500.

Potten, C. S. 1976. Identification of clonogenic cells in the epidermis and the structural arrangement of the epidermal proliferative unit (EPU). In: *Stem Cells of Renewing Cell Populations.* (Edited by Cairnie, A. B., Lala, P. K., and Osmond, D. G.), pp. 91–102. Academic Press, New York.

Potten, C. S., and Allen, T. D. 1976. A model implicating the Langerhans cell in keratinocyte proliferation control. *Differentiation* **5**, 43–47.

Prescott, D. M. 1976. *Reproduction of Eukaryotic Cells.* Academic Press, New York.

Robison, G. A., Butcher, R. S., and Sutherland, E. W. 1968. Cyclic AMP. *Annu. Rev. Biochem.* **37**, 149–174.

Rohrbach, R., Elgjo, K., Iversen, O. H., and Sandritter, W. 1972. Effects of methylcholanthrene on epidermal growth regulators. I. Variation in the M-factor. *Beitr. Pathol.* **147**, 21–27.

Rohrbach, R., and Laerum, O. D. 1974. Variations of mitosis-inhibiting chalone activity in epidermis and dermis after carcinogen treatment. *Cell Tissue Kinet.* **7**, 251–257.

Rytömaa, T. 1976. The chalone concept. *Int. Rev. Exp. Pathol.* **16**, 135–206.

Schluger, S., Yuodelis, R. A., and Page, R. C. 1977. *Periodontal Disease. Basic Phenomena, Clinical Management, and Occlusal and Restorative Interrelationships.* Lea and Febiger, Philadelphia.

Sun, T. T., and Green, H. 1977. Cultured epithelial cells of cornea, conjunctiva and skin: Absence of marked intrinsic divergence of their differentiated states. *Nature* **269**, 489–493.

Thornley, A. L. 1976. Chalone regulation of cell proliferation. *S. Afr. J. Med. Sci.* **41**, 239–254.

Thornley, A. L., and Laurence, E. B. 1975. The present state of biochemical research on chalones. *Int. J. Biochem.* **6**, 313–320.

Thornley, A. L., and Laurence, E. B. 1976. The specificity of epidermal chalone action: The results of in vivo experimentation with two purified skin extracts. *Dev. Biol.* **51**, 10-22.

Thornley, A. L., Spargo, D. J., and Laurence, E. B. 1977. A simple method for measuring DNA synthesis in epidermis and sebaceous glands and its application in chalone assays. *Br. J. Dermatol.* **97**, 11–23.

Tutton, P. J. 1973. Control of epithelial cell proliferation in the small intestinal crypt. *Cell Tissue Kinet.* **6**, 211–216.

Tutton, P. J., and Barkla, D. H. 1977. The influence of adrenoreceptor activity on cell proliferation in colonic crypt epithelium and in colonic adenocarcinomata. *Virchows Arch. (Cell Pathol.)* **24**, 139–146.

Uzuka, M., Adachi, K., Iizuka, H., Halprin, K. M., and Levine, V. 1977. Epidermal adenylate cyclase systems: The retention of hormone responsiveness after enzymatic separation of pure epidermis. *J. Invest. Dermatol.* **69**, 194–197.

Voaden, M. J. 1968. A chalone in the rabbit lens? *Exp. Eye Res.* **7**, 326–331.

Voaden, M. J. 1971. The effects of superior cervical ganglionectomy and/or bilateral adrenalectomy on the mitotic activity of the adult rat cornea. *Exp. Eye Res.* **12**, 328–336.

von Sallmann, L., and Grimes, P. 1974. Effects of isoproterenol and cyclic AMP derivatives on cell division in cultured rat lenses. *Invest. Opthalmol.* **13**, 210–218.

Voorhees, J. J., Duell, E. A., and Kelsey, W. H. 1972. Dibutyryl cyclic AMP inhibition of epidermal cell division. *Arch. Dermatol.* **105**, 384–386.

13

Cell Kinetics in Premalignancy

M. W. HILL

Dows Institute for Dental Research, College of Dentistry, University of Iowa, Iowa City, Iowa

A characteristic feature of all lining and covering epithelia is that they maintain their structural integrity by a system of cell renewal in which cells, produced by mitosis in the deepest layers, migrate to the surface from which they are shed. However, in any tissue there is a homeostasis whereby the rate at which new cells are produced is balanced by the rate at which cells die. In malignant lesions, the number of mitotic figures generally appears to be higher than in corresponding normal tissue; in fact it is commonly regarded as one of the features indicative of malignancy (Kramer et al. 1974; Johnson 1977). As cell production in a tumor exceeds cell loss (Iversen 1975), it is probable that the cell kinetics of such lesions are altered as part of the neoplastic process, possibly before any morphological changes are manifested. If this should prove to be the case, we would then have a technique to distinguish between lesions which were truly premalignant and those of a more benign nature.

In order to understand the possible interpretation and significance of cell kinetic data, it is first necessary to review briefly the most common methods by which such data have been obtained.

1. METHODS FOR THE ANALYSIS OF CELL KINETICS

Cell replication is a cyclical process (Fig. 1), and the techniques used to evaluate the rate at which cells pass through this cycle are dependent upon being able to identify cells in either the synthetic or mitotic phase.

Thus, information about the proliferative behavior of tissues can be obtained by a variety of methods, viz.:

1. Counting the numbers of cells in mitosis in biopsy or autopsy specimens.
2. Counting the number of cells which have been arrested in metaphase following the administration of stathmokinetic agents for a known period of time.
3. Determining the number of labeled cells or labeled mitotic figures following the administration of radioactively labeled thymidine.

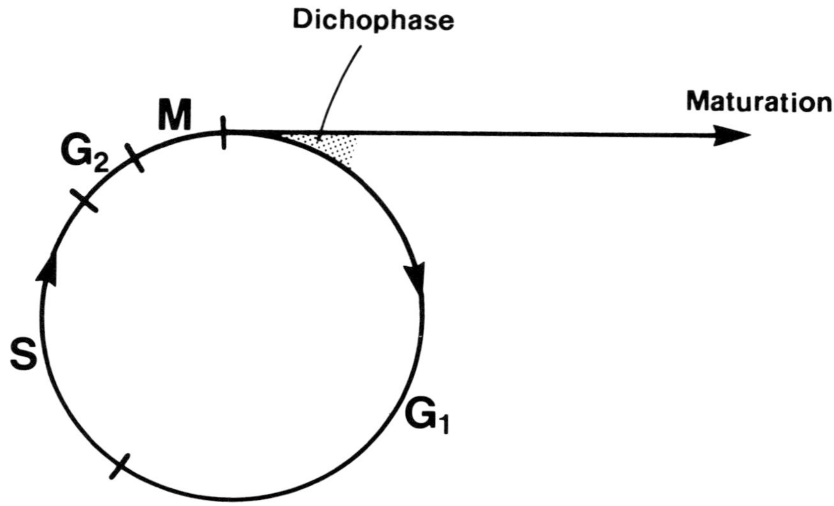

FIGURE 1. The cell cycle in mammalian cells. Cells in the progenitor compartment preparing to divide initially double their DNA content during the synthetic phase (S). After a short resting phase (G_2) cells enter the microscopically visible process of mitosis (M) to produce two daughter cells. When the tissue is in homeostasis one daughter cell on average enters the maturation compartment whilst the other enters the postmitotic presynthetic period (G_1).

4. Microspectrophotometric measurements of Feulgen stained cell suspensions to determine the cell DNA content and thus the distribution of cells in the cell cycle.

The simplest method is to count the number of naturally occurring mitotic figures. Although this method does not interfere with the proliferative process, such as may occur with the use of blocking agents or radioactively labeled substances, it does suffer from several major drawbacks. Unless the tissue has a high mitotic activity there are relatively few mitotic figures visible in sections of untreated tissues, and it can be difficult to recognize accurately cells in all phases of mitosis, especially early metaphase and late telophase. Further, the number of cells observed undergoing division is dependent on the rate at which cells pass through mitosis and, as Giacometti (1967) has noted, it cannot be assumed that mitotic duration remains constant under various conditions. As the penetration of fixative into biopsy specimens takes a measurable period of time, it is possible that mitoses, present in the tissues at the time of excision, may proceed through division before fixation is complete, thus resulting in an underestimate of proliferative activity.

Stathmokinetic (or cytostatic) drugs, such as colchicine or vinblastine, appear to interfere with the development and function of the spindle apparatus and thus arrest dividing cells at metaphase (Cutts 1961). The main advantage of this technique is that a time dimension is introduced; as these agents effectively inhibit cell division during a period of 4 to 6 hours, the number of cells entering mitosis per hour can be determined. The result is a measure of the rate at which cells pass through mitosis and is independent of the duration of the mitotic phase of the cell cycle. However, mitotic arrest agents have certain disadvantages; unless the dose level and duration of action of such drugs used is optimal, the number of dividing cells will be underestimated (Tannock 1967). Another problem is the differential responsiveness of animals and tissues to these agents. In particular, tissues of the Syrian hamster both in vivo and in vitro show a resistance to colchicine (Midgley et al. 1959), and different tissues may require different dosages of the same drug (Tannock 1967).

The administration of thymidine, usually labeled with tritium, and subsequent autoradiography has been widely used to determine the number of cells synthesizing DNA. However, in the same way that simple mitotic counts are influenced by the duration of the mitotic process, the number of labeled cells will depend on the duration of the DNA synthetic period (S-phase or T_S). It is therefore necessary to determine the duration of the S-phase, if the rate of new cell production is to be determined. Estimates of the duration of S-phase can be made either by the percentage labeled mitosis (PLM) method (Quastler and Sherman 1959) or by the use of double labeling techniques (Wimber and Quastler 1963).

The PLM method involves the single injection of radioactively labeled thymidine and sequential sampling to determine the percentage of labeled mitoses at different time intervals. Using this data, a graph can be plotted and the duration of the various phases of the cell cycle can be determined (Fig. 2); Cleaver (1967) suggests that the duration of the S-phase should be determined at the 50% intercept level, but in view of the fact that the duration of each phase of the cell cycle varies from cell to cell Quastler (1963) suggested estimating T_S at the 37% level. This complicates the interpretation of published data as both levels have been used in different studies to determine values for T_S.

The total cell cycle time (T_C) can also be determined from the PLM curve when a second wave of labeled mitoses is present, but it is most commonly determined from the initial labeling index (percentage of labeled cells) using Wright's hypothesis (Wright 1925), which states that the number of cells present at any stage in the cell cycle is proportional to the time spent in that phase. A weakness of this method is the need to know the size of the pool of potentially proliferative cells, i.e., the progenitor compartment, an estimate which cannot be based on any currently available reliable criteria, particularly in lesional tissue where there may be a disordered organization.

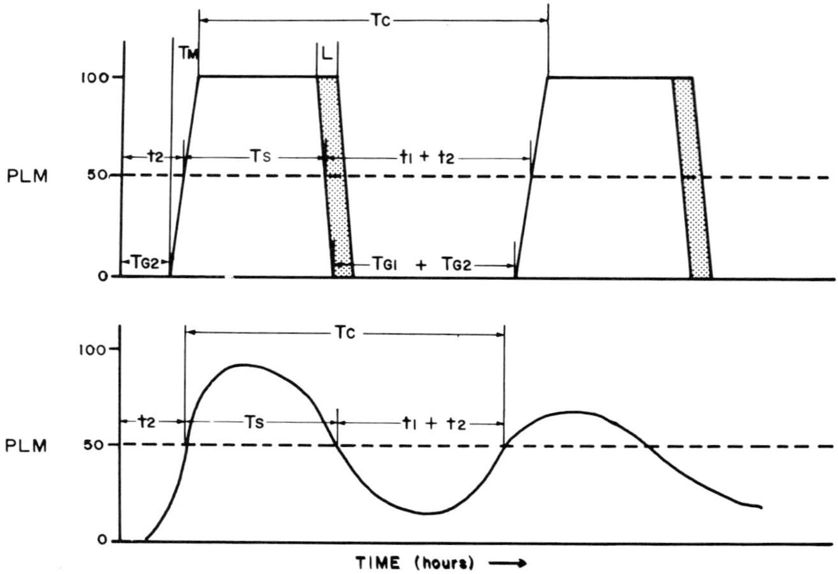

FIGURE 2. Determination of the duration of the phases of the cell cycle from the percentage labeled mitoses (PLM) curve. The *upper diagram* illustrates the ideal case in which each of the phases occupies the same time in all cells. If the period of labeling is significant T_S will be overestimated by the duration of labeling (L) with a consequent underestimate of $t_1 + t_2$. The *lower diagram* illustrates a typical PLM curve. The variations in T_{G2} result in a more gradual increase in labeled mitotic figures than the ideal case and it is not possible to estimate T_M from this curve. Similarly, a variation in T_S within the cell population causes the fall of the curve to be more gradual than the rise. For these reasons the values obtained for the duration of the various phases are by the PLM method median rather than mean. $t_1 = T_{G1} + \frac{1}{2}T_M$; $t_2 = T_{G2} + \frac{1}{2}T_M$.

The double labeling technique in its original form utilizes two separate pulses of thymidine, one labeled with H^3 and the other with C^{14}. Due to their different energies, these isotopes can be distinguished autoradiographically. The method involves administering a pulse of H^3 thymidine followed by a pulse of C^{14} thymidine after a known time interval equal to or less than G_2 (usually one hour). This results in two populations of labeled cells; the first a population of cells which corresponds to cells which were in DNA synthesis during the first pulse but have completed synthesis during the interval between the two pulses, and a second population of cells all of which will be labeled with C^{14} thymidine and some of which will also be labeled with H^3. Assuming no labeled cells have divided, T_S can be obtained by the ratio between the singly labeled H^3 cells and all the cells labeled with C^{14} (Wimber and Quastler 1963).

$$\text{i.e., } T_S = \frac{\text{number of cells labeled with second pulse}}{\text{number of cells labeled with first pulse}} \text{ x time between pulses}$$

More recently a number of papers have appeared using two pulses of tritium labeled thymidine at different dose levels (e.g., Galand and Chretien 1969; Heenen et al. 1973; Chopra and Forbes 1974; Hasegawa et al. 1976), assuming that a greater dose of thymidine will result in heavier labeling comparable with that of C^{14}. Whilst this method works in that two populations of cells can be distinguished (Chopra and Forbes 1974), its validity has not been proven. All the methods utilizing radio-labeled thymidine are subject to the effects that both the radiation and exogenous thymidine may have on the cell cycle (Gibbs and Casarett 1969; Møller et al. 1974). As these effects are probably concentration dependent (Greulich et al. 1961; Feinendegen 1967), caution must be exercised in the comparison of different studies in which thymidine of varying concentration and specific activity have been used.

An additional difficulty in the interpretation of data relating to phases of the cell cycle obtained from labeling studies is the necessity to make certain assumptions concerning the extent of the progenitor population and synchrony of cell division. All cell cycle analyses are based on the tissue being in a state of equilibrium (Cleaver 1967); under these circumstances the progenitor population will form a constant proportion of the total population at all sampling intervals. However, in neoplastic tissues the size of the progenitor compartment relative to the total cell population is likely to vary. This has led to the concept of a "growth fraction" (Mendelsohn 1962), but as Lamerton (1976) has pointed out, this is a term in wide use but the underlying concept of which is far from clear and the methods used in its determination involve an arbitrary decision. Nelson and Schiffer (1973) suggest that the presence of DNA primer-template and DNA dependent DNA-polymerase, which can be identified using an autoradiographic technique, may identify those cells in the replication cycle. This method is not contingent upon cells being in S-phase, but the relationship between the number of such cells and the growth fraction has not been established. However, the majority of workers have used a variety of theoretical mathematical models for cell cycle analysis; unfortunately the models used vary between studies, and frequently between normal and tumor tissues in the same study, making valid comparisons difficult.

The first major problem in applying these techniques to human patients is an ethical one—can we justify administering mitotic blocking agents or radioactively labeled materials to patients experimentally, and subsequently removing single or multiple biopsies? Whilst there have been a number of such studies on terminal cancer patients (e.g., Frindel et al. 1968; Bennington 1969; Averette et al. 1970; Friedman et al. 1973; Bresciani et al. 1974), there are few ethical committees that would approve the use of such methods in cases of presumptive premalignant lesions.

Local injection of isotope, which reduces the total radioactivity administered to the patient, would appear to be a satisfactory alternative (Hell and Hodgson 1966; LaChapelle 1969; LaChapelle and Gillman 1969; Hell and Maibach 1972; Johnson and Hopps 1974), but some workers have found that it causes local tissue damage, and the injection site may be difficult to locate accurately, even when marked (LaChapelle 1969).

These difficulties inevitably have led to the development of in vitro incubation techniques, and while Fabrikant and Wisseman (1968), Alvares et al. (1972), Heenen et al. (1973) and Rubio and Lagerlöf (1974a) have used the technique to study kinetics of human diseased epithelia, their usefulness and reliability have not been clearly established. Using 1 mm slices of skin incubated in vitro, LaChapelle and Gillman (1969) reported labeling to be "regular and widespread throughout the specimens" and to give results quantitatively similar to those obtained following local in vivo administration of tritiated thymidine. Denekamp and Kallman (1973), in a comparative study of in vivo and in vitro labeling of a variety of animal tumors, found the correspondence between individual labeling indices very variable; however, when groups of tumors were compared, there was no statistical difference between the methods. Other workers have reported that following in vitro incubation with tritiated thymidine, labeling of epithelial cell nuclei is restricted to the edges of the specimen (Feit and Staniček 1967; Powell 1967; Fabrikant and Cherry 1969; Alvares et al. 1972; Heenen et al. 1973; Mackenzie and Ettinger 1977). This complication frequently has been eliminated by restricting counts of labeled cells to the outer margins (150–300 μm) of the specimen (Alvares et al. 1972; Heenen et al. 1973). The lack of uniform labeling, frequently attributed to poor thymidine penetration, may be due to insufficient oxygen (Rajewsky 1965; Steel and Bensted 1965), and other workers have attempted to overcome this problem by using increased oxygen tensions during incubation (e.g., Fabrikant 1971). In vitro blocking with stathmokinetic agents has not been widely used but does not appear to be subject to this "edge-effect" (Hill 1978).

Microspectrophotometry estimates of DNA in the nucleus of individual cells combined with tritiated thymidine and autoradiography has been used to study tumor kinetics (e.g., Erbe et al. 1977), and is another possible method for cell cycle analysis of premalignant lesions (see chapter 21). Apart from the fact that it is very time consuming, it has the decided disadvantage in the study of tumors that the results are difficult to evaluate when aneuploidy and polyploidy are present.

There is an extensive literature on the determination of cell cycle parameters in a wide variety of both human and experimental tumors (see Baserga 1965; Gavosto and Pileri 1971; Tubiana an Malaise 1976a), which show extremely diverse patterns of behavior, but there is only limited data on human premalignant lesions. As both skin and the epithelium of the uterine cervix share a number of common morphological features with oral mucosa, it is proposed initially to examine the patterns of kinetic behavior of lesions in these tissues, in an attempt to determine whether there is any common pattern which is specifically related to the induction of malignancy.

2. CELL KINETICS OF NORMAL AND PATHOLOGICAL TISSUES

2:1 EPIDERMIS

Although there have been a number of studies of cell kinetic behavior in tumors of both animal and human skin, the majority of studies have investigated a limited number of parameters and frequently lack comparable controls (Table 1).

In a study of five skin tumors in humans using intravenous tritiated thymidine and sequential sampling of the lesions, Frindel et al. (1968) found a wide range in both the labeling index and the various phases of the cell cycle, but in the absence of any data from uninvolved skin, it is not possible to determine how the kinetic behavior of lesional tissue varies from that of normal tissue. Further, one of the patients examined in this study had been extensively treated with radiotherapy, surgery, and cytotoxic drugs, all of which could have modified the general metabolism as well as the behavior of the malignant tissues.

LaChapelle (1969, 1970), using an in vitro labeling technique, examined the labeling index (LI) of normal skin as well as a range of human skin lesions, and some interesting trends are apparent. In the benign condition, sebborrheic keratosis, there is an increased LI, but in the later study

TABLE 1 Cell Kinetic Parameters for Normal and Diseased Skin

Lesion	*MI*	*LI (%)*	T_c *(h)*	T_S *(h)*	T_{G2} *(h)*	T_M *(h)*	T_{G1} *(h)*	*Reference*
(a) *Human*								
Basal cell carcinoma	0.7	7.0	82.0	19.0	14.0			1
Squamous cell carcinoma	1.4	13.5	36.5	11.5	5.5			
Spindle cell carcinoma	1.4	7.0		21.0				
Normal skin		2.2						2
Normal skin		2.0–5.0						3
Seborrheic keratosis		0.9–8.7						
Solar keratosis		7.1–10.3						
Bowen's lesion		16.3						
Basal cell carcinoma		6.9–18.0						
Squamous cell carcinoma		9.8–15.0						
Seborrheic keratosis								
inflamed		1.6						4
noninflamed		6.7						
Kerato-acanthoma		6.6						
Solar keratosis		7.9						
Bowen's lesion		14.1						
Basal cell carcinoma		10.4						
Squamous cell carcinoma		11.3						
Basal cell carcinoma		9.2	217.0	20.0	7.0	1.5	188.5	5
Normal skin		5.8	184.0	10.3				6
Basal cell carcinoma		9.2	207.0	19.2				
Normal skin		4.5**		7.6			170.0	7
Seborrheic keratosis		1.4**		9.2			630.0	
Fibroepithelial tumor		8.4**		18.4			218.0	
Basal cell syndrome		8.2**		14.3			173.0	

(b) *Animal*						
Normal skin	rabbit	3.8**				8
Viral tumor	rabbit	25.0**	21.2	5.3		
Chemical tumor	rabbit	20.3**				
Normal skin	mouse	6.8		8.2		9
Hyperplastic skin	mouse	10.2		4.5		
Squamous cell carcinoma	mouse	19.0		3.1		

LI=the number of labeled cells as a percentage of all nucleated epithelial cells or ** as the percentage of basal cells.

REFERENCES

1. Frindel et al. (1968).
2. LaChapelle and Gillman (1969).
3. LaChapelle (1969).
4. LaChapelle (1970).
5. Weinstein and Frost (1970).
6. Heenen, Acten and Galand (1973).
7. Heenen et al. (1975).
8. Rashad and Evans (1968).
9. Chopra and Forbes (1974).

(LaChapelle 1970) it was found that in such lesions free of inflammation the LI is similar to that of normal skin; when inflammation was present, it was increased about three-fold, a level comparable with that found in the benign conditions of kerato-acanthoma and solar keratosis. However, lesions of Bowen's disease and both basal cell and squamous cell carcinomas displayed considerably higher labeling indices. Although Weinstein and Frost (1970) do not have any data for unaffected skin, their labeling index of 9.2% for basal cell carcinomas, obtained using a local injection of tritiated thymidine, agrees with the findings of Heenen et al. (1973) who, using an in vitro double labeling technique, found a 60% increase in the LI of basal carcinomas, when compared with normal skin.

The general trend of an increased labeling index in tumors has also been described in experimental lesions induced by viral and chemical agents in rabbits (Rashad and Evans 1968), and by ultraviolet irradiation of mice (Chopra and Forbes 1974).

There is little work on human skin indicating whether the change in labeling index is gradual and progressive, or whether there is a correlation between changes in labeling index and any histologically recognizable alteration in the tissues. However, Heenen et al (1975), in a limited study, have shown that in both the fibroepithelial tumor of Pinkus and epithelial pits in a patient with the basal cell nevus syndrome (both of which can evolve into basal cell carcinoma), the labeling index is higher than in normal epidermis.

As previously discussed, the labeling index alone is of limited value unless we know that the duration of S-phase remains constant. Although the data is far from complete, reference to Fig. 3 shows that the T_S shows little change in the nonmalignant conditions, and probably in squamous cell carcinoma, but is markedly increased in both the premalignant lesions and those of basal cell carcinoma. This would suggest that the higher labeling index in the basal cell carcinoma is largely a reflection of the increased duration of synthesis at the time of labeling, and that it is in squamous cell carcinoma alone that there is a marked increase in the rate at which cells are produced. Incidentally, it is interesting to note that in contrast with the increased duration of T_S observed in human skin lesions, in experimental carcinoma induced by ultraviolet light in animals (Chopra and Forbes 1974) there is a progressive decrease in the duration of T_S.

2:2 UTERINE CERVIX

As in the studies on skin, the available data on cell kinetics in the uterine cervix are mainly derived from labeling studies (Table 2). However, dysplasia and carcinoma in situ of the uterine cervical epithelium have clearly been demonstrated to progress, if left untreated, to squamous cell carcinoma (Chi et al. 1977); this provides a continuum against which changes in cell kinetics can be judged, i.e., early dysplastic changes can be regarded as being truly premalignant. In both experimental animals and humans, the labeling index increases with an increasing degree of dysplasia, a relationship which was originally described by Richart (1963) as being logarithmic. However, whilst this trend appears to hold true in all of the studies cited, it will be seen that the values for normal cervical epithelium vary greatly between different studies, and thus it is impossible to define premalignancy by a specific value of a labeling index. As T_S remains relatively constant, the increased labeling index in cervical epithelium suggests that there is an increased production of cells, an interpretation supported by the increased number of mitotic figures described by Feit and Staniček (1967), Hillemanns et al. (1968), and Hasegawa et al. (1976).

Probably the most significant fact to be derived from these studies is not simply the increased number of labeled cells but their distribution. In the normal cervical epithelium, cells both in DNA synthesis and in mitoses are restricted to the basal layer, but with increasing disturbance they are seen more frequently at higher levels (Richart 1963); Feit and Staniček 1967; Chi et al. 1977), probably indicating an increase in the size of the proliferative pool of cells.

2:3 ORAL MUCOSA

The most complete analysis of changes in cell cycle parameters is available for carcinoma of the hamster cheek pouch induced by topical application of dimethyl benzanthracene (DMBA). Further, the three principal studies, those of Reisken and Mendelsohn (1964), Reisken and Berry (1968), and Thilagaratnam and Main (1972) have not only reported the epithelial cell cycle values for control tissues and the induced carcinomas, but also the values obtained during the phase of hyperplasia which precedes the appearance of the histological features of carcinoma. The different studies show moderately close agreement in the values for different phases of the cell cycle for each of the histological categories (Table 3). It is, however, interesting to note that there is also a close similarity between the hyperplastic response to friction reported by Mackenzie and Miles (1973) and that induced by chemical carcinogens. Indeed, it appears that the increase in mitotic index is greater in the case of friction. As the experimental studies of oral carcinogenesis have been based on the same animal model (i.e., the hamster cheek pouch), the data is pooled in Fig. 3 and a striking trend is apparent; with the development of tumors, there is a marked reduction in all phases of the cell cycle (except G_2), and this is associated with increases in both labeling and mitotic indices.

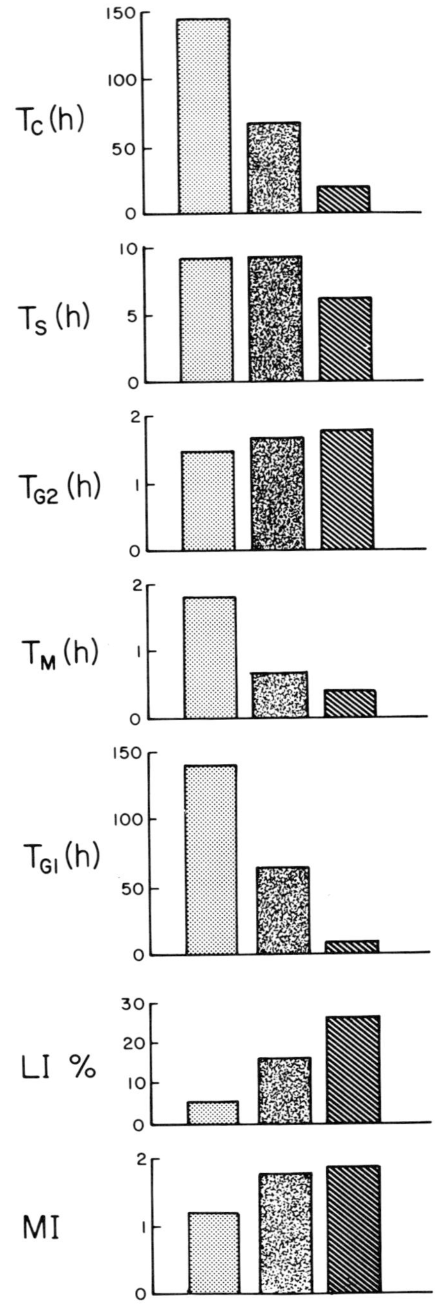

T_C (h)
150
100
50
0
T_S (h)
10
5
0
T_{G2} (h)
2
1
0
T_M (h)
2
1
0
T_{G1} (h)
150
100
50
0
LI %
30
20
10
0
MI
2
1
0

FIGURE 3. Changes in the duration of cell cycle parameters, labeling index and mitotic index in the hamster cheek pouch following topical application of DMBA. There is a marked reduction in T_C, T_S, T_M, and T_{G1} and on increase in T_{G2} as well as the labeling index and mitotic index.

normal control epithelium

squamous cell carcinoma

hyperplastic epithelium

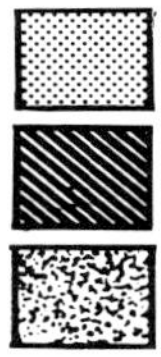

The pooled data have been derived from Brown and Berry (1968); Brown and Oliver (1968); Reisken and Berry (1968); Reisken and Mendelsohn (1964); Thilagaratnam and Main (1972); Toto and Swatske (1973).

Information on the cell kinetics of human leukoplakia and carcinoma of the oral cavity is far less complete (Fig. 5), and it is difficult to extrapolate from one study to another, because of the varying techniques and different indices used. Meyer et al. (1976) reported an increased mitotic index as compared with controls in leukoplakia induced by the use of tobacco products, and in a retrospective study of human biopsy material, El-Labban et al. (1971) found that the mitotic index was a useful discriminator between keratosis, leukoplakia, and lichen planus. Similarly, both Alvares et al. (1972) and MacDonald and Warnakulasuriya (1976) found the labeling index was increased in leukoplakia, which in the study of MacDonald and Warnakulasuriya, was not associated with a change in T_S.

Meyer and Donaldson (1969), Friedman et al. (1973), Bresciani et al. (1973), and Tubiana and Malaise (1976b) all report on various cell cycle parameters of oral tumors, but it is difficult to evaluate the significance of their findings, as comparable control values of normal oral mucosa are not available. Although there is an increased labeling or mitotic index in human oral leukoplakia comparable with that described in premalignant lesions of the skin and uterine cervical epithelium, the statement that "all precancerous changes in human pathology are distinguished by an increased proliferative activity in comparison with the tissue of origin" (Oehlert 1973) should not be taken to imply that it is a feature which discriminates between neoplastic and nonneoplastic tissues. Increased cell proliferation also occurs in regeneration (Bertalanffy 1969), wound healing (Winter 1972), hyperplasia (Mackenzie and Miles 1973), and in association with inflammation (Marwah et al. 1960; LaChapelle 1970; Hopps and Johnson 1974) and thus cannot be regarded as a tumor-specific feature. Indeed, inflammation associated with presumptive premalignant lesions and established neoplasms may itself drastically alter the behavior of the tissue.

TABLE 2 Cell Kinetic Parameters for Normal and Diseased Uterine Cervical Epithelium

Lesion	*MI*	*LI (%)*	T_c *(h)*	T_s *(h)*	T_{G2} *(h)*	T_M *(h)*	T_{G1} *(h)*	*Reference*
(a) *Human*								
Normal epithelium		4.6						10
Minimal dysplasia		5.6						
Mild dysplasia		10.3						
Moderate dysplasia		15.2						
Severe dysplasia		20.3						
Carcinoma in situ		46.5						
Normal epithelium		6.4						11
"Abnormal" epithelium		11.2						
Atypical epithelium		15.9						
Preinvasive carcinoma		23.2						
Normal epithelium	0.48							12
Carcinoma in situ	2.17							
Squamous cell carcinoma	2.2							
Squamous cell carcinoma	3.2	33.0	14.9	11.2	1.9	1.2	1.3	13
Normal cervical epithelium		8.2**	789.0	9.0	5.4	0.17		14
Normal epithelium		7.0						15
Slight dysplasia		11.0						
Moderate dysplasia		17.0						
Severe dysplasia		21.0						
Carcinoma in situ		26.0						
Carcinoma in situ with buds		35.0						

Normal epithelium		14.3	63.0	9.0	5.4	0.17	48.0	16
Squamous cell carcinoma		21.2	44.0	9.4	6.4	0.4	28.0	
Squamous cell carcinoma (invasive)		27.2	33.0	8.0	4.2	0.5	15.0	
(b) *Animal* (mouse)								
Normal		14.0						17
Grade I atypia		26.0						
Grade II atypia		38.0						
Grade III atypia		37.0						
Normal epithelium	1.2ø	10.5		5.4	4.6		22.8	18
Anaplastic epithelium	2.4ø	26.1		8.7	1.9		23.0	
Squamous cell carcinoma (early)	3.6ø	42.9		9.0				
Squamous cell carcinoma (invasive)	3.4ø	54.2		11.7	2.3		26.1	

LI=number of labeled cells as a percentage of all nucleated cells or ** as a percentage of basal cells.
MI=number of mitotic figures as a percentage of all nucleated cells.
ø=mitotic index not defined.

REFERENCES
10. Richart (1963).
11. Feit and Staniček (1967).
12. Hillemanns et al. (1968).
13. Bennington (1969).
14. Averette et al. (1970).
15. Rubio and Lagerlöf (1974a).
16. Averette et al. (1976).
17. Rubio and Lagerlöf (1974b).
18. Hasegawa et al. (1976).

TABLE 3 Cell Kinetic Parameters for Normal and Diseased Oral Epithelium

Lesion	*MI*	*LI (%)*	T_c *(h)*	T_s *(h)*	T_{G2} *(h)*	T_M *(h)*	T_{G1} *(h)*	*Reference*
(a) *Human*								
Normal epithelium	0.7*							19
Leukoplakia	1.2*							
Squamous cell carcinoma				4.6–39.0		0.28–1.53		20
Normal epithelium		3.5						21
Leukoplakia		4.4						
Lichen planus	1.0*							22
Keratosis	1.4*							
Leukoplakia	1.9*							
Squamous cell carcinoma			63–71	26.0				23
Normal epithelium		3.4**		6.0				24
Leukoplakia		6.0**		6.0				
Squamous cell carcinoma		19.8	65.0	23.4	17.2			25
Squamous cell carcinoma				18.0 (median value)	6.0 (median value)			26
Normal buccal mucosa		6.62						27
Leukoplakic buccal mucosa		5.53						
(b) *Hamster*								
Normal cheek pouch epithelium	0.85	4.8	140.0	8.6	1.4	0.8–1.2		28
Normal cheek pouch epithelium		4.4	135.0	8.6				29

Normal epithelium	1.7	7.2	142.0	10.2	1.6	2.6	128.0	30
Hyperplastic epithelium	1.5	24.6	42.0			0.5		
Squamous cell carcinoma	2.0	29.5	21.0	6.1	2.3	0.4	11.9	
Normal epithelium	1.1	6.0	155.0	9.3	1.1	2.2	142.4	31
Hyperplastic epithelium	1.8	15.7	61.1	10.4	1.6	0.1	47.4	
Squamous cell carcinoma	1.6	24.9	21.9	6.5	2.0	0.06	6.5	
Normal epithelium	1.1	6.1	163.9	10.0	1.9	1.8	150.0	32
Hyperplastic epithelium	2.0	11.0	90.8	8.3		1.6	80.9	
Preneoplastic epithelium			22.7	8.2	1.8	0.9	11.9	
Squamous cell carcinoma	2.0	21.7	15.4	6.2	1.4	0.7	7.1	
Normal epithelium		10.6						33
Preneoplastic epithelium		32.9						
Normal epithelium	3+*	7.5*		11.7				34
Hyperplastic epithelium (friction induced)	13+*	12.5*		12.8				

LI = labeling index = number of labeled cells as percentage of basal cells or ** as percentage of all nucleated cells.
* Calculated by the present author as the number of naturally occurring mitotic figures (or labeled cells)/100 basal cells from data in the original reference.
+ Per 4 hour after the administration of vinblastine.

REFERENCES

19. Meyer et al. (1967).
20. Meyer and Donaldson (1969).
21. Alvares et al. (1972).
22. El-Labban et al. (1971).
23. Friedman et al. (1973).
24. MacDonald and Warnakulasuriya (1973).
25. Bresciani et al. (1973).
26. Tubiana and Malaise (1976b).
27. Maidhof et al. (1977).
28. Brown and Berry (1968).
29. Brown and Oliver (1968).
30. Reisken and Mendelsohn (1964).
31. Reisken and Berry (1968).
32. Thilagaratnam and Main (1972).
33. Toto and Swatske (1973).
34. Mackenzie and Miles (1973).

It must therefore be concluded that a knowledge of cell cycle changes is of limited diagnostic and prognostic use. However, an understanding of cell cycle changes and their control may nevertheless provide one of the keys to understanding the process of carcinogenesis. As mentioned at the beginning of this chapter, the maintenance of a cell population is dependent upon an equilibrium between the rate of birth of new cells and their lifespan (or rate of death). Cell proliferation has been a natural candidate for investigation, because the increased number of mitotic figures in tumors can readily be observed. However, it might also be argued that it is a failure of the tumor cells to enter the maturation pathway at a rate proportional to mitosis which is the primary defect, thus increasing the relative number of cells capable of further division. Such a defect would be most likely to occur at that point of the cell cycle at which the daughter cells of mitosis have to "make the decision" as to whether to leave the cell cycle, i.e., at dichophase; therefore, perhaps future kinetic studies should be directed towards understanding the dichophase switch and the mechanisms controlling the rate of epithelial maturation.

REFERENCES

Alvares, O., Skougaard, M. R., Pindborg, J. J., and Roed-Petersen, B. 1972. In vitro incorporation of tritiated thymidine in oral homogeneous leukoplakias. *Scand. J. Dent. Res.* **80**, 510–514.

Averette, H. E., Weinstein, G. D., Ford, J. H., Girtanner, R. E., Hoskins, W. J., and Ramos, R. 1976. Cell kinetics and programmed chemotherapy for gynecologic cancer. I. Squamous-cell carcinoma. *Am. J. Obstet. Gynecol.* **124**, 912–923.

Averette, H. E., Weinstein, G. D., and Frost, R. 1970. Autoradiographic analysis of cell proliferation kinetics in human genital tissues. I. Normal cervix and vagina. *Am. J. Obstet. and Gynecol.* **108**, 8–17.

Baserga, R. 1965. The relationship of the cell cycle to tumor growth and control of cell division: A review. *Cancer Res.* **25**, 581–595.

Bennington, J. L. 1969. Cellular kinetics of invasive squamous carcinoma of the human cervix. *Cancer Res.* **29**, 1082–1088.

Bertalanffy, F. D. 1969. Comparison between the rates of proliferation of induced malignancies and their normal tissues of origin. In: *Recent Results in Cancer Research, Vol. 17. Normal and Malignant Cell Growth.* (Edited by Fry, R. J., Griem, M. L., and Kirsten, W. H.), pp. 136–146. Springer-Verlag, Berlin.

Bresciani, F., Paoluzi, R., Benassi, M., Nervi, C., Cosale, C., and Ziparo, E. 1974. Cell kinetics and growth of squamous cell carcinomas in man. *Cancer Res.* **34**, 2405–2415.

Brown, J. M., and Berry, R. J. 1968. The relationship between diurnal variation of the number of cells in mitosis and of the number of cells synthesizing DNA in the epithelium of the hamster cheek pouch. *Cell Tiss. Kinet.* **1**, 23–33.

Brown, J. M., and Oliver, R. 1968. A new method of estimating the cell cycle time in epithelial tissues of long generation time. *Cell Tiss. Kinet.* **1**, 11–21.

Chi, C. H., Rubio, C. A., and Lagerlöf, B. 1977. The frequency and distribution of mitotic figures in dysplasia and carcinoma in situ. *Cancer* **39**, 1218–1223.

Chopra, D. P., and Forbes, P. D. 1974. Analysis of cell kinetics during ultraviolet light-induced epidermal carcinogenesis in hairless mice. *Cancer Res.* **34**, 454–457.

Cleaver, J. E. 1967. *Thymidine Metabolism and Cell Kinetics*, p. 115. Elsevier/North Holland, Amsterdam.

Cutts, J. H. 1961. The effect of vincaleukoblastine on dividing cells in vivo. *Cancer Res.* **21**, 168–172.

Denekamp, J., and Kallman, R. F. 1973. In vitro and in vivo labelling of animal tumours with tritiated thymidine. *Cell Tiss. Kinet.* **6**, 217–227.

El-Labban, N., Lucas, R. B., and Kramer, I. R. H. 1971. The mitotic values for the epithelium in oral keratoses and lichen planus. *Br. J. Cancer* **25**, 411–416.

Erbe, W., Linden, W. A., Reddy, S. B., Zywoetz, F., and Baisch, H. 1977. Studies on the population kinetics of the Walker carcinoma by autoradiography and pulse cytophometry. *Cell Tiss. Kinet.* **10**, 269–277.

Fabrikant, J. I. 1971. The kinetics of cellular proliferation in normal and malignant tissues: A review of methodology and the analysis of cell population kinetics in human tissues. *Am. J. Roentgenol. Rad. Therp. Nucl. Med.* **111**, 700–711.

Fabrikant, J. I., and Cherry, J. 1969. The kinetics of cellular proliferation in normal and malignant tissues. III. Cell proliferation in the larynx. *Ann. Otol. Rhinol. Laryngol.* **78**, 326–341.

Fabrikant, J. I., and Wisseman, C. L. 1968. In vitro incorporation of tritiated thymidine in normal and neoplastic tissue. *Radiology* **90**, 361–363.

Feinendegen, L. E. 1967. *Tritium Labeled Molecules in Biology and Medicine*, pp. 250–255. Academic Press, New York.

Feit, J., and Staniček, J. 1967) Histoautoradiographical investigation of DNA synthesis in precancerous states and carcinomas of the uterine cervix in bioptical material. *Neoplasma* **14**, 499–505.

Friedman, M., Nervi, C., Casale, C., Starace, G., Arcangeli, G., Page, G., and Ziparo, E. 1973. Significance of growth rates, cell kinetics, and histology in the irradiation and chemotherapy of the squamous cell carcinoma of the mouth. *Cancer* **31**, 10–16.

Frindel, E., Malaise, E., and Tubiana, M. 1968. Cell proliferation kinetics in five human solid tumors. *Cancer* **22**, 611–620.

Galand, P., and Chretien, J. 1969. Is double-labeling with two levels of ^{3}H-thymidine a reliable method for evaluating mitotic parameters? *J. Nucl. Biol. Med.* **13**, 87–93.

Gavosto, F., and Pileri, A. 1971. Cell cycle of cancer cells in man. In: *The Cell Cycle and Cancer.* (Edited by Baserga, R.), pp. 99–128. Marcel Dekker, New York.

Giacometti, L. 1967. Healing of skin wounds in primates. 1. The kinetics of cell proliferation. *J. Invest. Dermatol.* **48**, 133–137.

Gibbs, S. J., and Casarett, G. W. 1969. Influences of a circadian rhythm and mitotic delay from tritiated thymidine on cytokinetic studies in hamster cheek pouch epithelium. *Radiat. Res.* **40**, 588–600.

Greulich, R. C., Cameron, I. L., and Thrasher, J. D. 1961. Stimulation of mitosis in adult mice by administration of thymidine. *Proc. Natl. Acad. Sci. USA.* **47**, 743–748.

Hasegawa, K., Matsuura, Y., and Tojo, S. 1976. Cellular kinetics and histological changes in experimental cancer of the uterine cervix. *Cancer Res.* **36**, 359–364.

Heenen, M., Achten, G., and Galand, P. 1973. Autoradiographic analysis of cell kinetics in human normal epidermis and basal cell carcinoma. *Cancer Res.* **33**, 123–127.

Heenen, M., Lambert, J. C., Achten, G., and Galand, P. 1975. Kinetics of cell proliferation in benign and premalignant tumors of the human epidermis. *J. Natl. Cancer Inst.* **54**, 825–827.

Hell, E., and Hodgson, C. 1966. The uptake of ^{3}H-thymidine by epidermal cells in normal and psoriatic subjects. *Br. J. Dermatol.* **78**, 262–268.

Hell, E., and Maibach, H. 1972. A comparison of in vivo and in vitro methods of identifying human epidermal cells in DNA synthesis. *Br. J. Dermatol.* **86**, 506–507.

Hill, M. W. 1978. Epithelial cell kinetics of rat palatal mucosa in organ culture. *Arch. Oral Biol.* **23**, 941–948.

Hillemanns, H. G., Fröhlich, D., and Prestel, E. 1968. Zellzahl und Mitosefrequenz bei entstehung des Cervix-carcinoms (zum Carcinoma in situ und Mikrocarcinom der Cervix). *Arch. Gynaek.* **206**, 292–319.

Hopps, R. M., and Johnson, N. W. 1974. Relationship between histological degree of inflammation and epithelial proliferation in macaque gingiva. *J. Periodont. Res.* **9**, 273–283.

Iversen, O. H. 1975. Kinetic characterization of malignant tumours. In: *International Symposium on the Biological Characterization of Human Tumours, 6th, Copenhagen, 1975. Biological Characterization of Human Tumours.* Advances in Tumour Prevention, Detection and Characterization, Vol. 3. (Edited by Davis, W., and Maltoni, C.), pp. 173–184. Excerpta Medica, Amsterdam.

Johnson, N. W. 1977. Histological and histochemical studies of oral cancer. *Int. Dent. J.* **27**, 25–34.

Johnson, N. W., and Hopps, R. M. 1974. Epithelial cell proliferation in gingiva of macaque monkeys studies by local injections of (^{3}H)thymidine. *Arch. Oral Biol.* **19**, 265–268.

Kramer, I. R. H., El-Labban, N. G., and Sonkodi, S. 1974. Further studies on lesions of the oral mucosa using computer-aided analyses of histological features. *Br. J. Cancer* **29**, 223–231.

LaChapelle, J. M. 1969. Isotopic labelling of cutaneous structures. A preliminary comparison of local in vivo and in vitro techniques applied to healthy and pathological human skin. *Br. J. Dermatol.* **81**, 299–305.

LaChapelle, J. M. 1970. Etude radioautographique de l' incorporation in vitro de thymidine tritiée dans la peau humaine normale et dans certaines proliferations epidermiques. *Pathol. Eur.* Suppl. 1, 1–197.

LaChapelle, J. M., and Gillman, T. 1969. Tritiated thymidine labelling of normal human epidermal cell nuclei. A comparison in the same subjects of in vivo and in vitro techniques. *Br. J. Dermatol.* **81**, 603–616.

Lamerton, L. F. 1976. Cell population kinetics in normal and malignant tissues. In: *Scientific Foundations of Oncology*. (Edited by Symington, T., and Carter, R. L.), Chap. 15, pp. 119–125. William Heinemann, London.

MacDonald, D. G., and Warnakulasuriya, K. A. A. S. 1976. Epithelial cell kinetics in leukoplakia. Abstract. *J. Dent. Res.* **55**, Special Issue D, 110.

Mackenzie, I. C., and Ettinger, R. L. 1977. Evaluation of in vitro cell labeling of mouse epithelia with tritiated thymidine. *Arch. Oral Biol.* **22**, 133–137.

Mackenzie, I. C., and Miles, A. E. 1973. The effect of chronic frictional stimulation on hamster cheek pouch epithelium. *Arch. Oral. Biol.* **18**, 1341–1349.

Maidhof, R., Hornstein, O. P., Schell, H., Rosenberger, H., and Prantl, F. 1977. Vergleichende histologische und histoautoradiographische Untersuchungen an benignen oralen Leukoplakien. *Arch. Dermatol. Res.* **259**, 71–82.

Marwah, A. S., Weinmann, J. P., and Meyer, J. 1960. The effect of chronic inflammation on the epithelial turnover of the human gingiva. *Arch. Pathol.* **69**, 147–153.

Mendelsohn, M. L. 1962. Autoradiographic analysis of cell proliferation in spontaneous breast cancer of the C3H mouse. III. The growth fraction. *J. Natl. Cancer Inst.* **28,** 1015–1029.

Meyer, J., Daftary, D. K., and Pindborg, J. J. 1967. Studies in oral leukoplakias. XI. Histopathology of leukoplakias in Indians chewing "pan" with tobacco. *Acta Odont. Scand.* **25**, 397–435.

Meyer, J. S., and Donaldson, R. C. 1969. Growth kinetics of squamous cell carcinoma in man. A study of four squamous cell carcinomas using stathmokinetic effect of vinblastine in vivo. *Arch Path.* **87**, 479–490.

Midgley, A. R., Pierce, B., and Dixon, F. J. 1959. Nature of colchicine resistance in golden hamster. *Science* **130**, 40–41.

Møller, U., Larsen, J. K., and Faber, M. 1974. The influence of injected tritiated thymidine on the mitotic circadian rhythm in the epithelium of the hamster cheek pouch. *Cell Tiss. Kinet.* **7**, 231–240.

Nelson, J. S. R., and Schiffer, L. M. 1973. Autoradiographic detection of DNA polymerase containing nuclei in sarcoma 180 ascites cells. *Cell Tiss. Kinet.* **6**, 45–54.

Oehlert, W. 1973. Cellular proliferation in carcinogenesis. *Cell Tiss. Kinet.* **6**, 325–335.

Powell, R. N. 1967. Gingival tissue physiology in vitro. I. Gingival organ cultures. *J. Periodont. Res.* **2**, 290–296.

Quastler, H. 1963. The analysis of cell population kinetics. In: *Cell Proliferation.* (Edited by Lamerton, L. F., and Fry, R. J.), pp. 18–36. F. A. Davis, Philadelphia.

Quastler, H., and Sherman, F. G. 1959. Cell population kinetics in the intestinal epithelium of the mouse. *Exp. Cell Res.* **17**, 420–438.

Rajewsky, M. F. 1965. In vitro studies of cell proliferation in tumours. II. Characteristics of a standardised in vitro system for the measurement of ^{3}H-thymidine incorporation into tissue explants. *Eur. J. Cancer* **1**, 281–287.

Rashad, A. L., and Evans, C. A. 1968. Radioautographic study of epidermal cell proliferation and migration in normal and neoplastic tissues of rabbits. *J. Natl. Cancer Inst.* **41**, 845–853.

Reiskin, A. B., and Berry, R. J. 1968. Cell proliferation and carcinogenesis in the hamster cheek pouch. *Cancer Res.* **28**, 898–905.

Reisken, A. B., and Mendelsohn, M. L. 1964. A comparison of the cell cycle in induced carcinomas and their normal counterpart. *Cancer Res.* **24**, 1131–1136.

Richart, R. M. 1963. A radioautographic analysis of cellular proliferation in dysplasia and carcinoma in situ of the uterine cervix. *Am. J. Obstet. Gynecol.* **86**, 925–930.

Rubio, C. A., and Lagerlöf, B. 1974a. Autoradiographic studies of dysplasia and carcinoma in situ in cervical cones. *Acta Pathol. Microbiol. Scand.* **82**, 411–418.

Rubio, C. A., and Lagerlöf, B. 1974b. Autoradiographic studies of experimentally induced atypias in the cervical epithelium of mice. *Acta Pathol. Microbiol. Scand.* **82**, 475–482.

Steel, G. G., and Bensted, J. P. 1965. In vitro studies of cell proliferation in tumours. I. Critical appraisal of methods and theoretical considerations. *Eur. J. Cancer* **1**, 275–279.

Tannock, I. F. 1967. A comparison of the relative efficiencies of various metaphase arrest agents. *Exp. Cell Res.* **47**, 345–356.

Thilagaratnam, C. N., and Main, J. H. 1972. Changes in cell cycle characteristics in hamster cheek pouch epithelium during treatment with D.M.B.A. *J. Oral Pathol.* **1**, 89–102.

Toto, P. D., and Swatske, C. 1973. Premalignant DNA synthesis in hamster pouch. *Oral Surg.* **36**, 393–396.

Tubiana, M., and Malaise, E. P. 1976a. Growth rate and cell kinetics in human tumours: Some diagnostic and therapeutic implications. In: *Scientific Foundations of Oncology.* (Edited by Symington, T. and Carter, R. L.), Chap. 16, pp. 126–136. William Heinemann, London.

Tubiana, M., and Malaise, E. 1976b. Comparison of cell proliferation kinetics in human and experimental tumors: Response to irradiation. *Cancer Treat. Rep.* **60**, 1887–1895.

Weinstein, G. D., and Frost, P. 1970. Cell proliferation in human basal cell carcinoma. *Cancer Res.* **30**, 724–728.

Wimber, D. E., and Quastler, H. A. 1963. A ^{14}C and ^{3}H-thymidine double labeling technique in the study of cell proliferation in Tradescantia root tips. *Exp. Cell Res.* **30**, 8–22.

Winter, G. D. 1972. Epidermal regeneration studies in the domestic pig. In: *Epidermal Wound Healing.* (Edited by Maibach, H. I., and Rovee, D. T.), Chap. 4, pp. 71–112. Year Book Medical Publications, Chicago.

Wright, G. P. 1925. The relative duration of the various phases of mitosis in chick fibroblasts cultivated in vitro. *J. Roy. Micr. Soc.* 414–417.

Discussion

Professor Smith asked Dr. Squier if there is any work which correlates the findings of physiological studies of permeability with morphological studies of permeability using tracers. Dr. Squier replied that physiologists have been mainly interested in movement of small particles such as ions whereas morphological studies tend to use larger molecules. The morphological approach most closely approximates the physiological when tracers such as lanthanum, which may be ionic at certain concentrations, are used. He felt that a more serious problem is the present lack of knowledge about permeability pathways of the lipid-soluble substances. Tracers such as horseradish peroxidase, ferritin, and lanthanum are all water soluble, and so diffuse in the aqueous phase and appear to pass across epithelia by an intercellular pathway. Croton oil and many carcinogens are, on the other hand, primarily lipid-soluble. Such substances may move in the membrane phase, but at present only bulk measurements of movement are possible and no method for tracing their pathways of penetration has been developed. This is a pity as it rules out studies specifically designed to prevent absorption.

Professor Kramer remarked on the high figure given by Landay and Schroeder's (1977) work for the relative volume occupied by tonofilaments in nonkeratinized oral mucosal cells. He asked whether the method of measurement adequately allowed for the interspace between the rather diffusely arranged small filaments of this tissue. Dr. Squier replied that the high magnification of the electron micrographs used in such studies would allow adequate resolution of the individual filaments. However, even if there were a considerable error, say as high as 25%, the findings were still quite remarkable.

Dr. Mashberg commented that about 96% of the lesions he had observed in the mouth occurred in three areas: the floor of the mouth, the ventral tongue, and the soft palate. He suggested that this distribution might relate to some common feature of epithelial structure. Dr. Squier added that the common features of these areas are nonkeratinization and a relatively thin epithelium. This might make them more permeable. Tracer experiments have demonstrated a permeability barrier in nonkeratinized epithelium, but the barrier appears to be rather frail and more susceptible to damage than that of a keratinizing epithelium. The epithelium of the cheek, which was also nonkeratinized, is considerably thicker than the epithelia of the regions referred to by Dr. Mashberg. Dr. Pindborg commented that the greater permeability of the mucosa of the floor of the mouth has been empirically known for many years and is a site recommended for rapid absorption for medicaments and, in India, is also the preferred site for absorption of chewing tobacco.

Dr. Van Scott asked whether the hydration of the oral mucosa affected permeability and whether cyclical changes of the oral mucosa occurred in women, similar to those observed in the vaginal epithelium. Dr. Squier pointed out that hydration of the skin by occlusive dressings increases its permeability: so the normal hydration of many regions of the oral mucosa may have a similar effect. Evidence for oral mucosal changes associated with the menstrual cycle is controversial and has been obtained primarily from studies using exfoliative cytology. However atrophic changes associated with hormonal imbalances in postmenopausal women are not uncommon.

Dr. Wilbanks asked Dr. Squier to comment on what he meant by squamous metaplasia. Dr. Squier answered that he meant, in this context, a change from a normally nonkeratinized epithelium to a keratinizing one. This implied more than just a change in the superficial strata, for Schroeder's ultrastructural studies have shown that differences between the cells of normal keratinized and nonkeratinized epithelia are apparent at all levels within the epithelium (Landay and Schroeder 1977). Electron microscopic studies of leukoplakias arising in normally nonkeratinizing regions show cellular features similar to those in keratinized epithelium in all strata including the basal cells (Klein-Szanto et al. 1976). A change in differentiation is therefore apparent throughout the tissue. Dr. Van Scott asked whether areas containing taste buds, where permeation is apparently instantaneous, form important sites for penetration of carcinogens. Dr. Binnie replied that it is interesting that the junction between the anterior two thirds and the posterior third of the tongue, where there are many taste buds, also formed a relatively common site for carcinoma.

Dr. Mackenzie asked Dr. Slavkin how he thought mechanisms of embryonic induction during embryogenesis were related to mechanisms maintaining normal adult epithelial structure and functions. Dr. Slavkin answered that these mechanisms should operate in both prenatal and postnatal periods; each stage of induction is apparently a single event and restricts the expression of the genome of the induced cells. In the usual sense of the term, a particular inductive step happens only once. For example, the phenotype of the oral mucosal cells is established at a certain time in development. Dr. Mackenzie commented that although the initial structure of the oral mucosa might be established at a given point in time, there appears to be considerable evidence from recombination experiments that a continuous and regionally-specific influence of the subepithelial connective tissue is necessary to maintain regional variation in epithelial structure during adult life (Billingham and Silvers 1963). He asked whether Dr. Slavkin would consider the nature of this continuous "message" or modulating influence to be similar to the type of the message transmitted upon induction. Dr. Slavkin replied that, as no inducer has been identified in a eukaryotic system, no concept based on reliable data could as yet be established. It could be that epithelial modulation acts at the level of reorganization of intracellular components rather than at the level of inducing new gene products.

Professor Pindborg illustrated a number of altered histological features of the connective tissue of human tissues showing actinic elastosis and submucous fibrosis. These conditions, which are considered likely to have a higher rate of malignant transformation than normal mucosa, are associated with epithelial atrophy. He wondered whether this epithelial atrophy might make the tissue more susceptible to the action of carcinogens and asked whether Dr. Smith thought the atrophy was the result of connective tissue changes leading to some failure of nutrition of the overlying epithelium. Dr. Smith replied that he imagined that the connective tissue might not be able to support the normal function of the epithelium. Dr. Mackenzie commented that the growth of epithelium appears to be stimulated by certain types of subepithelial connective tissue. Further, there is most probably a continuous specific modulating influence exerted by the connective tissue on the overlying epithelium. These effects probably arise from a certain type of cell, putatively a fibroblastic type of cell, which might be lost as a result of connective tissue damage. The epithelial changes observed could therefore be considered as perhaps a result of loss of the specific influence of connective tissue cells rather than an unfavorable nutritive environment. Dr. Smith remarked that, apart from studies of inflammatory cells, examination of changes in the cellular component of the connective tissue during carcinogenesis does not seem to have been done. Dr. Slavkin pointed out that the extensive fibrous connective tissue in the conditions Dr. Pindborg illustrated might arise as a result of decreased collagen breakdown rather than increased synthesis. He also added that epithelium is an avascular tissue and that there is a possibility of the existence of an angiogenic factor derived from epithelium similar to that obtained from cartilage, and that this is an aspect of the interaction between epithelium and connective tissue which is of particular relevance to carcinogenesis. Although not much work has been done on premalignant tissues, the possibility of identifying changing patterns of localization of such substances by immunofluorescent methods at the stage of early invasion might be a useful diagnostic tool.

Dr. Smith said that if diffusible factors from the epithelium and connective tissue have an important influence on epithelial mitotic rate, changes in the pattern of cell proliferation might be expected in a normal epithelium lying in close proximity to a malignant one which had invaded from a deeper surface. He had not observed such changes and asked whether there were any recorded observations concerning the behavior of normal epithelia lying in close proximity to malignancy. Dr. Solt referred to work by Argyris and Argyris (1962) which suggested a change in epidermis overlying experimentally implanted Ehrlich ascites tumors in mice. Dr. Mackenzie indicated that this work had demonstrated an increased mitotic rate in the normal epidermis, the opposite of what might be expected if chalones were escaping from the tumor, and that this stimulation is also seen in some nonepidermal tissues. Dr. Laurence referred to work which has shown that epidermal tumors in mice lead to a greatly reduced mitotic rate in the normal epidermis, although in this case it is difficult to clearly distinguish a chalone effect from a stress effect (Kariniemi and Rytömaa 1976).

Dr. Slavkin asked Dr. Laurence about the mechanism of action of chalones and whether there is any known similarity between the binding of chalone to epithelial cells and, for example, the binding of mitogens to lymphocytes. Dr. Laurence replied that, from preliminary work examining mitogens such as concanavalin, it does not appear that such agents affect the epidermis. However, the action of G_2 chalone is potentiated by adrenalin and hydrocortisone and appears to be associated with surface β receptors and mediated by cyclic AMP, thus they do seem to act at the cell surface. There appear to be two types of hyperplasia, one possibly resulting from modification of surface receptor sites, the other associated with greater cell membrane changes and perhaps leakage of chalone. For example, the hyperplastic epithelial tissue which results from gentle massage maintains its responsiveness to chalones, but hyperplasias associated with wounding or sellotape stripping are not responsive to chalones (Bertsch et al. 1976; Bullough 1969). Tumors are apparently responsive to chalones and the potentiation effect of adrenalin and therefore behave more like a friction or massage hyperplasia than a wound.

Dr. Mackenzie raised the point that biopsies of both normal and pathological human tissues are usually taken under conditions which, for the patient, are highly stressful and questioned how much influence stress prior to, and during, the surgical procedure might have on kinetic measurements made on the excised tissues. In response to a question from Dr. Van Scott, Dr. Laurence said that differentiating cells apparently have the ability to reenter the mitotic cycle upon stimulation. Some evidence of this was found in the observation that all of the basal layer of mouse ear epidermis, which normally contains some differentiating cells, could be found in the proliferative cycle two days after stimulation.

Dr. Mackenzie offered an alternative explanation for this observation, namely that such stimuli cause a more rapid loss of early differentiating cells from the basal layer and their replacement by newly formed cells which have not entered the differentiation phase. Dr. Slavkin asked about the connective tissue influence on epithelial mitotic activity, and asked Dr. Laurence why the concept of antichalones had been introduced. Dr. Laurence suggested that since the same chalone appeared to act on all regions of the epidermis, a connective tissue factor, termed antichalone, is apparently necessary to account for the observed differences in rates of mitosis, transit times, and thickness of the epidermis from region to region.

Dr. Slavkin referred to the work of William Rutter's group (Pictet et al. 1975) which has isolated and characterized a mesenchymal factor, a glycoprotein, which acts as a powerful mitogen for pancreatic epithelium and also amplifies amylase synthesis. Dr. Slavkin asked Dr. Laurence whether chalone has been localized topographically: is it normally found within the cell cytoplasm or localized on the cell membrane? Dr. Laurence replied that Elgjo's group (1973) had localized the sources of G_2 chalone to the basal, and of G_1 chalone to the suprabasal, levels of the epidermis, but commented that there is little information about the sites of chalone within the normal cell. It appears that granulocyte chalone could be extracted in higher concentrations from normal granulocytes than from the serum in which they are maintained, but that malignant granulocytes apparently leak large quantities of chalone into the serum (see Rytömaa 1976).

Dr. Smith commented that the rate of the type of epithelial cell death referred to as apoptosis would probably vary in pathological conditions and especially in malignant ones. He asked Dr. Hill how apoptosis would affect estimates of cell cycle time obtained by labeling studies and change the basic reference population for kinetic studies. Dr. Hill replied that if a labeled cell died and released label prior to sampling, it would clearly not be counted as a labeled cell. This might affect the overall labeling index in longer-term labeling studies, but would probably not greatly influence short-term ones. The question of the reference population, however, is a more important one. The numerical proportion contributed to the total epithelial population by the progenitor population is not known and, indeed, probably changes under different conditions. A measure of the proportion of the population undergoing maturation in each circumstance is needed, but is not available. This aspect of the problem was emphasized by Dr. Laurence who pointed out that even in a normal epithelium, where patterns of stratification allow exclusion of some cells as progenitor cells, it is still not possible to distinguish visually the basal progenitor cells from basally-positioned cells which are differentiating. In a malignant tissue, where the normal pattern of organization is lost to a greater or lesser extent, the problem of identifying the progenitor population is even more complicated. Dr. Laurence also pointed out that proliferative epidermal and oral epithelial cells are semisynchronous populations: little is known about synchrony in malignant tissues although they are perhaps more likely to be asynchronous. A further factor that did not seem to be considered in the labeling studies described by Dr. Hill is the possibility of differences between normal and malignant tissues in terms of access of thymidine to the nuclei and the sizes of the thymidine pools. Such differences would also markedly affect double-labeling studies.

Dr. Hill suggested that, given the problems presently associated with determination of cell cycles, the most productive way of looking at differences between malignant and normal tissues might be to examine differences in rates of production of cells by cell blocking. Dr. Mackenzie asked whether simple studies comparing the labeling or mitotic indices of normal and pathologically involved tissues might be expected to provide much information of diagnostic significance. It is necessary to make a wide range of assumptions, for example about comparability of synchrony, progenitor pool size, length of the DNA synthesis phase, steady state, and rates of cell death, in order to make such comparisons. Many of these assumptions are unacceptable, and even if this were not so, a labeling index could only rise, fall, or remain the same as normal. As such effects, or lack of them, could be found in a wide range of nonmalignant conditions, could they be in any way tumor-specific? Dr. Hill indicated that assumptions that tumor growth is associated with a higher than normal rate of cell production might well be unfounded, as increased tissue mass could result from a reduced rate of cell maturation and death as well as from increased cell proliferation.

REFERENCES

Argyris, T. S., and Argyris, B. F. 1962. Differential response of skin epithelium to growth-promoting effects of subcutaneously transplanted tumor. *Cancer Res.* **22**, 73–77.

Bertsch, S., Csontos, K., Schweitzer, J., and Marks, F. 1976. Effect of mechanical stimulation on cell proliferation in mouse epidermis and on growth regulation by endogenous factors (chalones). *Cell Tiss. Kinet.* **9**, 445–457.

Billingham, R. E., and Silvers, W. K. 1963. The origin and conservation of epidermal specificities. *N. Engl. J. Med.* **268**, 477–539.

Bullough, W. B. 1969. Epithelial repair. In: *Repair and Regeneration.* (Edited by Dunphy, J. E., and Van Winkle, W.), pp. 35–46. McGraw-Hill, New York.

Elgjo, K. 1973. Epidermal chalone: Cell cycle specificity of two epidermal growth inhibitors. *Natl. Cancer Inst. Monogr.* **38**, 71–76.

Kariniemi, A. L., and Rytömaa, T. 1976. Effect of the Hewitt keratinising epidermal carcinoma on cell proliferation in different organs of the host mouse and in human psoriatic skin cultured in diffusion chambers. *Br. J. Dermatol.* **94**, 512–522.

Klein-Szanto, A. J. P., Bánóczy, J., and Schroeder, H. E. 1976. Metaplastic conversion of the differentiation pattern in oral epithelia affected by leukoplakia simplex; a stereologic study. *Pathol. Eur.* **11**, 189–210.

Landay, M. A., and Schroeder, H. E. 1977. Quantitative electron microscopic analysis of the stratified epithelium of normal human buccal mucosa. *Cell Tiss. Res.* **177**, 383–405.

Pictet, R. L., Filesa, S., Phelps, P., and Rutter, W. J. 1975. Control of DNA synthesis in the embryonic pancreas: Interaction of the mesenchymal factor and cyclic AMP. In: *Extracellular Matrix Influences on Gene Expression.* Santa Catalina Island Colloquium, 2d., 1974. (Edited by Slavkin, H. C., and Greulich, R. C.), pp. 531–540. Academic Press, New York.

Rytömaa, T. 1976. The chalone concept. *Int. Rev. Exp. Pathol.* **16**, 135–206.

Slavkin, H. C., Trump, G. N., Brownell, A., and Sorgente, N. 1977. Epithelial-mesenchymal interactions: Mesenchymal specificity. In: *Cell and Tissue Interactions.* (Edited by Lash, J. W., and Burger, M. N.), pp. 29–46. Raven Press, New York.

Wahl, D. V., Chapman, W. H., Hellstrom, I., and Hellstrom, K. E. 1974. Transplantation immunity to individually unique antigens of chemically induced bladder tumors in mice. *Int. J. Cancer* **14**, 114–121.

14

Spatial Organization and Tissue Architecture in Normal Epithelia

I. C. MACKENZIE

Dows Institute for Dental Research, College of Dentistry, University of Iowa, Iowa City, Iowa

1. INTRODUCTION

The process of histopathological diagnosis typically involves the recognition of certain features within a specimen and a comparison of these features with those anticipated to be typical for normal tissue of the site of origin. Experience has led pathologists to associate increased diagnostic significance with certain alterations of appearance and, for oral lesions, the validity of these beliefs has been examined and extended by recent studies (see chapter 19).

Apart from artifacts produced during processing, the appearances observed in static histological preparations are reflections of cellular events taking place prior to the time of biopsy. The histological appearance of a tissue thus indirectly indicates changes which may have occurred in the behavior of cells within the tissue but normal diagnostic methods do not typically examine the nature of these changes at the cellular or molecular level. An attempt to understand the cellular basis for histologically-detectable changes of diagnostic interest appears to be worthwhile from two points of view. First, little is known about how such changes become established and such processes merit attention as they may indicate the underlying nature of the disorder. Secondly, it is conceivable that a variety of apparently unrelated changes observed at the histological level could have their common origin in a single cellular change. If this were so, perhaps diagnostic tests of increased sensitivity or reliability could be developed.

From what is currently known of the biology of epithelial cells, it does not appear that the altered histological features associated with oral premalignancy (Smith and Pindborg 1969) can be related to a single aspect of altered cellular behavior. However, the histological appearance of premalignant lesions indicates that several changes, such as altered rete-peg morphology and loss of polarity, represent changes in architectural features of the tissue and reflect changing interrelationships between cells.

Excellent detailed descriptions of the histological appearance of oral epithelia are to be found in the literature (Squier et al. 1976; Squier et al. 1975). Unlike the underlying connective tissue, an epithelium is an essentially cellular tissue. The region of the junction between the epithelium and the connective tissue varies from a relatively flat plane to a highly interdigitated surface. Maturation of the cells formed in the basal region leads to changes in their histological appearance as they pass from the basal region to the surface and so gives rise to a series of different cell layers. Stratified squamous epithelia therefore possess a distinct polarity of organization. The relative contribution of each stratum to the total epithelial thickness varies but, in general, there is a tendency for each of the strata to be thicker with increasing thickness of the epithelium as a whole. In addition to a marked polarity, many epithelial tissues show precise patterns of macroscopic and microscopic spatial organization. The exquisite detail of cellular architecture in feather (Sengel 1976) and hair (Mercer 1961) serve to illustrate the epithelial capacity for spatial organization, and similar, if less impressive, architectural organization is seen in many lining or covering epithelia. The way in which cells come to be precisely positioned within an epithelium is one of the basic problems in understanding the maintenance of epithelial structure.

2. INFLUENCE OF CHANGES IN RATES OF CELLULAR ACTIVITY ON EPITHELIAL APPEARANCE

Tissues may be classified as having renewing, expanding, or static cell populations (Leblond et al. 1964). Stratified squamous epithelia continuously renew their component cell populations and, in the absence of peturbations induced by influences such as mechanical or chemical irritation, the rate of formation of cells in the basal strata of an epithelium is balanced by the rate of loss of cells by desquamation from the surface. Epithelia are therefore conceived to exist in a steady state. This steady state of gain and loss applies not only to the epithelium as a whole but also to various distinguishable subcompartments within it; for example, the histologically recognizable strata.

Regional variations in the mass or thickness of epithelia are usually associated with differences in rates of cell proliferation, a higher rate being found in thicker epithelia (Christophers and Laurence 1973; Alvares and Meyer 1971). Many studies have shown that various stimuli, for example ultraviolet light (Fukuyama and Epstein 1966; Epstein et al. 1970), mechanical trauma (Mackenzie 1974a, 1974b), inflammation (Mackenzie and Miles 1973) and carcinogens (Iversen 1966) markedly increase normal rates of epithelial cell proliferation and are associated with epithelial thickening. An imbalance between the rates of formation and rate of loss of cells could clearly influence the total number of cells in an epithelium and thus affect its thickness. This factor initially may be of importance to the increased tissue thickness associated with hyperplasia, but in the normal steady state the factor primarily determining epithelial thickness is the relationship between the rate of cell formation and the rate of cell maturation. This relationship is illustrated in Figure 1. Rate of maturation of epithelial cells may be studied by observing the rate of passage of labeled cells sequentially through the epithelial strata (Mackenzie 1974c), or may be calculated by combining counts of the number of suprabasal cells with information about rates of proliferation (Meyer et al. 1960; Mackenzie 1974b). Rates of cell maturation have not been investigated as extensively as rates of cell proliferation, but there is evidence that rates of cell maturation are linked to rates of proliferation. For example, the reduced epidermal cell proliferation observed in starved mice is associated with a reduced rate of passage of cells through the suprabasal strata (Bullough and Ebling 1952). Conversely, the increased rate of proliferation resulting from mechanical trauma is associated with an increased rate of maturation. It has been observed that repeated stimulation of an epithelium can lead to the reestablishment of a steady state in the rates of cell formation and loss, but although a new steady state is established the epithelium is thicker as a result of the increase in the rate of cell proliferation being greater than the increase in the rate of cell maturation (Mackenzie 1974b).

A mechanism for achieving epithelial homeostasis has been proposed by Bullough and Laurence (1960), who have presented evidence that the rate of epithelial cell proliferation is primarily influenced by a diffusible inhibitor of mitosis (termed "chalone") which is produced by postmitotic maturing cells (see also chapter 12). Bullough (1972a, 1972b) has also proposed that "chalone" also acts to influence rates of cell maturation and death. An extensive review of "chalones" in epithelia and other tissues is given in Houck (1976).

3. EPITHELIAL POLARITY

Polarity is basic to the pattern of organization and function of most epithelia and can be seen, for example, in terms of the direction of secretory activity in glandular epithelia, in the distal position of cilia in ciliated columnar epithelia, and in the sequence of cell maturation in multilayered stratified squamous epithelia.

The establishment of a pattern of polarity in stratified squamous epithelia, has been attributed to a "nutritional" gradient established by the varying distance of cells from the underlying connective tissue. In such a scheme, the basal layer, being closest to the connective tissue source of nourishment, is the most active part of the epithelium. The cells here produced jostle for position and those squeezed out of the basal layer are pushed progressively further away from the vascular connective tissue and, as a result, undergo the sequence of supposedly degenerative changes recognized as keratinization. Such a concept fits the histological appearance of healing wounds, where restoration of basal cell density is a forerunner of stratification, and of experimentally-buried epithelia (Christophers 1972), which form cysts by growing out and polarizing away from the connective tissue. However, biochemical studies of keratinization (Mier and Cotton 1976) and autoradiographic studies of the incorporation of labeled isotopes (Fukuyama and Epstein 1975, 1977) have indicated that keratinization is not simply a degenerative process and that suprabasal cells, particularly granular cells, are metabolically highly active and the site of specific syntheses. A simple concept of cell "degeneration" with increasing distance from the connective tissue does not therefore seem plausible.

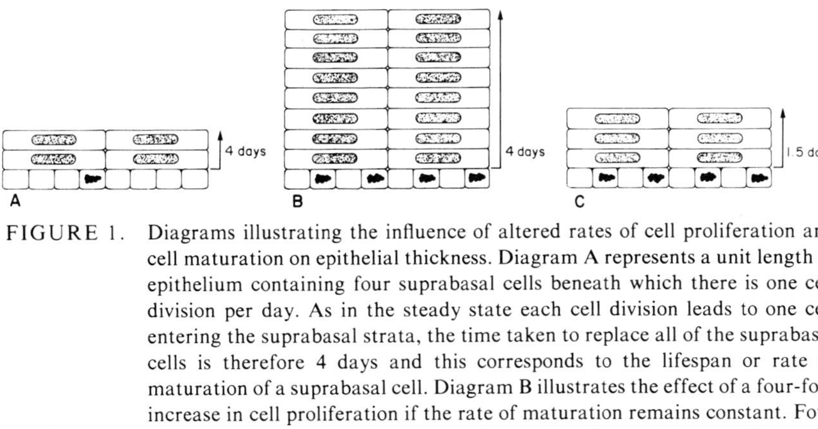

FIGURE 1. Diagrams illustrating the influence of altered rates of cell proliferation and cell maturation on epithelial thickness. Diagram A represents a unit length of epithelium containing four suprabasal cells beneath which there is one cell division per day. As in the steady state each cell division leads to one cell entering the suprabasal strata, the time taken to replace all of the suprabasal cells is therefore 4 days and this corresponds to the lifespan or rate of maturation of a suprabasal cell. Diagram B illustrates the effect of a four-fold increase in cell proliferation if the rate of maturation remains constant. Four cells enter the suprabasal strata per day, and as they each have a lifespan of 4 days, a total of 16 suprabasal cells would be present. Diagram C shows the experimentally observed effect (Mackenzie 1972b) of a stimulus which produces a four-fold increase in cell proliferation. Here the number of suprabasal cells increases by only 50% indicating that the rate of cell maturation is approximately 2.5 times faster. The link between rates of cell proliferation and maturation tends to reduce the effects of changing rates of cell proliferation on epithelial thickness.

A number of tissue culture studies (Jepsen 1974; Fusenig and Worst 1975) have demonstrated that it is possible to grow pure, or nearly pure, populations of epithelial cells in culture and that the tissue so formed shows patterns of polarity and keratinization comparable to an epithelium growing in vivo. Here, however, the direction of cell movement with maturation is away from the culture dish and towards the tissue culture medium which is the source of nutrients. These observations seem to indicate, first, that epithelial polarity is determined not by gradients associated with metabolic substances but may be primarily determined by the attachment of the epithelium to its substrate and secondly that polarity is a basic property of the epithelium itself. The connective tissue may not influence it, apart from acting as a point of attachment. Some evidence, however, suggests that factors in serum or dermis may tend to stimulate basal epithelial proliferation by inactivation of epithelially-produced mitotic inhibitors (Elgjo and Edgehill 1973; Laurence et al. 1972). The gradient established by such substances might augment epithelial polarity (Bjerknes and Iversen 1974).

4. THE INTERFACE BETWEEN EPITHELIUM AND CONNECTIVE TISSUE

The contour of the interface between the epithelium and the connective tissue differs in normal tissues from region to region, and pathologically-involved tissues often show deviations from the normal regional pattern. Normal human tissue from the same anatomical region of different subjects may show quite marked differences. There is a marked tendency for the contour of the epithelial-connective tissue junction to be regionally dependent, both in terms of the frequency and depth of interdigitations of the epithelium with the connective tissue (Squier et al. 1975; Klein-Szanto and Schroeder 1977), but the epithelial-connective tissue junction at a particular anatomical region can vary between subjects (Karring and Löe 1970). The contour of the epithelial-connective tissue junction may be functionally significant in providing a greater attachment of the epithelium to the connective tissue (Scapino 1967), or providing a greater proliferative pool (MacDonald 1971). In some tissues the position of such epithelial-connective tissue interdigitations forms a regular anatomical pattern; in the epithelium of the midline raphe of rat palate, the number, size, and proportion of rete ridges is quite consistent and appears to contribute to the surface form of the tissue.

The mechanisms leading to rete peg formation and to the changes in shape which occur in epithelial disorders and after certain experimental procedures are obscure, but the form of the junction appears to be influenced by patterns of epithelial cell proliferation, both in terms of rate

(Bullough 1972a, 1972b) and local grouping of mitosis (Löe et al. 1972), and also by patterns of cell maturation (Meyer and Schroeder 1975). Differential patterns of cell proliferation and maturation are clearly related to the papillary contour of structurally organized units such as tongue papillae (Cameron 1966).

An epithelium is generally considered to grow outwards, i.e., away from the connective tissue (Pinkus 1954; Van Scott 1964), but Ryan (1966), discussing the "direction" of epithelial growth, has raised some points which are of interest when the mechanisms controlling epithelial polarity and the contour of the epithelial-connective tissue junction are to be considered. The stated purpose of Ryan's (1966) discussion was to indicate that "*it is not reasonable to separate the phenomenon of epithelial budding* [during embryogenesis] *and invasion* [of malignant lesions] *from normal growth on account of apparent differences of direction of growth.*" He suggests that the direction of epithelial growth is always towards the connective tissue, but that normal connective tissue acts as a barrier to this attempted ingrowth. A connective tissue influence producing an altered contour of the dermo-epidermal junction in psoriasis has been suggested to be the result of changes in the "texture" of the subepithelial connective tissue (Braun-Falco and Christophers 1974; Van Scott and Ekel 1963).

Van Scott (1964) suggests that epithelial proliferation produces crowding and pressure within the basal layer and that epithelial cells are pushed in the direction of least resistance, normally, that is, outwards. Leblond et al. (1964) also suggested that basal cells are subjected to competition for space on the basement membrane and are squeezed out randomly from the basal layer. The findings of Iversen et al. (1968), however, suggest that emigration from the basal layer is restricted to the oldest G_1 cell in the vicinity of a mitosis, implying, perhaps, that some form of preparatory period is necessary before a basal cell is ready to undertake the maturation phase.

If population pressure is not the cause of loss of cells from the basal layer, alternative mechanisms must be sought to explain why particular cells should choose to enter the maturation pathway. Bullough (1972a, 1972b) has proposed a system which combines both an effect of pressure and of preparedness for emigration. He suggests that the decision taken by a basal cell, whether to enter the maturation pathway or return to the proliferative cycle, is influenced by the level of mitotic inhibitor present in the epithelium. In an epithelium with a flat epithelial-connective tissue junction, the pressure generated by mitosis may be relieved by the extrusion of neighboring post-mitotic cells, but when the mitotic rate has risen to the point where all basal cells are in the mitotic cycle, the lateral pressure generated leads to a folding of the basal layer.

Two recent studies indicate that emigration of basal cells into the stratum spinosum may have little to do with the generation of pressure by basal cell crowding. Changes in basal cell density were examined by Etoh et al. (1975) following irradiation, and by Potten and Allen (1975a) following removal of the surface layers with adhesive tape. In both studies it was observed that during the initial phases of the epithelial response the rate of emigration of basal cells into stratum spinosum was faster than their rate of replacement by proliferation. There was thus a phase of reduced basal cell density during which emigration continued. The observation that basal cell emigration can continue in the absence of crowding seems to indicate that emigration is an active process and not the result of squeezing out of cells. The driving force for this movement is uncertain but might be associated with development of a preferentially increased adhesion to overlying cells relative to the basal lamina, which could lead to the cell being pulled out of the basal layer in a way comparable to the "zipping" together of cells suggested by Mercer (1961) to account for cell movement during hair formation.

5. THE CELLULAR ARCHITECTURE OF EPITHELIA

It has been known for many years that keratinized epithelia are capable of producing structures showing regular and precise patterns of microarchitecture. The pattern of cellular organization in a number of structures such as feather (Sengel 1976), hair (Mercer 1961), and tongue papillae (Cameron 1966; Cane and Spearman 1969), has been described in detail and the role of cell-to-cell interactions and epithelial-mesenchymal interactions in the establishment of such structures in the embryo has been investigated (Mercer 1961; Sengel 1976). The interfollicular epidermis has also been shown to possess a pattern of alignment of the more superficial cells into columnar units of structure which are associated with nonrandom patterns of cell division in the underlying basal strata (Mackenzie 1969, 1975). These observations suggest the idea that such patterns may be basic features of epithelial organization, and that units of organization may also be present even in epithelia where such patterns are not morphologically identifiable by present techniques. Furthermore, the mechanisms leading to the more complex patterns of epithelial spatial organization may differ in complexity, but perhaps not in type from those present in simpler epithelia.

The mechanisms leading to precise patterns of cellular architecture in epithelial tissue are at present unknown. It is not clear whether the cell alignment seen in various epithelial structures is established primarily by cell packing, or by cell contact phenomena at the level at which it is first morphologically identifiable, or whether cell alignment is the first morphologic evidence of spatially-ordered activity established at a deeper level. In structures such as tongue papillae, probably both types of organization occur, but any attempt to explain the establishment of ordered structure serves principally to emphasize how little direct evidence is available to serve as a basis for speculation.

5:1 THE ESTABLISHMENT OF PATTERNS OF CELLULAR ARCHITECTURE IN EPITHELIA

In the epidermis (Fig. 2), the flattened cells of the spinous, granular, and cornified layers are stacked and aligned to form a series of hexagonal units of structure 30-40 μm across (Mackenzie 1969). A number of studies of this pattern serve to illustrate the features associated with the development of epithelial organization. The observable events which occur during the formation of columnar units of structure (Mackenzie 1975) are that a cell formed by division in the basal layer enters the stratum spinosum where, at a level which varies with epidermal thickness, it flattens and moves laterally in relation to adjacent cells. An aligned stack of flattened cells having, within a particular column, a closely similar polygonal shape is thus formed.

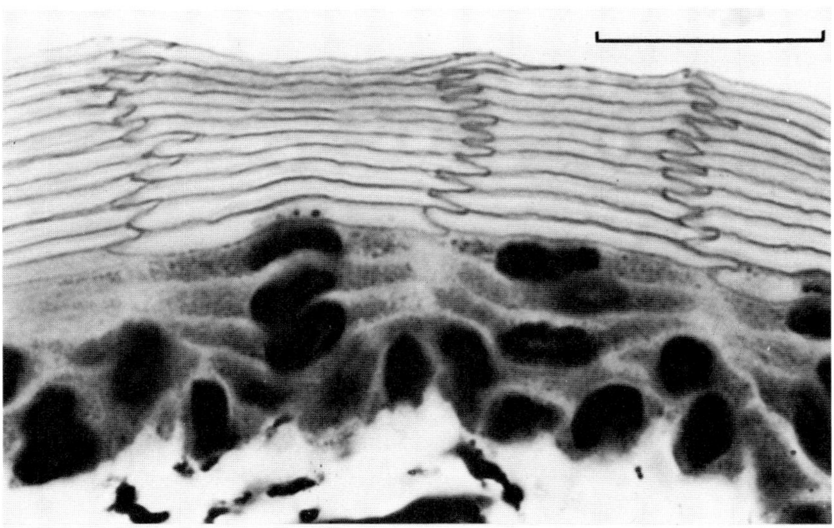

FIGURE 2. Photomicrograph of a frozen section of mouse ear epidermis stained with methylene blue and mounted in buffer at pH 12.5. Units of structure are clearly visible. Three layers of nucleated suprabasal cells are aligned beneath the columns of cells in the stratum corneum. (Scale = 0.03 mm).

Christophers (1971a, 1971b) has suggested that alignment of cells into columns may depend upon the sequence of addition of cells to adjoining columns. When a cell which is to flatten moves up toward the granular layer, the presence of a step-like boundary formed by the edge of a previously flattened overlying cell may tend to guide it away, or limit its lateral expansion, into the territory of the column to which the previous cell had been added. It therefore flattens into line beneath an adjacent column and as, after flattening, it lies slightly below previously flattened cells, it reestablishes a step which determines the position of further cell addition. A repetition of this sequence can be sustained with a two-dimensional model but, when the third dimension is considered, it is apparent that each column has not two, but five or six boundaries. It would require a regular and complex sequential addition of squames to a group of columns to result in each column in turn presenting the necessary boundaries.

Hexagonal close packing of cells is often found in both plant and animal tissues. Examples of its occurrence and the physical principles governing its establishment were discussed over fifty years ago by D'Arcy Thompson (1961). When uniformly-sized circular discs are packed closely together in the same plane, the six points of contact of each disc flatten and each disc tends to assume a hexagonal outline. The outlines which are formed have a similar appearance to the stained outlines of squames in sheets of stratum corneum. Menton (1976) has discussed the concept of hexagonal packing and minimal surface energy in relation to the formation of epidermal cell columns. Comparing packed soap bubbles with epidermal cells, he has demonstrated a similarity of the shape established by both and suggested that flattened epidermal cells are tetrakaidecahedra, which fill space with a minimum surface area. However, this model also demonstrates that simple physical packing does not produce a vertical alignment similar to that of the stratum corneum. An analogy between the formation of polygonal columns of squames and the mechanical packing together of circular bodies may also be inappropriate in other ways. First, epithelial cells are not bodies of a constant volume which are compressed into shape; rather they are initially bodies of relatively small size which expand laterally to acquire a polygonal shape. Secondly, desmosomes act as areas of attachment between epithelial cells and, although such cell attachments are probably lost and reestablished quite rapidly during normal epidermal turnover (Mishima and Pinkus 1968), the presence of desmosomes at the cell surface suggests that there is not a free sliding of adjacent cell surfaces over one another. In order for cells to expand laterally, it seems necessary that desmosomal contact be actively broken and reestablished.

The maintenance of columnar structure also normally appears to depend on a slow rate of formation and maturation of epidermal cells. The most precisely ordered stacking of squames is found in epidermis from regions such as the rodent ear in which the mitotic rate is normally relatively low (Mackenzie 1969; Christophers 1971a). In tissues with a somewhat higher mitotic rate, such as the general body epidermis of primates, the pattern tends to be less regular. Plantar and palmar epidermis and oral mucosa have a high rate of turnover (Mackenzie 1972) and show no evidence of column formation. A relationship between a low mitotic rate and the formation of columns is suggested by the finding that stacking of squames is lost from guinea pig ear epidermis during the period of increased mitotic activity which follows Scotch tape stripping but is reestablished when the rate of cell regeneration has returned to a low level after about ten days (Christophers 1971b). A complete explanation of the mechanism by which such structure is established should therefore presumably account not only for its presence at many epithelial sites but also for its loss at such sites after damage and for its absence from sites such as palmar and plantar epidermis.

Cell flattening is a common feature of all keratinizing epithelia, and it is perhaps in the factors producing and controlling lateral expansion of cells during flattening that the immediate mechanisms for establishment of alignment should be sought. Branson (1968) has described orthogonal arrays of microtubules in flattening cells of the granular layer of newborn rat epidermis and suggested that their presence is related to the changes in cell shape occurring at this level. Although the mechanism is uncertain, the finding that flattening occurs during the keratinization of foci of cultured cells and outgrowths of epidermis (Karasek 1975; Delescluse et al. 1976) suggests that the ability to flatten is an active property of individual epithelial cells, rather than the result of cell population pressure. It has been suggested (Mercer 1961) that an enhancement of intercellular adhesion may, during hair formation, play an active role in molding the shapes of cells, and that an area of contact between two epidermal cells, by spreading in a zipper-like fashion, could produce relative movement and cell flattening.

5:2 PATTERNS OF CELL PROLIFERATION AND EMIGRATION RELATED TO EPITHELIAL ARCHITECTURE

Foci of mitotic activity are observed in structures such as hair and tongue papillae (Cameron 1966), but until recently it was generally assumed that mitotic activity occurred randomly amongst the basal cells of interfollicular epidermis and lining epithelia (Leblond et al. 1964). However, a nonrandom pattern of mitosis has been shown to be related to epidermal cell columns, and there is also evidence for units of proliferation in other epithelia, such as oral mucosa.

About ten smaller, unflattened basal cells lie beneath each unit of structure in the epidermis, and it was shown that cells in mitosis are found principally beneath the periphery of such units (Mackenzie 1970). It was initially proposed (Mackenzie 1970) that the nonproliferative cells beneath the center of each cell column represent cells which, as described by Iversen et al. (1968), are older G_1 cells preparing for emigration into the suprabasal strata. It was thus conceivable that mitotic activity in the ring of cells beneath the column periphery produces cells that move centrally to migrate from the basal layer in alignment with the overlying cell stacks. This arrangement might have proved somewhat analogous to the situation in intestinal villi where cells migrate laterally along the basement membrane after leaving the crypt, but Christophers (1972), using a method of differential staining of maturing cells with fluorescein isothyocyanate, showed that cell migration into the suprabasal strata occurs principally from the peripheral region beneath the cell column.

Potten (1974) examined both sections of mouse skin and sheets of mouse epidermis by autoradiography following either flash or continuous labeling with tritiated thymidine. In sheet preparations, he scored the epidermal nuclei as labeled or unlabeled and as central or peripheral to the overlying epidermal cell columns. He found that compared with peripheral cells, central cells tend to label less frequently following pulse labeling, and that central cells accumulate label less rapidly under conditions of continuous labeling. Karatschai et al. (1971) similarly reported a preferential position of labeled cells in relation to the periphery of the overlying cell columns, and postulated a fairly complex pattern of cell production and proliferation. Potten and coworkers have proposed a role of the central, nonmitotically-active cells as stem cells for the epidermis. Potten and Hendry (1973) analyzed published data (Withers 1967a, 1967b; Emery et al. 1970) for the cell numbers (extrapolated from split-dose survival curve data) from which epidermal regeneration initially occurs following irradiation. As the number of cells from which regeneration occurred was considerably lower than the normal basal cell density, they concluded that these data provide evidence for a subpopulation of epidermal cells which behave similarly to the stem cells identified in other tissues (Lajtha 1970). One stem cell per columnar unit was proposed and in further papers Potten and Allen (1975a, 1975b) and Potten (1976) have extended the epidermal stem cell model to postulate a slow stem cell cycle and an eight-fold amplification of an initial stem cell division, with the amplification division being related to a sequence of central or peripheral positions beneath the cell columns. Such suggestions are interesting, but at present there is only very limited experimental evidence pointing to the existence of epidermal stem cells.

This work on epidermis points to spatially organized patterns of interaction between cells during the maintenance of normal structure. Units of tissue architecture similar to those of the epidermis have not, as yet, been demonstrated in the majority of oral mucosal epithelia, but there are some indications that cell division may not occur randomly among the basal cells of mucosal epithelia. Evidence exists for nonrandom patterns of cell division in a number of internal epithelia (Purnell and Stowers 1977) and, in oral mucosa, nonrandom patterns of cell proliferation have been observed in hamster cheek pouch epithelium (Gibbs and Casarett 1972) and in murine mucosa (Burns et al. 1976). In gingival epithelium, mitotic figures have been described to occur preferentially in the most basal (deepest) part of the rete ridges (Löe et al. 1972). The morphometric work of Meyer and Schroeder (1975) has characterized the cytoplasmic contents of the cells in contact with the basal lamina at the tips of the connective tissue papillae as being more typical of stratum spinosum cells than that of basal cells lying in the deeper part of the rete ridges. The pattern of blood group antigen staining of the surface of these cells also corresponds more to a pattern of spinous than of basal cells (Mackenzie and Dabelsteen, unpublished observations). It therefore seems probable that the epithelial rete ridge acts as a unit of proliferation for the overlying epithelial strata, even though no corresponding demarcation of the suprabasal region into units is apparent.

Hume and Potten (1976) have examined the structure of lingual papillae of the mouse and described the associated patterns of cell proliferation. The pattern of cell labeling found suggests the existence of a stem cell zone from which cells are produced, possibly with an asymmetric pattern of division. They also suggest that each papilla corresponds to a group of columnar units such as are found in epidermis, and that postmitotic cells move laterally along the basement membrane, from their point of origin at the base of the papillae, to enter the stratum spinosum at the tip. These findings are of particular interest as they indicate the ability of mucosal epithelium to form spatially ordered structures, and furthermore they suggest that quite complex structures may be derived by reorganization of simpler structural units of the type found in epidermis.

6. INFLUENCES OF SUBEPITHELIAL CONNECTIVE TISSUE ON EPITHELIAL STRUCTURE

In the adult animal, epithelium occurs in a wide variety of functional and morphological forms, and the mechanisms whereby structures as diverse as skin, mucosa, hair, feathers, salivary glands, and teeth can result from a single embryonic tissue, with an apparently uniform genetic constitution, have been the subject of several extensive reviews (Fleischmajer and Billingham 1968; Slavkin and Bavetta 1972). Epithelial-mesenchymal interactions appear to play an important role in the morphogenesis of epithelial structures, and the mesenchyme appears to act in two ways (Sengel 1976): (a) it may act to differentiate, or to modulate continuously, the state of differentiation of its associated epithelium, and (b) it facilitates the growth of an associated epithelium in a way which allows the expression of an established epithelial phenotype (Wessels 1962). From several studies it can be concluded that the primary induction of embryonic morphogenesis of epithelial structure, whether it be of feathers (Sengel 1976), scales (Rawles 1963), or hair (Kollar 1970, 1972), is dependent on an influence from the underlying mesoderm.

The specific regional differences in structure of the epithelia of oral mucosae and skin, which are established during development, normally remain stable for the rest of the lifespan, despite a continuous replacement of structure by cell proliferation. Investigations of the role of the underlying connective tissue in contributing to the maintenance of organization and behavior of oral epithelia in the adult animal are limited, but suggest a continuing influence of subepithelial connective tissue on both epithelial survival and the pattern of structure developed during its continuous histogenesis. Karring et al. (1975), from an experimental study of monkey oral mucosa, consider that gingival connective tissue is capable of inducing keratinization in the normally nonkeratinized alveolar epithelium. These findings are supported by the work of Heaney (1977) on pig, and Stambaugh and Gordon (1973) on human tissue. However, it might be postulated that in these studies the epithelium was not actively remodulated by the connective tissue but only reverted to a basic pattern of unmodulated differentiation which was that of keratinization.

Billingham and Silvers (1967) suggested that conservation of epithelial specificity may be due either to (a) basal cells of different epithelia being intrinsically different due to their differing developmental origin, or (b) all germinal epithelial cells being equipotential, with the particular pathway of cytodifferentiation that they pursue being determined by the underlying connective tissues. A limited histological evaluation of heterotypic recombinant grafts of skin epithelium and connective tissue from the sole of the foot, the ear, and the trunk which were transplanted to full thickness beds prepared in the chest wall of syngeneic hosts, suggested that the dermis was responsible for the phenotypic expression of the overlying epidermis (Billingham and Silvers 1967). However, after recombination of the epithelial component of tongue, esophagus, and hamster cheek pouch with ear or sole dermis, these mucosae conserved their epithelial specificity. Beer and Billingham (1972) have interpreted these results as indicating that the generative cells of skin epithelium are equipotential, the phenotypic character of the tissue being determined by the continuous influence of distinctive and regionally different stimuli from the underlying dermis. The specific differentiative behavior found for oral mucosae suggests either that these tissues are more fixed in character than epidermis, have a reduced capacity for modulation, or perhaps require a quantitatively stronger or more specific stimulus.

Beer and Billingham (1970) have described an interesting system for evaluating the inherent properties of different epithelia by implanting a variety of epithelia and their supporting connective tissues into the uterus of adult rats. When animals so implanted are subjected to chronic estrogen stimulation, the epithelium of the implant grows off its own connective tissue to replace the native endometrial surface. The structure of the epithelium growing on the uterine connective tissue is thus reorganized in the absence of any site specific message that may have been provided by the original connective tissue. This provides a useful model for examining the maintenance of various adult epithelia removed from their normal environment, and gives a measure of the epithelial potential for self-determination of structure. Beer and Billingham (1970) found that epithelia growing in association with their site-specific connective tissue maintained their specific pattern of differentiation. However, epidermis of the tail failed to develop any of its characteristic pilosebaceous appendages when on the uterine connective tissue, and when suspensions of tail epidermal cells were injected into an estrogen-primed uterus a stratified squamous epithelium lacking the organization of tail was formed. Migrating lingual epithelium appeared to maintain some of its architectural features.

Mackenzie and Smith (1976) using the uterine implantation method of Beer and Billingham (1970) have examined tongue mucosa and skin, tissues which show characteristic patterns of keratinization and tissue architecture. Autografts of intact tissues, or of their EDTA-separated pure epithelia, were implanted, unilaterally or bilaterally, into the uteri of ovarectimized, estrogen-treated rats. Two to four months later, the uteri were removed for frozen sectioning. Observations from over fifty implants and their outgrowths showed that the structure of epithelia growing in the uterus was essentially normal in the presence of the originally transplanted connective tissue. However, epithelial outgrowths from the original implant and implants of pure epithelium showed that epithelia growing on the uterine connective tissue continued to keratinize but invariably lost specific patterns of spatial organization and tissue architecture. Outgrowths of ear epidermis growing on the uterine connective tissue failed to develop a normal columnar structure and no appendages were formed (Fig. 3).

Implants of tongue showed an interesting pattern (Fig. 4). With continuing keratinization into the lumen of the uterus, the uterine cavity became distended and appeared to stretch the basal layer of the implanted specimen, and the foci of epithelium, which were producing the "hard" keratin, normally associated with the dorsal aspect of the papillae, became spaced. The stream of layers of "hard" keratin produced from individual tongue papillae during this accumulation of keratin in the lumen led to an appearance somewhat like the spokes of a cartwheel suggesting that new foci for producing papillae were not formed and that, as the existing foci became spaced, the intervening epithelium was replaced by a keratinized epithelium, but of a "nonspecific" type. Pure sheets of lingual epithelium implanted into the uterus in the absence of lingual connective tissue produced only a single type of keratin similar to that of the interpapillary region.

These observations suggest that the subepithelial connective tissue markedly affects the overlying epithelium. Although a site-specific connective tissue influence is not necessary to maintain a basic pattern of keratinization, a site-specific influence appears to be necessary for the expression of regionally specific patterns of keratinization and spatial organization of epithelia.

7. SUMMARY

The continuous process of histogenesis of epithelia in the adult animal is associated with events which are in some ways similar to those occurring during the initial differentiation and histogenesis of tissues in the embryo. Bonner (1974), discussing embryogenesis, suggests that it may be helpful to separate in one's mind three kinds of events: the synthesis of substances, the timing of their synthesis, and their localization in space. A similar concept may also be of value when classifying the factors associated with the maintenance of epithelial structure, and this process may be considered in terms of (a) the types of cellular synthetic activity occurring, (b) the rate at which various synthetic activities occur, and (c) the disposition in space of the resulting cells and cellular products. Many factors have been identified which may influence specific patterns of epithelial structure but, at present, little is known about the mechanisms by which such factors operate.

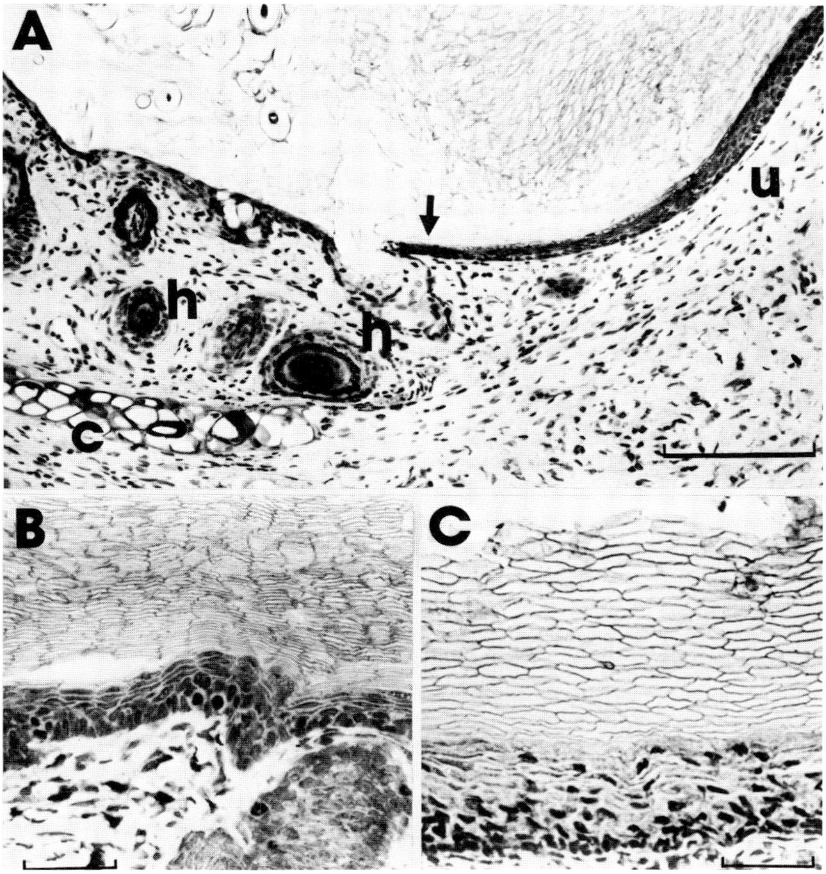

FIGURE 3. Photomicrographs of frozen sections of the wall and lumen of a rat uterus implanted 10 weeks previously with an autogenous fragment of ear. A. To the left is the implant, which can be identified by the presence of the cartilaginous plate (c), and in this region the epidermis is relatively normal and there are hair follicles (h). The region of the junction between ear and uterus connective tissues is marked by an arrow and to the right, the epidermis of the ear has grown out to replace the columnar epithelium of the uterine lining. Here the ear epidermis growing on the uterine connective tissue (u) is somewhat thicker than normal and no appendages are formed. (Scale 0.15 mm). B. Treatment with buffer at pH 12.5 displays the columnar pattern of arrangement of the epidermis over the original implant and of the keratinized cells piled up in the uterine lumen. C. No columnar pattern is seen in epidermis growing on the uterine connective tissue. (Scales for B and C = 0.05 mm).

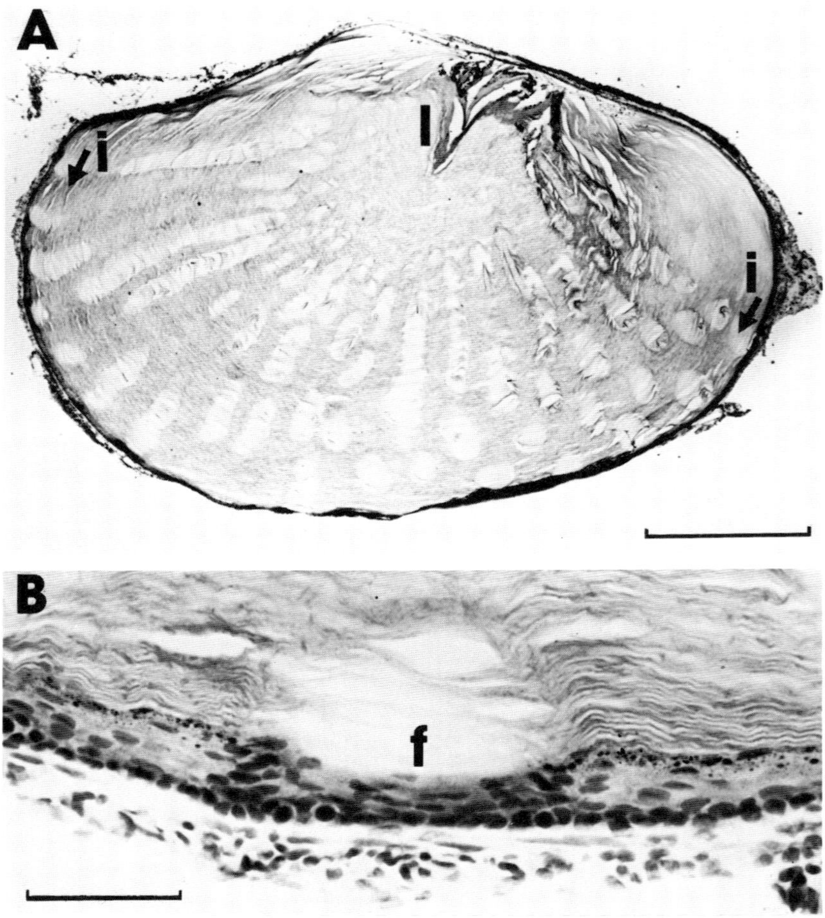

FIGURE 4. Photomicrographs of a frozen section of a uterus implanted 12 weeks previously with an autogenous fragment of tongue mucosa. A. The lumen of the uterus has been greatly distended by the continued production of keratinized cells by the implanted epithelium. The region presumed to correspond to the original implant with its connective tissue lies between the arrows marked I. Here a dual pattern of keratinization corresponding to the pattern of hard and soft keratin of the tongue papillae is conserved and, with distention of the uterus, the epithelial foci producing hard keratin have become increasingly separated so that streams of keratin radiate out from the original position of the lumen (l) as the spokes of wheel. Judging from the amount of keratin accumulated, the tongue epithelium in association with its original connective tissue has been more active then the epithelium which has grown out onto the uterus. (Scale = 0.6 mm). B. A higher power of one of the epithelial foci (f) producing hard keratin. (Scale = 0.01 mm).

The existing evidence suggests that the particular type of synthesis undertaken by an epithelium is partly the consequence of inductive interactions, which take place during embryogenesis, and partly the effect of a continuing influence of the subepithelial connective tissue which modulates, to a significant but uncertain degree, regional variations in the type of synthesis occurring. The mechanism by which the dermis modulates its associated epithelium and the cellular or stromal origin of the modulating influence are unknown.

The balance between rates of various cellular activities, for example rates of cell formation and cell maturation, is the primary factor determining epithelial mass. Investigations of mechanisms controlling rates of various epithelial activities appear to point to some form of intraepithelial negative feedback mechanism as the most probable form of control. In so far as regional variations occur in rates of epithelial proliferation, it seems probable that subepithelial connective tissues play some role in establishing the "setting" of this homeostatic mechanism.

Factors such as growth pressure and constraints imposed by the close packing of cells probably play a part in the establishment of spatial patterns of organization of epithelial cells. Attempts have been made to explain simple patterns of columnar structure solely in terms of cell packing, but evidence for active migration of cells from the basal region, and for an origin of the more complex epithelial structures from simpler ones, suggest that a more active biological mechanism should be sought. Possibly it may be found in the type of cell surface recognition properties and differential patterns of cell adhesion which are currently believed to be of importance in embryonic morphogenesis. Such a concept is attractive in that modulation of the synthesis of cell surface components by subepithelial connective tissue could explain the influence of connective tissue on epithelial architecture. As yet however, there have been few investigations of differences in epithelial cell surfaces from region to region or with maturation.

REFERENCES

Alvares, O. F., and Meyer, J. 1971. Variable features and regional differences in oral epithelium. In: *Current Concepts of the Histology of Oral Mucosa.* (Edited by Squier, C. A., and Meyer, J.), pp. 97–113. Charles C Thomas, Springfield, Illinois.

Beer, A. E., and Billingham, R. E. 1970. Implantation, transplantation, and epithelial-mesenchymal relationships in the rat uterus. *J. Exp. Med.* **132**, 721–736.

Beer, A. E., and Billingham, R. E. 1972. *In vivo* approaches to the analysis of the conservation of epidermal specificities. In: *Epidermal Wound Healing.* (Edited by Maibach, H. I., and Rovee, D. T.), pp. 187–202. Year Book Medical Publishing, Chicago.

Billingham, R. E., and Silvers, W. K. 1967. Studies on the conservation of epidermal specificities of skin and certain mucosas in adult mammals. *J. Exp. Med.* **125**, 429–446.

Bjerknes, R., and Iversen, O. H. 1974. "Antichalone": A theoretical treatment of the possible role of antichalone in the growth control system. *Acta Pathol. Microbiol. Scand. [A]* Suppl. 248, pp. 33–42.

Bonner, J. T. 1974. *On Development.* Harvard University Press, Cambridge, Massachusetts.

Branson, R J. 1968. Orthogonal arrays of microtubules in flattening cells of the epidermis. *Anat. Rec.* **160**, 109–121.

Braun-Falco, O., and Christophers, E. 1974. Structural aspects of initial psoriatic lesions. *Arch. Dermatol. Forsch.* **251**, 95–110.

Bullough, W. S. 1972a. The control of epidermal thickness. Part I. *Br. J. Dermatol.* **87**, 187–199.

Bullough, W. S. 1972b. The control of epidermal thickness. Part II. *Br. J. Dermatol.* **87**, 347–354.

Bullough, W. S., and Ebling, F. J. 1952. Cell replacement in the epidermis and sebaceous glands of the mouse. *J. Anat.* **86**, 29–34.

Bullough, W. S., and Laurence, E. B. 1960. The control of epidermal mitotic activity in the mouse. *Proc. R. Soc. Lond. [Biol.]* **151**, 517–536.

Burns, E. R., Scheving, L. E., Fawcett, D. F., Gibbs, W. M., and Galatzan, R. E. 1976. Circadian influence on the frequency of labeled mitoses method in the stratified squamous epithelium of the mouse esophagus and tongue. *Anat. Rec.* **184**, 265–274.

Cameron, I. L. 1966. Cell proliferation, migration and specialization in the epithelium of the mouse tongue. *J. Exp. Zool.* **163**, 271–284.

Cane, A. K., and Spearman, R. I. 1969. The keratinized epithelium of the house-mouse (Mus musculus) tongue, its structure and histochemistry. *Arch. Oral Biol.* **14**, 829–841.

Christophers, E. 1971a. Cellular architecture of the stratum corneum. *J. Invest. Dermatol.* **56**, 165–169.

Christophers, E. 1971b. The architecture of stratum corneum after wounding. *J. Invest. Dermatol.* **57,** 241–246.

Christophers, E. 1972. Kinetic aspects of epidermal healing. In: *Epidermal Wound Healing.* (Edited by Maibach, H. I., and Rovee, D. T.), pp. 53–69. Year Book Medical Publishers, Chicago.

Christophers, E., and Laurence, E. B. 1973. Regional variations in mouse skin: Quantitation of epidermal compartments in two different body sites. *Virchows Arch. Abt. B. Zellpath.* **12**, 212–222.

Delecluse, C., Fukuyama, K., and Epstein, W. L. 1976. Dibutyryl cyclic AMP-induced differentiation of epidermal cells in tissue culture. *J. Invest. Dermatol.* **66**, 8–13.

Elgjo, K., and Edgehill, W. 1973. Epidermal growth inhibitors (chalones) in dermis and serum. *Virchows Arch. [Cell Pathol.]* **13**, 14–23.

Emery, E. W., Denekamp, J., Bale, M. M., and Field, S. B. 1970. Survival of mouse skin epithelial cells following single and divided doses of x-rays. *Radiat. Res.* **41**, 450–466.

Epstein, J. H., Fukuyama, K., and Fye, K. 1970. Effects of ultraviolet radiation on the mitotic cycle and DNA, RNA and protein synthesis in mammalian epidermis *in vivo. Photochem. Photobiol.* **12**, 57–65.

Etoh, H., Taguchi, Y. H., and Tabachnick, J. 1975. Movement of beta-irradiated epidermal basal cells to the spinous-granular layers in the absence of cell division. *J. Invest. Dermatol.* **64**, 431–435.

Fleischmajer, R., and Billingham, R. E. (eds.) 1968. *Epithelial-Mesenchymal Interactions.* Williams and Wilkins, Baltimore.

Fukuyama, K., and Epstein, W. L. 1966. Epidermal keratinization: Localization of isotopically labeled amino acids. *J. Invest. Dermatol.* **47**, 551–560.

Fukuyama, K., and Epstein, W. L. 1975. A comparative autoradiographic study of keratohyalin granules containing cystine and histidine. *J. Ultrastruct. Res.* **51**, 314–325.

Fukuyama, K., and Epstein, W. L. 1977. Quantitative autoradiographic studies of proteins in keratohyalin granules. In: *Biochemistry of Cutaneous Epidermal Differentiation.* (Edited by Seiji, M., and Bernstein, I. A.), pp. 253–273. Baltimore, University Park Press.

Fusenig, N. E., and Worst, P. K. 1975. Mouse epidermal cell cultures. II. Isolation, characterization and cultivation of epidermal cells from perinatal mouse skin. *Exp. Cell Res.* **93**, 443–457.

Gibbs, S. J., and Casarett, G. W. 1972. Spatial distribution of cells in mitotic and DNA-synthetic phases of the cell cycle in hamster cheek pouch epithelium. *J. Dent. Res.* **51**, 30–38.

Heaney, T. G. 1977. A histological investigation of the influence of adult porcine gingival connective tissues in determining epithelial specificity. *Arch. Oral Biol.* **22**, 167–174.

Houck, J. (ed.) 1976. *Chalones.* Elsevier/North Holland, Amsterdam, and New York.

Hume, W. J., and Potten, C. S. 1976. The ordered columnar structure of mouse filiform papillae. *J. Cell Sci.* **22**, 149–160.

Iversen, O. H. 1966. Kinetics of epidermal reaction to carcinogens and other skin irritants. In: *Carcinogenesis. Advances in Biology of the Skin*, Vol. 7. (Edited by Montagna, W., and Dobsin, R. A.), pp. 37–54. Macmillan, New York.

Iversen, O. H., Bjerknes, R., and Devik, F. 1968. Kinetics of cell renewal, cell migration and cell loss in the hairless mouse dorsal epidermis. *Cell Tiss. Kinet.* **1**, 351–367.

Jepsen, A. 1974. An *in vitro* model of an oral keratinizing squamous epithelium. *Scand. J. Dent. Res.* **82**, 144–146.

Karasek, M. A. 1975. *In vitro* growth and maturation of epithelial cells from postembryonic skin. *J. Invest. Dermatol.* **65**, 60–66.

Karatcshai, M., Kinzel, V., Goerttler, K., and Suss, R. 1971. "Geography" of mitoses and cell divisions in the basal cell layer of mouse epidermis. *Z. Krebsforsch.* **76**, 59–64.

Karring, T., Lang, N. P., and Löe, H. 1975. The role of gingival connective tissue in determining epithelial differentiation. *J. Periodont. Res.* **10**, 1–11.

Karring, T., and Löe, H. 1970. The three-dimensional concept of the epithelial-connective tissue boundary of gingiva. *Acta Odontol. Scand.* **28**, 917–933.

Klein-Szanto, A. J., and Schroeder, H. E. 1977. Architecture and density of the connective tissue papillae of the human oral mucosa. *J. Anat.* **123**, 93–109.

Kollar, E. J. 1970. The induction of hair follicles by embryonic dermal papillae. *J. Invest. Dermatol.* **55**, 374–378.

Kollar, E. J. 1972. The development of the integument: Spatial, temporal and phylogenetic factors. *Am. Zoologist* **12**, 125–135.

Lajtha, L. G. 1970. Stem cell kinetics. In: *Regulation of Hematopoiesis*, Vol. I. (Edited by Gordon, A. S.), pp. 111–131. Appleton-Century-Crofts, New York.

Laurence, E. B., Randers Hansen, E., Christophers, E., and Rytömaa, T. 1972. Systemic factors influencing epidermis mitosis. *Europ. J. Clin. Biol. Res.* **17**, 133–139.

Leblond, C. P., Greulich, R. C., and Pereira, J. P. 1964. Relationship of cell formation and cell migration in the renewal of stratified squamous epithelia. In: *Wound Healing.*

Advances in Biology of the Skin, Vol. 5. (Edited by Montagna, W., and Billingham, R. E.), pp. 39–67. Macmillan, New York.

Löe, H., Karring, T., and Hara, K. 1972. The site of mitotic activity in rat and human oral epithelium. *Scand. J. Dent. Res.* **80**, 111–119.

MacDonald, D. G. 1971. Cell renewal in oral epithelium. In: *Current Concepts of the Histology of Oral Mucosa.* (Edited by Squier, C. A. and Meyer, J.), pp. 61–79. Charles C Thomas, Springfield, Illinois.

Mackenzie, I. C. 1969. The ordered structure of the stratum corneum of mammalian skin. *Nature* **222**, 881–882.

Mackenzie, I. C. 1970. Relationship between mitosis and the ordered structure of the stratum corneum in mouse epidermis. *Nature* **226**, 653–655.

Mackenzie, I. C. 1972. The ordered structure of mammalian epidermis. In: *Epidermal Wound Healing.* (Edited by Maibach, H. I., and Rovee, D. T.), pp. 5–25. Year Book Medical Publishing, Chicago.

Mackenzie, I. C. 1974a. The effects of frictional stimulation on mouse ear epidermis. I. Cell proliferation. *J. Invest. Dermatol.* **62**, 80–85.

Mackenzie, I. C. 1974b. The effects of frictional stimulation on mouse ear epidermis. II. Histologic appearance and cell counts. *J. Invest Dermatol.* **63**, 194–198.

Mackenzie, I. C. 1974c. The effects of oral administration of chlorhexidine on the rate of regeneration of epithelia of the oral mucosa and skin of mice. *J. Periodont. Res.* **9**, 181–187.

Mackenzie, I. C. 1975. Ordered structure of the epidermis. (Proceedings of the 24th Annual Symposium on the Biology of Skin.) *J. Invest Dermatol.* **65**, 45–51.

Mackenzie, I. C., and Miles, A. E. 1973. The effect of chronic frictional stimulation on hamster cheek-pouch epithelium. *Arch. Oral Biol.* **18**, 1341–1349.

Mackenzie, I. C., and Smith, M. L. 1976. Organization and differentiation of epithelia transplanted to the uterus. Abstract. *J. Dent Res.* **55**, Special issue B, B218.

Menton, D. N. 1976. A minimum-surface mechanism to account for the organization of cells into columns in the mammalian epidermis. *Am. J. Anat.* **145**, 1–22.

Mercer, E. H. 1961. *Keratin and Keratinization. An Essay in Molecular Biology.* Pergamon Press, Oxford, England.

Meyer, J. Medak, H., and Weinmann, J. P. 1960. Mitotic activity and rates of growth in regions of oral epithelium differing in width. *Growth* **24**, 29–46.

Meyer, M., and Schroeder, H. E. 1975. A quantitative electron microscopic analysis of the keratinizing epithelium of normal human hard palate. *Cell Tiss. Res.* **158**, 177–203.

Mier, P. D., and Cotton, D. W. 1976. *The Molecular Biology of Skin.* Blackwell Scientific Publications, Oxford, England.

Mishima, Y., and Pinkus, H. 1968. Electron microscopy of keratin layer stripped human epidermis. *J. Invest. Dermatol.* **50**, 89–102.

Pinkus, H. 1954. Biology of epidermal cells. In: *Physiology and Biochemistry of Skin.* (Edited by Rothman, S.), pp. 584–600. University of Chicago Press, Chicago.

Potten, C. S. 1974. The epidermal proliferative unit: The possible role of the central basal cell. *Cell Tiss. Kinet.* **7**, 77–88.

Potten, C. S. 1976. Identification of clonogenic cells in the epidermis and the structural arrangement of the epidermal proliferative unit (EPU). In: *Stem Cells of Renewing Cell Populations.* (Edited by Cairnie, A. B., Lala, P. K., and Osmond, D. G.), pp. 91–102. Academic Press, New York.

Potten, C. S., and Allen, T. D. 1975a. The fine structure and cell kinetics of mouse epidermis after wounding. *J. Cell Sci.* **17**, 413–447.

Potten, C. S., and Allen, T. D. 1975b. Control of epidermal proliferative units (EPUs). An hypothesis based on the arrangement of neighbouring differentiated cells. *Differentiation* **3**, 161–165.

Potten, C. S., and Hendry, J. H. 1973. Clonogenic cells and stem cells in epidermis. *Int. J. Radiat. Biol.* **24**, 537–540.

Purnell, D. M., and Stowers, D. J. 1977. Nonrandom frequency distribution of mitoses in rat lobuloalveolar mammary gland epithelium. *Am. J. Pathol.* **88**, 267–276.

Rawles, M. E. 1963. Tissue interactions in scale and feather development as studied in dermal-epidermal recombinations. *J. Embryol. Exp. Morphol.* **11**, 765–789.

Ryan, T. J. 1966. The direction of growth of epithelium. *Br. J. Dermatol.* **78**, 403–415.

Scapino, R. P. 1967. Biomechanics of prehensile oral mucosa. *J. Morphol.* **122**, 89–114.

Sengel, P. 1976. *Morphogenesis of Skin.* Cambridge University Press, Cambridge.

Slavkin, H. C., and Bavetta, L. A. (eds.) 1972. *Developmental Aspects of Oral Biology.* Academic Press, New York.

Smith, C., and Pindborg, J. J. 1969. *Histological Grading of Oral Epithelial Atypia by the use of Photographic Standards.* WHO International Reference Centre for Oral Precancerous Conditions, Copenhagen.

Squier, C. A., Johnson, N. W., and Hackemann, M. 1975. Structure and function of normal human oral mucosa. In: *Oral Mucosa in Health and Disease.* (Edited by Dolby, A. E.), pp. 1–112. Blackwell Scientific Publications, Oxford, England.

Squier, C. A., Johnson, N. W., and Hopps, R. M. 1976. *Human Oral Mucosa: Development, Structure and Function.* Blackwell Scientific Publications, Oxford, England.

Stambaugh, R., and Gordon, H. P. 1973. Connective tissue influence on mucosal keratinization. Abstract. *J. Dent. Res.* **52**, Special issue, 147.

Thompson, D'Arcy W. 1961. *On Growth and Form.* (Abridged edition edited by Bonner, J. T.) Cambridge University Press, Cambridge, England.

Van Scott, E. J. 1964. Definition of epidermal cancer. In: *The Epidermis.* (Edited by Montagna, W., and Lobitz, W. C.), pp. 573–586. New York Academic Press.

Van Scott, E. J., and Ekel, T. M. 1963. Kinetics of hyperplasia in psoriasis. *Arch. Dermatol.* **88**, 373–381.

Wessels, N. K. 1962. Tissue interactions during skin histodifferentiation. *Dev. Biol.* **4**, 87–107.

Withers, H. R. 1967a. The dose-survival relationship for irradiation of epithelial cells of mouse skin. *Br. J. Radio.* **40**, 187–194.

Withers, H. R. 1967b. Recovery and repopulation *in vivo* by mouse skin epithelial cells during fractionated irradiation. *Radiat. Res.* **32**, 227–239.

15

Quantitative Evaluation of Normal, Hyperplastic, and Premalignant Epithelium by Stereological Methods

C. D. FRANKLIN, K. GOHARI, C. J. SMITH, and F. H. WHITE

Department of Oral Pathology, University of Sheffield, Sheffield, England

1. INTRODUCTION

A small proportion of oral mucosal lesions with particular clinical features subsequently become malignant (see chapters 1 and 2). The main problem for both the clinician and the pathologist is to decide, from the clinical and microscopical features, how the lesion will behave in the future; this process is almost entirely subjective and depends significantly on training and experience. Gradually, however, certain clinical and histopathological features are being shown to be indicative of premalignancy in oral lesions (see chapters 2, 18, and 19). Computer-aided studies (Kramer et al. 1970a and b) have brought greater direction to a consideration of the relative importance of various histopathological and cytopathological characteristics, but the initial recognition of these abnormalities remains subjective. Thus, there is a need for more objective methods to be applied to the evaluation of normal and abnormal epithelium, both for diagnostic reasons and to enhance our understanding of the biological and pathological changes occurring in epithelium.

Stereological techniques have been applied to biological problems for some 15 years and have provided valuable quantitative descriptions of many different organs and tissues. Most of this work has been performed by anatomists rather than pathologists, probably because the sampling of diseased tissue can be more of a problem than it is for normal tissue. Human oral epithelium has been analyzed by stereological methods at the ultrastructural level (Schroeder and Münzel-Pedrazzoli 1970; Meyer and Schroeder 1975; Klein-Szanto el al. 1976; Landay and Schroeder 1977; Bernimoulin and Schroeder 1977), but not at the histological level. In our laboratory, stereological techniques have been applied to histological sections of oral epithelium in an attempt to quantify cell and tissue parameters that may in some way be related to the features of epithelial atypia described in chapter 3. These studies have been confined to normal, hyperplastic, premalignant, and malignant hamster cheek pouch epithelium (Franklin 1977; Franklin and Craig 1978a and b). Stereological methods have also been applied at the ultrastructural level to similar hamster material (White and Squier 1974; White and Gohari 1976; White and Gohari 1977; White 1978; Gohari 1977).

2. STEREOLOGICAL PRINCIPLES

Stereological methods allow mathematical extrapolation of 3-dimensional structural information to be made from measurements performed on random 2-dimensional flat images. In histology, the flat images are obtained from sections of finite thickness. The profiles of the cut tissue elements are measured or counted within representative sections and from the data thus obtained, conclusions are drawn about the geometrical properties of the original 3-dimensional objects (Weibel and Gomez 1962; Weibel 1963; Weibel et al. 1966; Weibel 1969; Elias et al. 1971). Stereology depends upon the presence of identifiable structures in sections and is often based on the assumption that individual component parts of an organ, tissue, or cell are similar to each other in size and shape. Whilst this latter assumption is often held to be true for the more homogeneous tissues, some tissues contain varying proportions of components and cells which differ in size and shape. In certain tissues the cells or components, although differing in size and shape, still make up an ordered structure; such tissues are said to be anisotropic, and common examples are stratified epithelium, cerebral cortex, kidney, and muscle. When this occurs the regularity of the structure must be taken into account, usually by careful and adequate random sampling within, for example, each stratum, and by correct application of appropriate stereological test systems. Also, the variation in size and shape of tissues, cells and organelles as well as section thickness must be taken into consideration by the application, where necessary, of mathematical correction formulae.

Stereological techniques are based on the 'Delesse Principle' (Delesse 1848). This states that the fractional area of a section occupied by a given component is approximately equal to the volume proportions of that same component in its containing volume. Glagoleff (1934) found that the problem of estimating area could be resolved by superimposing a regular point lattice on the section and counting the points which lay on transections of the structures. This is based on the rationale that areas may be represented by points and that the area of a square, for example, can be represented by a point at the center of that square.

Many procedures have now been evolved from areal analysis; these include linear analysis in which area fractions of sectional components are estimated by measuring the intercept lengths of a series of test lines superimposed onto the section (Chalkley et al. 1949; Loud 1962) and point counting analysis in which volume proportions are related to the proportion of points falling on a given sectional component (Chalkley 1943; Hally 1964; Weibel 1969).

To determine the number of particles (i) in a given volume (i.e., volume density) of a cube (Fig. 1), a number of infinitely thin slices are first removed from the cube (Fig. 2); a regular point test lattice is then superimposed on each slice (Fig. 3). The number of points falling on the particles (Pi) is proportional to the area of these particles (Ai) and hence to their volume (Vi). This procedure is carried out for randomly selected slices and the average of all the volume density values is then calculated to find an expression for the whole cube. If a structure with a well-defined surface is contained within a tissue, the *surface density* is defined as the surface area of the structure present in unit volume of tissue. As a relationship has been established between area and volume, the number of structural profiles counted per unit area can be used to derive the number of structures per unit volume *(numerical density)*. However, this relationship also depends upon the size and shape of the structures, as well as section thickness. The volume to surface ratio of a structure is often of biological interest. This can be calculated from the data given by volume density and surface density determinations or alternatively, a combination of point and intersect counting can be employed using an interrupted test system with lines of equal length (Fig. 4).

Although these stereological parameters provide meaningful information, data obtained for an integrated functional unit (organ or cell) would be of additional value. Methods are available for this purpose (Loud 1968; Weibel et al. 1969; Rowden 1975). Nuclear diameters are directly measured and, by assuming them to be a particular shape such as a sphere or an ellipsoid, the volume is calculated by simple substitution of the mean diameter into a geometric formula. This provides an estimate of mean nuclear volume. The ratio of nucleus to cytoplasm is estimated stereologically and from this the volume of cytoplasm, and hence the mean cell volume, is calculated.

These principles may be similarly applied to electronmicrographs or light photomicrographs.

2:1 SAMPLING FOR STEREOLOGICAL PROCEDURES

Stereological measurements are based on geometrico-statistical principles; they are derived from the probability with which section profiles of structures coincide with an appropriate test system. The tissue sample must be confronted with the test system in a random manner (Weibel 1969), for which the method of systematic random sampling is preferable to simple random sampling (Ebbeson and Tang 1967; Hennig 1967).

2:2 DETERMINATION OF MINIMAL SAMPLE SIZE

Several methods exist for the determination of minimal sample size (Chalkley 1943; Hally 1964; DeHoff 1968; Weibel and Gnagi 1968; Burri et al. 1968); these rely on the fundamental principle that as sample size increases so the sampling error decreases.

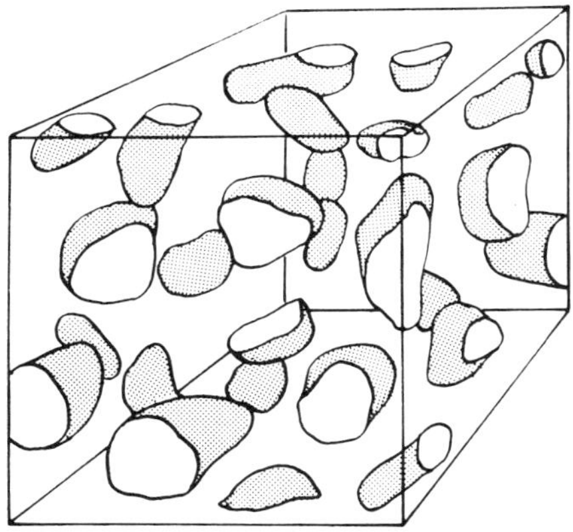

FIGURE 1. Cube containing a number of particles (i) for stereological analysis (modified from Weibel et al. 1966).

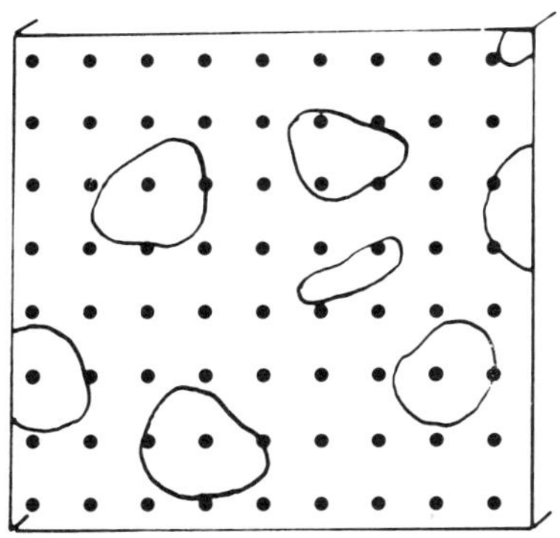

FIGURE 2. Infinitely thin section removed from cube (Fig. 1) for volumetric analysis by differential point counting (modified from Weibel et al. 1966).

3. APPLICATION OF AUTOMATED EQUIPMENT IN STEREOLOGY

During the last few years several sophisticated automatic and semiautomatic image analyzing computer systems have become available (Quantimet 720, Cambridge Instruments, England; Texture-Analyzing System, Leitz, West Germany; Manual Optical Image Analyzing System, Kontron, West Germany). In principle, the more sophisticated instruments operate by being able to distinguish varying shades of gray through to black in order to trace object area or perimeter on a computerized basis. They can operate directly by use of a television scanner through the microscope draw-tube or by examination of photomicrographs or drawings using an epidiascope attachment. These instruments function most efficiently when the objects under examination are isolated from each other and are clearly distinguishable as different shades of gray to black. This requirement can sometimes be achieved by using accessory electronic aids which "dilate" or "erode" the image. The advantage of these automatic systems is that they can provide rapid evaluation of data and can incorporate the various stereological correction procedures, thereby reducing the laborious process of manual counting. Unfortunately, neither ultrastructural nor histological staining techniques can produce electron micrographs, histological sections, or photomicrographs which show staining of identical structures in the same shade of gray. For example, electron micrographs may show several different structures with the same shade of gray, and the computer cannot then distinguish between them unless the operator traces the outline of the particular structure on the computer screen with a special light pen; this reintroduces the manual element. It is possible that these automatic systems can be improved and adapted for use in biological work, at which time they may become a valuable tool for rapid stereological and morphometric analysis.

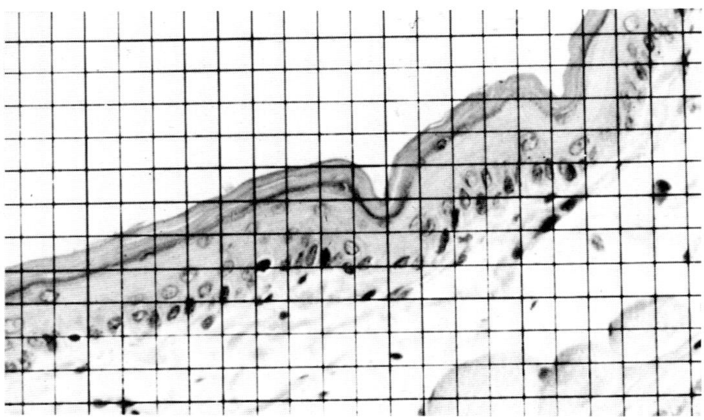

FIGURE 3. Normal hamster cheek pouch epithelium with centimeter square lattice superimposed. The intersections of lines serve as points for counting. The number of points falling on a component (i.e. nuclear profiles) is proportional to their volume fraction. Hematoxylin and eosin. X 330.

4. APPLICATION OF STEREOLOGICAL METHODS TO ORAL EPITHELIUM

Most biological work using stereology has been performed at the ultrastructural level because many cytological organelles can be evaluated.

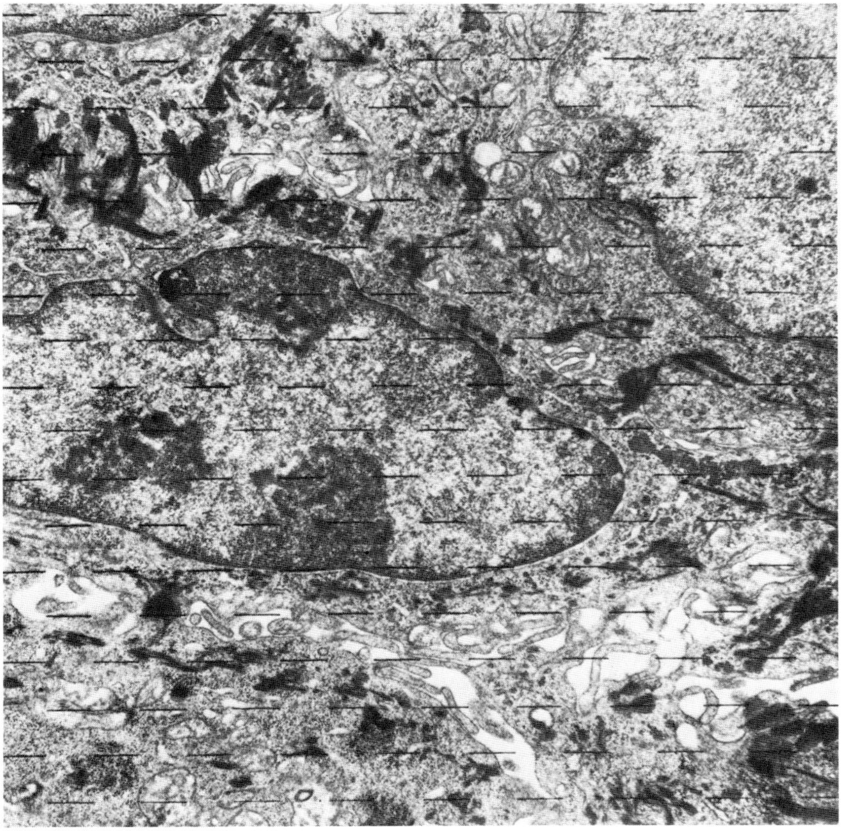

FIGURE 4. Electron micrograph of spinous cell with multipurpose test system superimposed for the estimation of volume to surface ratios.

Analysis of oral stratified squamous epithelium requires particular sampling techniques coupled, at the ultrastructural level, with certain assumptions, such as the existence of structural homogeneity within different strata (Schroeder and Münzell-Pedrazzoli 1970; Landay and Schroeder 1977). The aims of such studies have been to "(1) characterize the gradient of structural differentiation at different sites, (2) to compare the differentiation pattern of normal and pathologically altered epithelia, and (3) to establish a basis for correlating structure with chemistry and function of the various epithelial types" (Schroeder 1978). The stereological techniques used by Schroeder are based on analyses within histologically defined strata facilitated by specific computer programs (Hammer and Schroeder 1977).

Although stereological techniques are well established for use in electron microscopy, there have been only a few reports in which stereology has been applied to epithelia at the light microscope level (Sauter and Weibel 1971; Dunnill and Whitehead 1972; Underwood 1972; Risdon 1974; Risdon and Keeling 1974; Gerstl et al. 1976). This is probably due to the limited resolution of light microscopy for evaluating cytological details, and the difficulties that may be encountered in identifying profile boundaries in histological sections of finite thickness.

Our own recent work has been aimed at evaluating the potential of stereological techniques for the diagnosis and prognosis of oral epithelial lesions as well as for gaining more understanding of the biological changes and behavior of diseased epithelium. It was therefore decided to apply stereological techniques to histological sections in order to estimate parameters that may contribute to the various manifestations of epithelial atypia previously described (chapter 3).

The hamster cheek pouch was chosen as the experimental model because the early lesions produced often bear some resemblance to human oral leukoplakia (Salley 1954, 1957; Morris 1961; Smith 1968; and Smith, chapter 7). The main focus of our interest has been on the premalignant epithelial dysplasia and the preceding stage of epithelial hyperplasia, in which few atypical features are seen. Of particular concern has been the necessity to compare epithelial hyperplasia in the carcinogenesis model, which has to be considered premalignant though showing no overt features of such a potential, with epithelial hyperplasia that is known not to have premalignant connotations. Although a frictional model for producing epithelial hyperplasia in the cheek pouch mucosa is available (Mackenzie and Miles 1973), it was considered that chemically-induced epithelial hyperplasia would be more strictly comparable with the carcinogenesis model. Consequently, in one group of animals 50% oil of turpentine in liquid paraffin (TLP50) was used to produce a reversible epithelial hyperkeratosis (Craig and Franklin 1977). Carcinomas were produced in another group of animals by using the carcinogen 7–12 dimethylbenz (α) anthracene (DMBA) as a 0.5% solution in liquid paraffin.

After several weeks the DMBA-treated animals showed a range of pathological stages including epithelial hyperplasia, epithelial dysplasia, and invasive carcinoma. A stratified systematic random sampling procedure (Fig. 5) was used to obtain tissue from both groups of animals for analysis by light microscopy (Franklin and Craig 1978a). All the randomly selected sections from the DMBA-material were evaluated to determine the stages present and, with the exception of the carcinoma group, microscope fields of full thickness of epithelium were evaluated. Only invasive islands were analyzed in the carcinoma group.

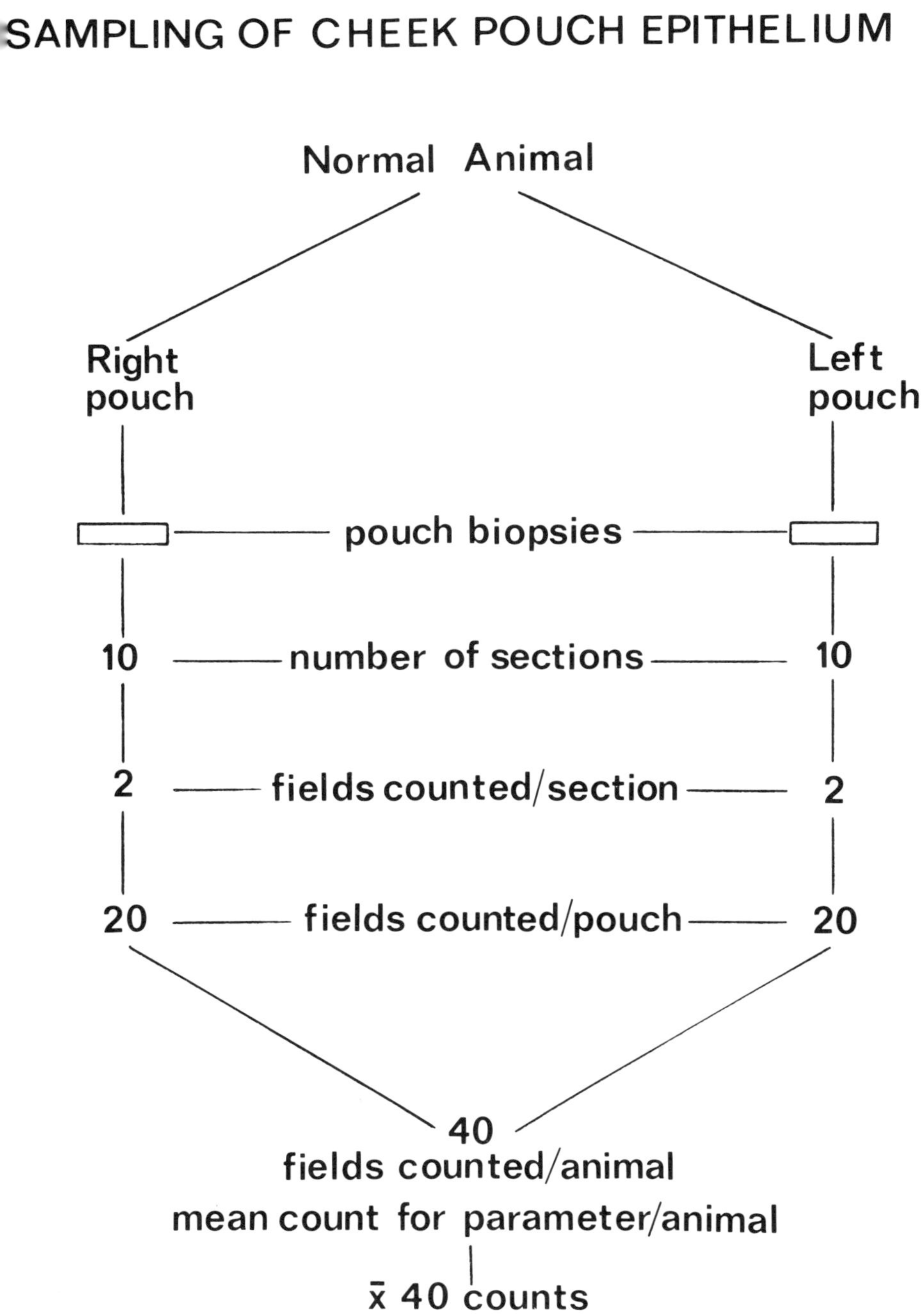

FIGURE 5. Scheme for systematic stratified random sampling of normal cheek pouch epithelium.

For electron microscopy, animals were selected from each of the normal, hyperplasia, dysplasia, and carcinoma groups.

A total of 10 parameters were evaluated at the light microscopic level (Table 1). The following provide illustrative examples of results that can be obtained from these methods:

1. Nuclear-cytoplasmic ratio.

The results (Fig. 6) showed a progressive increase in nuclear/cytoplasmic ratio through the DMBA-stages. However, the TLP50-hyperplasia has a value lower than control and hence quite different from the DMBA-hyperplasia. The differences in nuclear/cytoplasmic ratio between each stage were highly significant at $p < 0.001$ (t-test). When the figures were corrected for section thickness and nuclear diameter the trend was maintained.

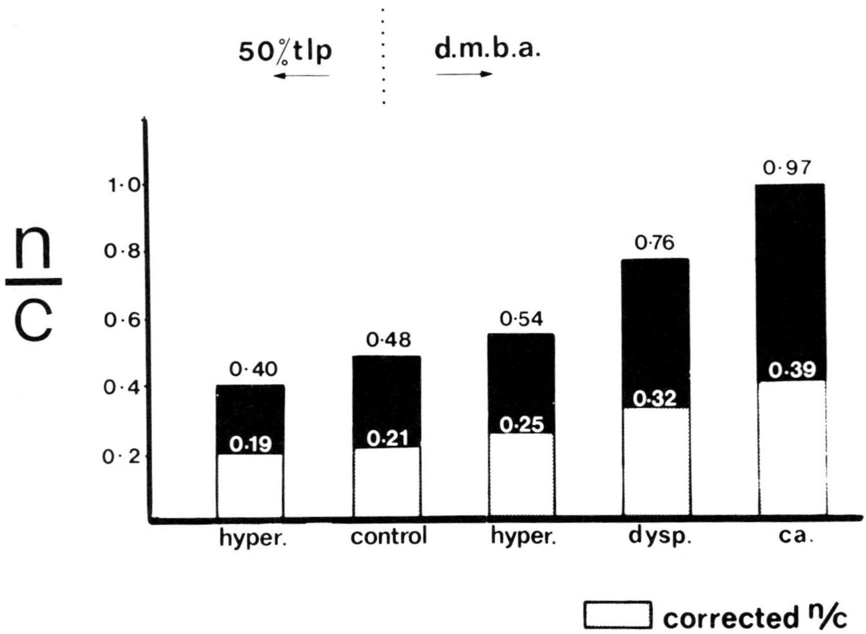

FIGURE 6. Histogram showing uncorrected and corrected values for nuclear-cytoplasmic ratio.

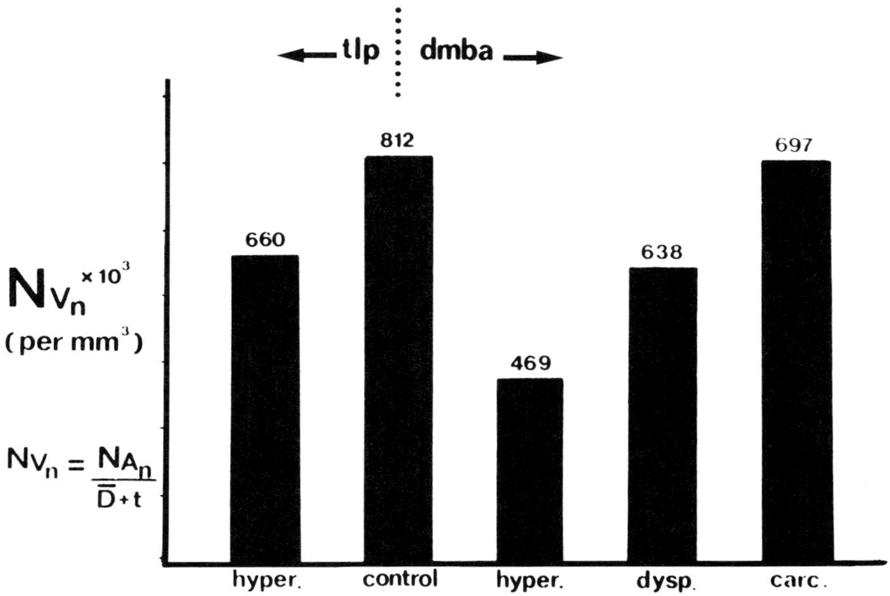

FIGURE 7. Histogram showing value for nuclei per unit volume (nuclear density) obtained using a correction factor which takes account of section thickness (t) and nuclear size ($\bar{D}$).

2. Nuclear numerical density (numbers of nuclei per unit volume).

The values for turpentine-hyperplasia were significantly different ($p < 0.001$) from those of DMBA-hyperplasia (Fig. 7).

3. Interface ratios of epithelium.

Using a Weibel grid of the type shown in Figure 8, it is possible to determine the volume to interface ratio for each interface. Furthermore, since the reference volume remains constant for each field it is possible to relate the interface surface areas directly by a simple numerical ratio.

As would be expected for normal hamster cheek pouch epithelium where there are no rete-ridges, the interface ratios were in a one to one relationship (Fig. 9). Unexpectedly, the TLP50-hyperplasia and dysplasia showed reduced ratios of 0.78 and 0.59 respectively. The TLP50-hyperplasia and DMBA-hyperplasia interface ratios were significantly different from the DMBA-dysplasia value ($p < 0.05$) but not from each other.

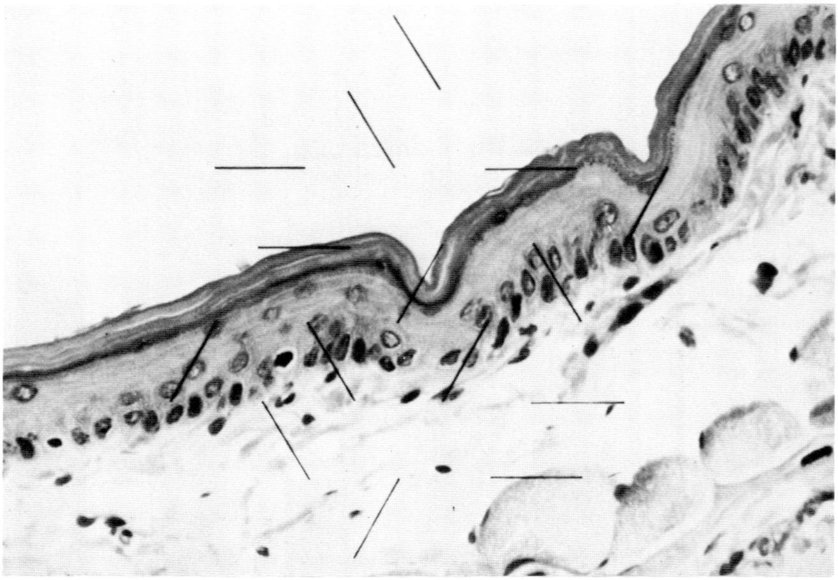

FIGURE 8. Normal hamster cheek pouch epithelium with Weibel grid superimposed. The end points of lines lying on the epithelium serve as volumetric points and the intersections of lines with the epithelial interfaces are proportional to interface area. Hematoxylin and eosin. X 360. Reprinted by permission from Franklin and Craig, 1978a.

At the ultrastructural level, estimations were made of many cell organelle parameters. In the spinous layer, for example, the numerical density of mitochondria in cytoplasm gradually decreased through the stages of carcinogenesis (Table 2). Although there was no significant difference between DMBA-hyperplasia and DMBA-dysplasia, these were both significantly different from the normal and carcinoma groups. On the other hand, cytochemically-positive lysosomal volume density decreased at first but in the carcinoma stage was double the normal value (Table 3). The number of desmosomes per unit area of cell surface decreased from normal through to carcinoma. This has been suspected for some time, but with these techniques it has been established on a firm quantitative basis (Table 4).

4:1 COMMENTS ON LIGHT MICROSCOPIC APPLICATIONS

At present, there is little work which has accurately quantified histological parameters in oral epithelium. Some comparison may be made with quantitative work undertaken on the human uterine cervix, but this has comprised mostly planimetric and simple mensurative studies performed on exfoliated whole cells. Nuclear and cellular area have been estimated for these cells either by planimetric estimation of projected areas or computed from direct microscope measurement of cell and nuclear diameters (Foraker and Reagan 1956; Reagan and Hamonic 1956; Reagan et al. 1957; Hillemanns et al. 1968a; Hillemanns et al. 1968b; Hillemanns and Prestel 1968; Meyer-Arendt and Humphries 1972). The results from these studies all show a trend towards an increase in nuclear size from normal through squamous metaplasia, atypical hyperplasia, dysplasia or carcinoma in situ, where the changes appear to be maximal. With invasive carcinoma the nuclear size diminishes slightly but is still greater than normal. The cell size is largest in normal cells and gradually reduces through the above stages, being at its smallest in invasive carcinoma. The nuclear/cytoplasmic ratio therefore increases through all the stages in much the same way as occurs in hamster cheek pouch carcinogenesis. A stereological analysis of bladder tumors (Fulker et al. 1976) has shown that relative nuclear volume (nucleus to cell ratio) increases as the tumors become less well-differentiated.

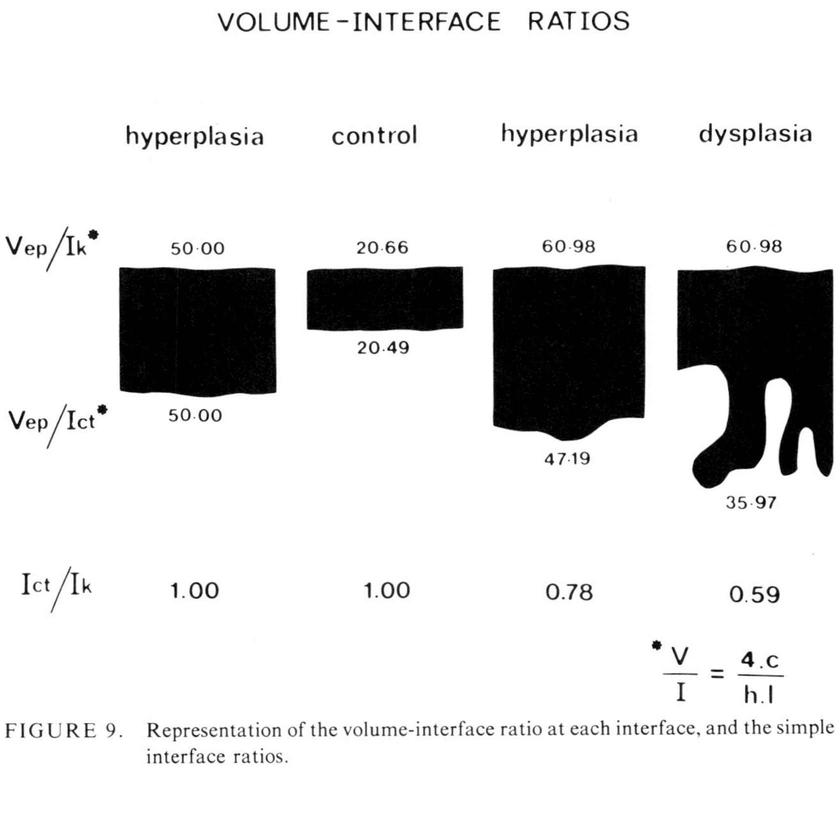

FIGURE 9. Representation of the volume-interface ratio at each interface, and the simple interface ratios.

TABLE 1 Parameters developed for analysis of histological material.

STEREOLOGICAL PARAMETERS

Cytological

- nuclear - cytoplasmic ratio
- Nuclear volume fraction
- mean nuclear diameter
- nuclei/ unit volume
- nuclear and cytoplasmic volume of 'average cell'
- 'average cells' / unit volume

Epithelial

- volume of epithelium
- volume - interface ratios (keratin interface)
  (connective tissue interface)
- interface ratio (keratin/ connective tissue)

TABLE 2

MITOCHONDRIA/ UNIT VOLUME CYTOPLASM

($N_{V_{mit}}$)

spinous layer

	DMBA - induced		
normal	hyperplasia	dysplasia	carcinoma
2.36 ± 0.45	1.60 ± 0.27	1.52 ± 0.37	1.08 ± 0.31

5 animals each group - mean value ± s.d.

TABLE 3

VOLUME DENSITY: LYSOSOMES IN CYTOPLASM

($V_{V_{ly}}$)

spinous layer

normal	DMBA - induced hyperplasia	DMBA - induced dysplasia	DMBA - induced carcinoma
0.0004 ± 0.0002 (0.04%)	0.00022 ± 0.0001 (0.02%)	0.00016 ± 0.00008 (0.016%)	0.0009 ± 0.0004 (0.09%)

5 animals each group - mean value ± s.d.

TABLE 4

DESMOSOMES/UNIT SURFACE AREA PLASMA MEMBRANE

($N_{S_{des}}$)

spinous layer

normal	DMBA - induced hyperplasia	DMBA - induced dysplasia	DMBA - induced carcinoma
1.41 ± 0.36	1.14 ± 0.06	0.87 ± 0.13	0.47 ± 0.06

5 animals each group - mean value ± s.d.

Two studies of human uterine cervix have evaluated cell counts per unit area (Castano-Almendral and Beato 1968; Hillemanns et al. 1968a). It is not quite clear what has actually been counted, but the estimates are probably based on counting nuclear profiles. These studies suggest that there is an increased cell count/unit area with increasing severity of dysplasia, which reaches its maximum in carcinoma in situ (278% of the normal); it has been suggested by Hillemanns et al. (1968b) that this is the "critical cell number" necessary for infiltration. The cell count/unit area falls in micro-invasive carcinomas to 128% of normal and to 95% of normal in invasive carcinoma; with advanced carcinoma the value rises again to 140% of normal. Similar changes were noted in hamster cheek pouch experiments (Franklin 1977).

4:2 COMMENTS ON ELECTRON MICROSCOPIC APPLICATIONS

Quantitative methods have been used at the ultrastructural level by Schroeder and his colleagues to provide relative (or percentage) values rather than absolute values and thus to provide comparative data in relation to unit volumes of epithelial stratum or of epithelial cytoplasm within a given stratum (see chapter 9). Similar techniques have been applied to biopsies of homogeneous oral leukoplakias (Klein-Szanto et al. 1976) from which it could be shown that leukoplakic epithelium from floor of mouth had a composition similar to that of leukoplakic cheek mucosa, but the epithelium of clinically normal floor of mouth was strikingly different. In leukoplakia epithelium, for example, nuclear, mitochondrial, and membrane-bound organelle volume densities decreased gradually from the basal layer to the granular layer, whereas in normal floor of mouth epithelium the volume density of tissue components changed in a stepwise fashion rather than forming continuous gradients.

Quantitative data obtained at the ultrastructural level can be usefully compared with biochemical information which is available for both normal and pathological conditions. The results obtained for the numerical density of mitochondria per unit volume of epithelium in premalignant and malignant hamster cheek pouch mucosa provide an example of the potential value of such comparisons. Warburg (1931) first suggested that malignant cells modify fermentation glycolytic mechanisms and a correlation has also been found between growth rate and glycolytic activity in malignant tissues (Burk et al. 1967; Johnson, chapter 20). Furthermore, an increase in lactate dehydrogenase activity and decrease in succinate dehydrogenase activity have been reported in hamster cheek pouch epithelium during carcinogenesis (Shklar 1965), and similar observations have been made on premalignant and malignant lesions of human oral mucosa (Cabrini 1973). The observed depletion of epithelial mitochondria in hamster cheek pouch carcinogenesis may be correlated with the reduced activity of mitochondrial enzymes.

Similarly, the increase in volume density of lysosomes supports previous biochemical and histochemical findings in malignant tumors (Smith 1972;

Poole 1973; Allison 1974). It may be, also, that lysosomal hydrolases are responsible for cell surface modifications that could interfere with intercellular attachment mechanisms (Weinstein et al. 1976; Poste and Weiss 1976), and the increased volume density of lysosomes may be related to the reduced frequency of desmosomes observed during hamster cheek pouch carcinogenesis.

5. CONCLUSIONS

Stereological methods can be used to provide reliable and accurate quantitative information. At the ultrastructural level these methods may find most value in comparison of normal site variation and patterns of differentiation; they will also be able to define baselines for pathological studies not primarily directed towards diagnosis. However, future developments may make electron microscopical techniques more amenable for diagnosis. At the histological level some studies have already shown diagnostic potential (Dunnill and Whitehead 1972; Risdon and Keeling 1974). In the histological studies performed on hamster cheek pouch the aim was to obtain quantitative values for parameters that may be related to the cytological and histological features of atypia described by Pindborg et al. (1963) and Kramer et al. (1970a and b). Of all the stereological parameters investigated at the light microscopic level, the nuclear/cytoplasmic ratio, nuclear density, and the interface ratios were best able to distinguish between benign and premalignant epithelium. These parameters would therefore seem to have the most diagnostic potential for evaluation of human oral mucosal lesions, and work along these lines is currently being undertaken in our laboratory. Since a pathologist's subjective impression of a particular feature may vary from day to day, and different pathologists evaluating the same feature may not agree on its severity or the extent to which it is present, this new possibility to obtain reproducible data may be a useful advance.

Stereological analysis of epithelium can be useful not only in the evaluation of parameters of special interest suggested by other observations, be they morphological, histochemical or biochemical, but also the results obtained from such an approach may point the way towards further specific nonmorphological investigations of biological and pathological problems. Before any stereological parameter can be considered of definitive value as a marker of malignant change or in diagnosis however, other disease processes in epithelium must also be evaluated. Consideration should also be given to the inherent biological and site variations which exist in normal epithelium.

ACKNOWLEDGEMENTS

The authors are grateful for financial support provided by the Medical Research Council (CJS, CDF, and FW), the Wellcome Trust (FW), the Yorkshire Branch of the Cancer Research Campaign (KG), and the Council of Europe (CDF). We are also grateful to Dr. T. M. Mayhew for advice on the application of stereological methods, and to Mr. M. Rudland and the technical staff of the Department of Oral Pathology, University of Sheffield, for the high quality of their technical assistance.

REFERENCES

Aherne, W. 1967. Methods of counting discrete tissue components in microscopical sections. *J. Roy. Micr. Soc.* **87**, 493–508.

Allison, A. C. 1974. Lysosomes in cancer cells. *J. Clin. Pathol.* Suppl. **7**, 43–50.

Alvares, O. F., and Meyer, J. 1971. Variable features and regional differences in oral epithelium. In: *Current Concepts of the Histology of Oral Mucosa.* (Edited by Squier, C. A., and Meyer, J.), Chap. 5, pp. 97–113. Charles C Thomas, Springfield, Illinois.

Barka, T., and Anderson, P. J. 1962. Histochemical methods for acid phosphatase using hexzonium pararosanalin as coupler. *J. Histochem. Cytochem.* **10,** 741–753.

Bernimoulin, J. P., and Schroeder, H. E. 1977. Quantitative electron microscopic analysis of the epithelium of normal human alveolar mucosa. *Cell Tiss. Res.* **180**, 383–401.

Burk, D., Woods, H., and Hunter, J. 1967. On the significance of glucolysis for cancer growth, with special reference to Morris rat hepatomas. *J. Natl. Cancer Inst.* **38**, 839–863.

Burri, P. H., Giger, H., Gnägi, H. R., and Weibel, E. R. 1968. Application of stereologic methods to cytophysiologic experiments on polarized cells. In: *Electron Microscopy 1968: Pre-Congress Abstracts of Papers Presented at the Fourth European Regional Conference Held in Rome.* (Edited by Bocciarelli, D. S.), Vol. 1, pp. 593–594. Tipographia Poliglotta Vaticana, Rome.

Cabrini, R. L. 1973. Histochemistry of early oral cancer. *Int. Dent. J.* **23**, 101–107.

Castano-Almendral, A., and Beato, M. 1968. Die Frühstadien des Plattenepithelcarcinoms des Collum uteri. II. Histometrische Untersuchungen. *Arch. Gynaek.* **205**, 428–451.

Chalkley, H. W. 1943. Method for quantitative morphologic analysis of tissues. *J. Natl. Cancer Inst.* **4**, 47–53.

Chalkley, H. W., Cornfield, J., and Park, H. 1949. A method for estimating volume-surface ratios. *Science* **110,** 295–297.

Craig, G. T., and Franklin, C. D. 1977. The effect of turpentine on hamster cheek pouch mucosa: A model of epithelial hyperplasia and hyperkeratosis. *J. Oral Path.* **6**, 268–277.

DeHoff, R. T. 1968. Quantitative metallography. In: *Techniques of Metals Research. Volume 11: Techniques for the Direct Observation of Structure and Imperfections, Part 1.* (Edited by Bunshah, R. F.), pp. 221–253. John Wiley, New York.

DeHoff, R. T., and Rhines, F. N. 1961. Determination of the number of particles per unit volume from measurements made on random plane sections: The general cylinder and the ellipsoid. *Tr. Metall. Soc. AIME* **221**, 975–982.

Delesse, M. A. 1848. Procede mechanique pour determines la composition des roches. *Ann. des Mines* **13**, 379–388.

Dunnill, M. S., and Whitehead, R. 1972. A method for the quantitation of small intestinal biopsy specimens. *J. Clin. Pathol.* **25**, 243–246.

Ebbesson, S. O., and Tang, D. H. 1967. A comparison of sampling procedures in a structured cell population. In: *Stereology. Proceedings of the Second International Congress for Stereology, Chicago, Apr. 8–13, 1967.* (Edited by Elias, Hans), pp. 131–132. Springer-Verlag, New York.

Elias, H., Henning, A., and Schwartz, D. E. 1971. Stereology: Applications to biomedical research. *Physiol. Rev.* **51**, 158–200.

Elze, C., and Hennig, A. 1956. Die inspiratorische Vergrösserung von Volumen und innererOoberfläche der menschlichen Lunge. *Ztschr. Anat.* **119**, 457–469.

Foraker, A. G., and Reagan, J. W. 1956. Nuclear size and nuclear-cytoplasmic ratio in the delineation of atypical hyperplasia of the uterine cervix. *Cancer* **9**, 470–479.

Franklin, C. D. 1977. Development of experimental hyperplasia and neoplasia in hamster cheek pouch epithelium: A stereological investigation. Ph.D. dissertation, University of Sheffield.

Franklin, C. D., and Craig, G. T. 1978a. Stereological quantification of histological parameters in normal hamster cheek pouch epithelium. *Arch. Oral Biol.* **23**, 337–345.

Franklin, C. D., and Craig, G. T. 1978b. Stereological quantification of histological parameters in turpentine-induced hyperplasia of hamster cheek pouch epithelium. *Arch. Oral Biol.* **23**, 347–353.

Fulker, M. J., Adamthwaite, S. J., and Anderson, C. K. 1976. Stereological measurements of bladder tumour morphology. *Eur. J. Cancer* **12**, 575–579.

Gerstl, B., Wong, S., and Yesner, R. 1976. Quantitative microscopy of epidermoid lung carcinoma: Correlation with survival time. *J. Natl. Cancer Inst.* **56**, 463–469.

Glagoleff, A. A. 1934. Quantitative analysis with the microscope by the "point" method. *Engineering & Mining J.* **135**, 399–400.

Gohari, K. 1977. A quantitative and cytochemical study of the synthetic metabolic apparatus in hamster cheek pouch epithelium during chemical carcinogenesis. Ph.D. dissertation, University of Sheffield.

Gomori, G. 1952. *Microscopic Histochemistry: Principles and Practice*, pp. 189–197. University of Chicago Press, Chicago.

Hally, A. D. 1964. A counting method for measuring the volumes of tissue components in microscopical sections. *Quart. J. Microscop. Sci.* **105**, 503–517.

Hammer, B., and Schroeder, H. E. 1977. Stereologic system and on/off-line computer program for analysing oral epithelia, based on a model of stratification. *Arch. Oral Biol.* **22**, 337–341.

Haug, H. 1967. Probleme und methoden der strukturzählung im Schnittpräparat. In: *Quantitative Methods in Morphology.* (Edited by Weibel, E. R., and Elias, H.), pp. 58–78. Springer-Verlag, Berlin.

Hennig, A. 1967. Fehlerbetrachtungen zur Volumenbestimmung aus der Integration ebener Schnitte. In: *Quantitative Methods in Morphology.* (Edited by Weibel, E., and Elias, H.), pp. 99–129. Springer-Verlag, Berlin.

Hillemanns, H. G., and Prestel, E. 1968. Karyometrie mit dem Teilchengrössenanalysator (TGZ) am Beispiel des Cervixcarcinoms und seiner Vorstufen. *Z. Krebsforsch.* **71**, 316–319.

Hillemanns, H. G., Fröhlich, D., and Prestel, E. 1968a. Zellzahl und Mitosefrequenz bei entstehung des Cervixcarcinoms (zum Carcinoma in situ und Mikrocarcinom der Cervix). *Arch. Gynaek.* **206**, 292–319.

Hillemanns, H. G., Sixtux-Klug, B., and Prestel, E. 1968b. Cytoplasmakernrelationen der Malignitätsstufen des Cervixepithels, gemessen mit dem Integrationsocular. I. Zum Carcinoma in situ und Mikrocarcinom der Cervix. *Arch. Gynaek.* **206**, 82–97.

Karnovsky, M. J. 1965. A formaldehyde-glutaraldehyde fixative of high osmolarity for use in electron microscopy. *J. Cell Biol.* **27**, 137A–138A.

Klein-Szanto, A. J., Bánóczy, J., and Schroeder, H. E. 1976. Metaplastic conversion of the differentiation pattern in oral epithelia affected by leukoplakia simplex. A stereologic study. *Pathol. Eur.* **11,** 189–210.

Kramer, I. R. H., Lucas, R. B., El-Labban, N., and Lister, L. 1970a. A computer-aided study on the tissue changes in oral keratoses and lichen planus, and an analysis of the groupings by subjective and objective criteria. *Br. J. Cancer* **24**, 407–424.

Kramer, I. R. H., Lucas, R. B., El-Labban, N., and Lister, L. 1970b. The use of discriminant analysis for examining the histological features of oral keratoses and lichen planus. *Br. J. Cancer* **24**, 673–683.

Landay, M. A., and Schroeder, H. E. 1977. Quantitative electron microscopic analysis of the stratified epithelium of normal human buccal mucosa. *Cell Tiss. Res.* **177**, 383–405.

Loud, A. V. 1962. A method for the quantitative estimation of cytoplasmic structure. *J. Cell Biol.* **15**, 481–487.

Loud, A. V. 1968. A quantitative stereological description of the ultrastructure of normal rat liver parenchymal cells. *J. Cell Biol.* **37**, 27–46.

Mackenzie, I. C., and Miles, A. E. 1973. The effect of chronic frictional stimulation on hamster cheek pouch epithelium. *Arch. Oral Biol.* **18**, 1341–1349.

Meyer-Arendt, J. R., and Humphreys, D. M. 1972. Quantitative morphology of cancer cells. *Acta Histochem.* **44**, 41–48.

Meyer, M., and Schroeder, H. E. 1975. Quantitative electron microscopic analysis of the keratinizing epithelium of normal human hard palate. *Cell Tiss. Res.* **158**, 177–203.

Morris, A. L. 1961. Factors influencing experimental carcinogenesis in the hamster cheek pouch. *J. Dent. Res.* **40**, 3–15.

Pindborg, J. J., Renstrup, G., Poulsen, H. E., and Silverman, S., Jr. 1963. Studies in oral leukoplakias. V. Clinical and histologic signs of malignancy. *Acta Odont. Scand.* **21**, 407–414.

Poole, A. R. 1973. Tumour lysosomal enzymes and invasive growth. In: *Frontiers of Biology, Vol. 29. Lysosomes in Biology and Pathology.* (Edited by Dingle, J. T.), Vol. 3, pp. 303–337. Elsevier/North Holland, Amsterdam, American Elsevier, New York.

Poste, G., and Weiss, L. 1976. Some considerations on cell surface alterations in malignancy. In: *Fundamental Aspects of Metastasis.* (Edited by Weiss, L.), pp. 25–47. Elsevier/North Holland, Amsterdam.

Reagan, J. W., and Hamonic, M. J. 1956. The cellular pathology in carcinoma in situ, cytohistopathological correlation. *Cancer* **9**, 385–402.

Reagan, J. W., Hamonic, M. J., and Wentz, W. B. 1957. Analytical study of the cells in cervical squamous-cell cancer. *Lab. Invest.* **6**, 241–250.

Reynolds, E. S. 1963. The use of lead citrate at high pH as an electron opaque stain in electron microscopy. *J. Cell. Biol.* **17**, 208–212.

Risdon, R. A. 1974. Quantitation of histological changes in the glomeruli in renal biopsy specimens from children: Total and different glomerular cell counts. *J. Pathol.* **114,** 185–197.

Risdon, R. A., and Keeling, J. W. 1974. Quantitation of the histological changes found in small intestinal biopsy specimens from children with suspected coeliac disease. *Gut* **15,** 9–18.

Rowden, G. 1975. Ultrastructural studies of keratinized epithelia of the mouse. III. Determination of the volumes of nuclei and cytoplasm of cells in murine epidermis. *J. Invest. Dermatol.* **64**, 1–3.

Salley, J. J. 1954. Experimental carcinogenesis in the cheek pouch of the Syrian hamster. *J. Dent. Res.* **33**, 253–262.

Salley, J. J. 1957. Histologic changes in the hamster cheek pouch during early hydrocarbon carcinogenesis. *J. Dent. Res.* **36**, 48–55.

Sauter, L. S., and Weibel, E. R. 1971. Morphometric evaluation of skin structures by stereologic methods. Application to testosterone-treated rats. *Dermatologica* **143**, 174–183.

Schroeder, H. E. 1978. Mucous membranes. In: *Stereological Principles for Biomorphometry.* (Edited by Weibel, E. R.) Academic Press, New York, London. In press.

Schroeder, H. E., and Münzel-Pedrazzoli, S. 1970. Application of stereologic methods to stratified gingival epithelia. *J. Microsc.* **92**, 179–198.

Shklar, G. 1965. Metabolic characteristics of experimental hamster cheek pouch carcinomas. *Oral Surg.* **20**, 336–339.

Smith, C. J. 1968. Experimental carcinogenesis in the hamster cheek pouch: A histochemical investigation. Ph.D. dissertation, University of London, England.

Smith, C. J. 1972. Variations in histochemical properties of hydrolytic enzymes in oral precancerous conditions. *J. Dent. Res.* **51**, 308–318.

Underwood, J. C. 1972. A morphometric analysis of human breast carcinoma. *Br. J. Cancer* **26**, 234–237.

Warburg, O. 1931. *The Metabolism of Tumours.* R. Smith, New York.

Weibel, E. R. 1963. Principles and methods for the morphometric study of the lung and other organs. *Lab. Invest.* **12**, 131–155.

Weibel, E. R. 1969. Stereological principles for morphometry in electron microscopic cytology. *Int. Rev. Cytol.* **26**, 235–302.

Weibel, E. R., and Gnägi, H. R. 1968. Improvements in efficiency of stereologic methods in electron microscopic cytology. In: *Electron Microscopy.* (Edited by Bocciarelli, D. S.), Vol. I, pp. 601–602. Tipografia Poliglotta Vaticana, Rome.

Weibel, E. R., and Gomez, D. M. 1962. A principle for counting tissue structures on random sections. *J. Appl. Physiol.* **17**, 343–348.

Weibel, E. R., Kistler, G. S., and Scherle, W. F. 1966. Practical stereological methods for morphometric cytology. *J. Cell Biol.* **30**, 23–38.

Weibel, E. R., Stäubli, W., Gnägi, H. R., and Hess, F. A. 1969. Correlated morphometric and biochemical studies on the liver cell. I. Morphometric model, stereologic methods, and normal morphometric data for rat liver. *J. Cell Biol.* **42**, 68–91.

Weinstein, R. S., Merk, F. B., and Alroy, J. 1976. The structure and function of intercellular junctions in cancer. *Adv. Cancer Res.* **23**, 23–89.

White, F. H. 1978. A stereological study of hamster cheek pouch epithelium: Ultrastructural changes in differentiation and chemical carcinogenesis. Ph.D. dissertation, University of Sheffield, England.

White, F. H., and Gohari, K. 1976. The ultrastructure of differentiation in hamster cheek pouch epithelium. II. Quantitative studies. Abstract. *J. Dent Res.* **55**, D147.

White, F. H., and Gohari, K. 1977. An ultrastructural quantitative study of chemically-induced carcinomas in hamster cheek pouch epithelium. Abstract. *J. Dent. Res.* **56**, D101.

White, F. H., and Squier, C. A. 1974. A quantitative study of the intercellular and basal attachment apparatus in hamster cheek pouch epithelium during carcinogenesis. Abstract. *J. Dent. Res.* **53**, 1072.

16

Immunological Aspects of Chemical Carcinogenesis

H. C. OUTZEN

The Jackson Laboratory, Bar Harbor, Maine

Interest in the relationship between neoplasia and immunity has been present since tumors were shown to carry tumor-related neoantigens recognizable by the host (Prehn and Main 1957; Klein et al. 1960). The exact role of the hosts' immune response on tumor induction and progression has yet to be resolved—is it stimulatory, inhibitory, or neither?

The question of whether or not the immune response may help regulate the growth of a tumor is based on the premise that a tumor is able to induce an immune response. It is becoming apparent that many tumors, particularly those occurring spontaneously, do not stimulate an immunologic reaction (Hewitt et al. 1976; Prehn and Main 1957). There is no question, however, that the majority of the tumors induced by chemical and viral oncogens, at least in the laboratory, do elicit a strong immune response.

Past investigations of the relationship between antigenicity, latent period, and tumor incidence suggest that there is an immunologic effect on tumor growth and progression (Prehn and Lappé 1971). Early studies in tumor immunology determined that some carcinogen induced tumors were highly antigenic while others were only weakly or nonantigenic. The dosage of carcinogen was shown to correlate directly with the tumor latent periods, higher doses of carcinogen producing tumors with shorter latent periods (Bryan and Shimkin 1943; Prehn 1975; Stutman 1975b). Tumors of relatively high immunogenicity generally had shorter latent periods (Prehn 1975; Bartlett 1972; Old et al. 1962). A direct relationship between tumor immunogenicity and carcinogen dose occurred when tumors induced with high or low doses of carcinogen but with similar latent periods were compared (Prehn 1975). This relationship, however, was not seen when a different antigenicity test system, a different method of carcinogen application, and another mouse strain were used (Stutman 1975b).

Tumor induction experiments with methylcholanthrene (MCA) (Outzen et al. 1975; Stutman 1975a) or urethane (Stutman 1975a) have not demonstrated any differences in tumor incidence between nude (nu/nu) mice,[1] heterozygous (nu/+) mice or normal (+/+) mice in either germfree (Outzen et al. 1975) or conventional (Stutman 1975a) mouse colonies. The spontaneous tumor incidence also was not significantly different between these groups of mice (Outzen et al. 1975; Stutman 1975a; Rygaard and Povlsen 1976), with the exception that old nude mice tended to develop a much higher incidence of lymphoreticular tumors than their haired littermates (Outzen et al. 1975; Giovanella, B. 1977, personal communication).

Growth inhibition of allogeneic or xenogeneic grafts of normal tissues in nude mice has not been detected, yet tumor transplants, xenogeneic ones in particular, tend to grow slower and show less invasion and metastasis in nude mice than in their syngeneic strain of origin (Maguire et al. 1976). This growth resistance to xenogeneic tumor transplanted subcutaneously in nude mice is radiosensitive and can be deleted by X-irradiation (Irvin et al. 1975; Prehn and Outzen 1977). Highly immunogenic MCA-induced sarcomas also grew much better when transplanted subcutaneously into X-irradiated nude mice than in nonirradiated nude controls, however MCA-induced tumors with little or no immunogenicity grew equally well in both groups of nude mice (Prehn and Outzen 1977). These reports using transplantable malignant sarcomas suggest that the nude mouse retains some ability to recognize tumor related antigens that are immunogenic in normal mice, and this response can be greatly depressed by X-irradiation of the nude mouse.

Studies on skin tumor induction in nude mice have shown that nude mice develop fewer tumors than heterozygous (nu/+) mice (Holland et al. 1977; Reed 1974), than nude (nu/nu) mice restored with thymus tissues (Holland et al. 1977; Reed 1974), or than hairless (hr/hr) mice (Schjerven et al. 1974). In these studies the carcinogen was directly applied to the host animal's skin and the immunosuppressive effect of the carcinogen (Prehn 1963; Stjernswärd 1965) may possibly have influenced the interpretation of the results. Since most carcinogens are immunosuppressive, experiments comparing carcinogen treated mice which originally were believed to be immunologically different may be difficult to interpret; in reality the immunological differences may not be as great as thought.

Papilloma induction in MCA-treated skin grafts (Lappé 1968), however, lends itself to tumor progression studies. This technique permits the

[1] The nude mouse (nu/nu) is a hairless congenitally athymic mouse mutant (Pantelouris 1968). The nude gene *nu* is recessive and in the heterozygous (nu/+) state causes no major immunological defects but when homozygous (nu/nu) the cellular immune system is deleted. Due to the congenital absence of the thymus, the nude mouse cannot raise a cell-mediated immune response and will accept permanently grafts of allogeneic and xenogeneic normal and tumor tissue (Rygaard 1969, 1974a, 1974b, 1974c, Rygaard and Povlsen 1969). The immune reactivity can be restored in nude mice by thymus transplants.

inductive steps of neoplastic transformation to occur in a donor mouse away from the recipient. As the tumor induction phase occurred in donor mice the systemic immunosuppressive effects of MCA were isolated and could not play a major role in affecting the immunologic status of the recipients.

Cell transfer experiments have shown that thymus-dependent immunity in nude mice may be restored using thymus or spleen cell grafts obtained from normal donors (Kindred and Wiler 1972; Schmidt and Good 1975). The thymus, spleen, and other peripheral lymphoid tissues contain a large number of thymus derived cells (T-cells) which are the cells responsible for maintaining cell-mediated immune functions in an animal. Bone marrow, however, is essentially free of T-cells, but contains all the other hematopoietic elements. Partial or complete restoration of the T-cell dependent immune function could be demonstrated by transplanting various numbers of T-cells into nude mice (Kindred 1975).

Papillomas induced on MCA-treated skin grafted onto recipient mice which range in a series of discrete steps in their immunologic capacity could be used to test whether or not the immune system can influence the rate benign skin papilloma progress towards malignancy. Immunodeficient nude mice, which were either X-irradiated or not, were altered immunologically by injecting them intraperitoneally with various numbers of spleen cells obtained from immunologically normal (+/+) donors. MCA-treated skin grafted onto these recipients developed numerous papillomas within a short period of time. The incidence, latent period, and progression of these papillomas in these preliminary experiments was markedly affected by the immune status of the recipients. Nonirradiated nude mice that had received moderate numbers (10^5) of spleen cells developed as many papillomas (13 tumors/15 mice) as the immunologically normal heterozygous (nu/+) controls (13 tumors/15 mice). Nonrestored nude mice, however, developed fewer papillomas (6 tumors/15 mice). Papilloma induction in 300 R X-irradiated nude mice restored with 10^2, or 10^7 immunologically normal spleen cells followed a similar pattern. X-irradiated nude mice receiving 10^2 spleen cells developed more papillomas (12 tumors/18 mice) than either those mice receiving no spleen cells (8 tumors/18 mice) or those receiving 10^7 spleen cells (4 tumors/18 mice). The average papilloma survival times were longer and their latent periods shorter in the nude mice restored with low to moderate numbers of spleen cells than in any of the other groups of mice.

Nonmutant normal mice were thymectomized, lethally X-irradiated and bone-marrow repopulated (TXB)[2] to produce another type of T-cell immunodeficient mouse that could be used instead of the nude mouse.

These TXB mice were tested to determine whether or not the results observed were restricted to nude mice or were a general phenomena that only depended on the modulation of the recipients immunologic parameters. The TXB mice that received 10^2 spleen cells also developed more skin tumors (36 tumors/31 mice) than TXB mice reconstituted with 10^7 spleen cells (19 tumors/23 mice) or mice that were not given spleen cells (20 tumors/23 mice). The average time that the grafts were tumor free was longer in the mice reconstituted with 10^7 spleen cells (52.9 days) than in those reconstituted with 10^2 spleen cells (33.3 days) or not reconstituted (47.8 days).

A random sample of the tumors developing in the immunomodulated mice was examined histologically for a dermal inflammatory response, cellular anaplasia and malignant carcinomatous invasion. Carcinomatous invasion was histologically confirmed more frequently in mice restored with spleen cells (7/18) than in those not restored (3/18). Mice restored with low numbers of spleen cells demonstrated more cellular anaplasia histologically than did either of the other groups (Table 1). No significant correlation was seen between the amount of dermal inflammatory response and the number of spleen cells the mice received. Histologic signs of malignant carcinomatous invasion, however, tended to correlate with the presence of a stromal inflammatory response ($p < 0.1$). In these tumors it appeared that the dermal infiltrate, as it was generally associated with carcinomatous invasion, was acting in a stimulatory fashion on tumor progression. This is contrary to the generally recognized viewpoint that an infiltrate is associated with immunosurveillance (Ioachim 1976) but Prehn (1977b) recently has refuted this argument.

Partial immunorestoration of nude mice apparently does influence tumor occurrence and progression. The studies reported in this paper, though preliminary, all show a trend in the same direction. Highly immunodepressed mice, whether they are nude, X-irradiated nude, or thymectomized, X-irradiated, bone-marrow repopulated, normal (+/+) mice, develop more tumors with reduced latent periods and more malignant characteristics when partially restored with moderate numbers of spleen cells than either nonrestored or restored immunodeficient mice. Using a different method of approach Prehn (1977a) has also shown that mice exposed to a high oncogenic stimulus (multiple MCA pellets) developed

[2] Mice, when thymectomized, lethally X-irradiated, and repopulated with syngeneic bone marrow, are severely depleted in their T-lymphocyte population. The bone marrow cells are essentially free of T-cell contamination and will protect the irradiated mice from the lethal effects of the X-irradiation by repopulating their bone-marrow cavities with all of the non-T-cell hematopoietic precursors.

more sarcomas when they had received small numbers of spleen cells than when they had either received none or large numbers of spleen cells. This immunostimulatory effect was not seen when a low oncogenic stimulus (single MCA pellet) was used.

As a direct correlation between dosage of carcinogen and immunogenicity of the resultant tumors has been demonstrated (Prehn 1975), it may be postulated that the results observed were dependent on the relatively greater immunogenicity of the tumors induced by the higher carcinogen dose. In both of these experiments where high carcinogen doses were used, the results as obtained are in agreement with the predictions of the immunostimulation hypothesis.

TABLE 1 Histologic Survey of Papillomas Induced in Immunomodulated Mice

Group	*Dermal Reaction*			*Number of Mice*	*Malignant Invasion*	*Cellular Anaplasia*
	±	+	++			
I	4	10	4	18	3	5
II	5	5	1	11	4	6
III	0	4	3	7	3	2

All groups were adult thymectomized, lethally X-irradiated (800 R) BALB/cJ mice repopulated with 1×10^7BALB/cJ (+/+) bone marrow cells IV the day after irradiation.

GROUP I —Received no additional treatment.
II —Received 1×10^2 BALB/cJ (+/+) spleen cells IP 5 days after skin grafting.
III—Received 1×10^7 BALB/cJ (+/+) spleen cells IP 5 days after skin grafting.

The dermal inflammatory reaction was:
± if there was little or no dermal infiltration of various types of mononuclear cells in the dermis at the base of the papilloma;
+ if the mononuclear infiltrate was moderate;
++ if the mononuclear infiltrate was very dense and could on occasion extend into the epithelial layers of the papilloma.

SUMMARY AND CONCLUSIONS

Immunodeficient mice restored with low numbers of normal spleen cells developed carcinogen induced skin tumors earlier than mice that either were not restored or were restored with large numbers of spleen cells. The gross appearance of these tumors suggested that carcinoma occurred most frequently in the mice restored with low numbers of spleen cells. More frequently carcinomatous invasion was histologically confirmed in the animals restored with spleen cells than in those that were not restored, and malignant dyskeratosis was observed more frequently in mice restored with low numbers of spleen cells. Histologic signs of malignant invasion in these preliminary experiments appear to correlate with the amount of stromal inflammatory response that was seen. These preliminary results, suggesting that the immune response is able to modulate tumor induction and progression, conform with the predictions of the immunostimulation hypothesis.

ACKNOWLEDGEMENTS

Part of this work was conducted at the Institute for Cancer Research in Philadelphia and was completed at the Jackson Laboratory, Bar Harbor, Maine. Support was provided by PHS grant CA–20920, ACS grant IM–83 and an appropriation from the Commonwealth of Pennsylvania.

REFERENCES

Bartlett, G. L. 1972. Effect of host immunity on the antigenic strength of primary tumors. *J. Natl. Cancer Inst.* **49**, 493–504.

Bryan, W. R., and Shimkin, M. B. 1943. Quantitative analysis of dose response data obtained with three carcinogeneic hydrocarbons in strain C3H male mice. *J. Natl. Cancer Inst.* **3**, 503–531.

Burnet, F. M. 1971. Immunological surveillance in neoplasia. *Transplant. Rev.* **7**, 3–25.

Hewitt, H. B., Blake, E. R., and Walder, A. S. 1976. A critique of the evidence for active host defence against cancer, based on personal studies of 27 murine tumours of spontaneous origin. *Br. J. Cancer* **33**, 241–259.

Holland, J. M., Perkins, E. H., and Gipson, L. C. 1977. Resistance of germfree athymic nude mice to two-stage epidermal carcinogenesis. (Abstract.) *Proceedings of the American Association for Cancer Research*, **18**, 10, No. 40.

Ioachim, H. L. 1976. The stromal reaction of tumors: An expression of immune surveillance. *J. Natl. Cancer Inst.* **57**, 465–475.

Irvin, A. D., Brown, C. G. D., Kanhai, G. K., and Stagg, D. A. 1975. Comparative growth of bovine lymphosarcoma cells and lymphoid cells injected with *Theileria parva* in athymic (nude) mice. *Nature* **255**, 713–714.

Kindred, B. 1975. The inception of the response to SRBC by nude mice injected with various doses of congenic or allogeneic thymus cells. *Cell. Immunol.* **17**, 277–284.

Kindred, B., and Wiler, E. 1972. The response to SRBC by nude mice injected with lymphoid cells other than thymus cells. *J. Immunol.* **109**, 382–387.

Klein, G. H., Sjögren, H. O., Klein, E., and Hellström, K. E. 1960. Demonstration of resistance against methycholanthrene-induced sarcomas in the primary autochthonous host. *Cancer Res.* **20,** 1561–1572.

Lappé, M. A. 1968. Evidence for the antigenicity of papillomas induced by 3-methycholanthrene. *J. Natl. Cancer Inst.* **40**, 823–846.

Maguire, H., Outzen, H. C., Custer, R. P., and Prehn, R. T. 1976. Invasion and metastasis of a xenogeneic tumor in nude mice. *J. Natl. Cancer Inst.* **57, 439–442.**

Old, L. J., Boyse, E. A., Clark, D. A., and Carswell, E. A. 1962. Antigenic properties of chemically induced tumors. *Ann. N.Y. Acad. Sci.* **101,** 80–106.

Outzen, H. C., Custer, R. P., Eaton, G. J., and Prehn, R. T. 1975. Spontaneous and induced tumor incidence in germfree "nude" mice. *J. Reticuloendothel Soc.* **17,** 1–9.

Pantelouris, E. M. 1968. Absence of thymus in a mouse mutant. *Nature* **217,** 370–371.

Prehn, R. T. 1963. Function of depressed immunologic reactivity during carcinogenesis. *J. Natl. Cancer Inst.* **31**, 791–805.

Prehn, R. T. 1975. Relationship of tumor immunogenicity to concentration of the oncogen. *J. Natl. Cancer Inst.* **55**, 189–190.

Prehn, R. T. 1977a. Immunostimulation of chemical oncogenesis in the mouse. *Int. J. Cancer* **20**, 918–922.

Prehn, R. T. 1977b. Immunostimulation of the lymphodependent phase of neoplastic growth. *J. Natl. Cancer Inst.* **59**, 1043–1049.

Prehn, R. T., and Lappé, M. A. 1971. An immunostimulation theory of tumor development. *Transplant Rev.* **7**, 26–54.

Prehn, R. T., and Main, J. M. 1957. Immunity to methycholanthrene-induced sarcomas. *J. Natl. Cancer Inst.* **18**, 769–778.

Prehn, L. M., and Outzen, H. C. 1977. Primary tumor immunity in nude mice. *Int. J. Cancer* **19**, 688–691.

Reed, N. D. 1974. Comment during discussion in: *Proceedings of the First International Workshop on Nude Mice.* (Edited by Rygaard, J., and Povlsen, C. O.), p. 268. Gustav Fischer Verlag, Stuttgart.

Rygaard, J. 1969. Immunobiology of the mouse mutant "nude". Preliminary investigations. *Acta Pathol. Microbiol. Scand.* **77**, 761–762.

Rygaard, J. 1974a. Skin grafts in nude mice. 1. Allografts in nude mice of three genetic backgrounds (BALB-c, C3H, C57-BL). *Acta Pathol. Microbiol. Scand. [A]* **82**, 80–92.

Rygaard, J. 1974b. Skin grafts in nude mice. 2. Rat skin grafts in nude mice of three genetic backgrounds (BALB-c, C3H, C57-BL). The effects after preparation by thymus grafts. *Acta Pathol Microbiol. Scand. [A]* **82**, 93–104.

Rygaard, J. 1974c. Skin grafts in nude mice. 3. Fate of grafts from man and donors of other taxonomic classes. *Acta Pathol. Microbiol Scand. [A]* **82**, 105–112.

Rygaard, J., and Povlsen, C. O. 1969. Heterotransplantation of a human malignant tumour to "nude" mice. *Acta Path. Microbiol. Scand.* **77**, 758–760.

Rygaard, J., and Povlsen, C. O. 1976. The nude mouse vs. the hypothesis of immunological surveillance. *Transplant. Rev.* **28**, 43–61.

Schmidt, M., and Good, R. A. 1975. Transplantation of human cancers to nude mice and effects of thymus grafts. *J. Natl. Cancer Inst.* **55**, 81–87.

Schjerven, L., Elgjo, K., Iversen, O. H., and Palbo, J. 1974. Skin carcinogenesis in nude mice. A preliminary study. In: *Proceedings of the First International Workshop on Nude Mice.* (Edited by Rygaard, J., and Povlsen, C. O.), pp. 265–268. Gustav Fischer Verlag, Stuttgart.

Stjernswärd, J. 1965. Immunodepressive effect of 3-methylcholanthrene. Antibody formation at the cellular level and reaction against weak antigenic homografts. *J. Natl. Cancer Inst.* **35**, 885–892.

Stutman, O. 1975a. Immunodepression and malignancy. In: *Proceedings of the XI International Cancer Congress; Cell Biology and Tumor Immunology.* (Edited by Bucalossi, P., Veronesi, U., and Cascinelli, N.), Vol. I, pp. 275–279. Excerpta Medica, Amsterdam, American Elsevier, New York.

Stutman, O. 1975b. Immunodepression and malignancy. *Adv. Cancer Res.* **22**, 261–422.

17

Introduction to Tumor Immunology and Immunological Aspects of Oral Premalignant and Malignant Lesions

E. DABELSTEEN

Departments of Oral Pathology and Oral Diagnosis, The Royal Dental College, Copenhagen, Denmark

The immune system was orginally considered only a protection mechanism against foreign invaders such as bacteria and virus. However, this concept has been modified and it seems established that host macromolecules and cells, including cancer cells, although not foreign invaders, can activate the immune system. Immunological reactions consequently seem to play an important role in cancer biology (Prehn and Main 1957).

Most studies of cancer immunology have been based on the belief that there is something unique about a cancer cell that distinguishes it from normal cells, and that this difference can be recognized by the body's immune system. In agreement with this, the infiltrate of lymphocytes, plasma cells, and macrophages seen in many tumors is usually regarded to reflect the host's immunological defense reaction toward the tumor, and several reports have supported this by showing a correlation between the intensity of the infiltrates in the tumor and improved survival of the patient (Black and Speer 1958; Berg 1959; Black et al. 1972; Black et al. 1974; Lund et al. 1975).

1. IMMUNOLOGICAL ASPECTS OF ANIMAL TUMORS

1:1 TUMOR-ASSOCIATED ANTIGENS

The initiation of an immunological reaction which may lead to tumor destruction requires that the tumor cell membranes be different from those of normal cells. Such cell surface structures that distinguish cancer cells from normal cells will in this chapter be termed "tumor-associated antigens."

Several different tumor-associated antigens have been described.

1:1:1 *Oncogenic viral antigens*

All tumors induced by a given virus carry the same surface viral antigens irrespective of the species in which they are expressed (Sjögren et al. 1961).

1:1:2 *Unique antigens*

Tumors induced by chemical agents possess transplantation antigens which in contrast to the virally induced antigens are unique, not only to the species, but also to the individual tumors induced by the same carcinogen (Prehn and Main 1957; Baldwin 1973).

1:1:3 *Oncofetal antigens*

Oncofetal antigens are macromolecules normally present during embryonic life, absent in adult life, but reexpressed during neoplasia. These antigens are present on virally as well as chemically induced tumors and crossreact widely within different tumors and within species. These antigens may sometimes only be antigenic in species other than the host (Alexander 1972; Baldwin and Embleton 1974; Steele and Sjögren 1974).

1:2 ANTIGENS IN SPONTANEOUS TUMORS

"Spontaneous" tumors in animals, i.e., tumors that arise without the apparent intervention of an etiologic agent, tend to have little or no antigenicity (Prehn and Main 1957; Hewitt et al. 1976). It has been shown that tumors induced by low levels of chemical carcinogen develop slowly and also have low antigenicity. Prehn (1975) suggested that the tumors arising sporadically and with low frequency in a population may also result from low levels of carcinogen and have little or no antigenicity. If this hypothesis holds, it will mean that many human tumors and especially those which are preceded by a long period of preneoplastic cell populations will have low or no antigenicity.

1:3 ANTIGENS IN EXPERIMENTAL PREMALIGNANT LESIONS

Only a limited amount of experimental work has dealt with tumor antigens in premalignant lesions (Lappé 1969; Halpin et al. 1972). From the data presented here it is seen that antigenic properties of preneoplastic cell populations are carried over into the resulting tumors, and that antigenicity or lack of antigenicity is a property that is already established in the preneoplastic stages of tumor development.

1:4 DEMONSTRATION OF TUMOR-ASSOCIATED ANTIGENS

Tumor-associated antigens were first studied in inbred mice where many experimental tumors can be shown by transplantation techniques to process antigens which can elicit tumor rejection response in the host (Foley 1953; Prehn and Main 1957; Klein et al. 1960; Old and Boyse 1964). This is true whether the tumor is induced by chemical carcinogen, virus, or radiation. A tumor antigen which elicits an immune response resulting in rejection of a tumor cell graft must, as mentioned previously, be a cell membrane antigen. Molecular changes located in the interior of the tumor cells are believed to be inaccessible to humoral or cell-mediated immunity and therefore of little significance to the immunological tumor-host relationship.

As transplantation techniques only can be used in studies of reactions to tumors in inbred animals and therefore are of little value in studies of human tumors, several in vitro techniques have been developed (Hellström 1967; Takasugi and Klein 1970; Halliday et al. 1975; Vánky et al. 1975; Bloom and David 1976). By these techniques immunity has been demonstrated to a range of virus- and carcinogen-induced animal tumors (Hellström 1967; Taranger et al. 1972; Baldwin 1973; Herberman et al. 1974), and some human tumors (Andersen et al. 1970; Hellström et al 1970, 1971; Halliday 1975; Perlmann et al. 1977), and it is generally believed that the in vitro assay illustrates the transplantation rejections seen in animal experiments. However, although they are tumor-associated antigens and they elicit a specific immune response which can be demonstrated in in vitro systems, they do not necessarily function as effective rejection antigens, and the value of the in vitro test systems is not clear yet (Klein et al. 1976; Perlmann et al. 1977).

1:5 REACTIONS TO TUMOR-ASSOCIATED ANTIGENS

From animal studies it is generally believed that cell-mediated immune reactions to tumor-associated antigens play a major role when rejection of tumors are observed. Thymus-derived (T) lymphocytes appear to be the most important effector cells in these reactions, but other subpopulations of lymphocytes and macrophages seem to be involved as well. Antibodies to tumor antigens may, in the presence of complement, be cytotoxic to neoplastic cells, but they may also destroy tumor cells in concert with other inflammatory cells (Wood and Morton 1970; Perlmann et al. 1972; Evans 1973; Hellström and Hellström 1974; Bakács et al. 1977).

Although tumor-associated antigens elicit a specific immune response in the tumor-bearing host, it is recognized that this reponse does not always lead to rejection of the tumor (Baldwin and Robins 1976). It is thus becoming increasingly apparent that under certain circumstances the immune system may induce enhancement of tumor growth rather than tumor destruction (Baldwin 1973; Hellström and Hellström 1974; Kirkwood and Gershohn 1974; Herberman 1974; chapter 16), and that the mechanism that prevents tumor destruction probably is a facet of the same mechanism that prevents autoimmune diseases (Coggin et al. 1974; Coggin and Anderson 1974; Prehn and Prehn 1975).

From the growing understanding of the complexity of the tumor-host relationship, it seems that no simple mechanism exists in tumor immunology, and it is therefore not surprising that, although tumor-specific reactivities are demonstrated in many test systems, the results bear no correlation with the clinical situation. It also seems unlikely that the pathologist will be able to predict the nature of the immunological response to a tumor by examining histological preparations alone.

2. IMMUNOLOGICAL ASPECTS OF HUMAN TUMORS WITH SPECIAL REFERENCE TO ORAL PREMALIGNANT AND MALIGNANT LESIONS

2:1 GENERAL ASPECTS

Immunological studies involving mainly in vitro tests but also cutaneous delayed hypersensitivity tests have indicated the occurrence of a tumor-specific host response in many human tumor patients (Andersen et al. 1970; Hellström et al. 1971; Perlmann et al. 1973, 1977; Vánky et al. 1974; Troye et al. 1977). The significance of the response and the nature of the antigens involved are at present largely unknown, and unlike the animal studies no unique tumor antigens have yet been identified. However, several different fetal products associated with human neoplasia have been isolated and characterized, and some authors have suggested that human tumor-associated antigens are mainly oncofetal antigens (Hellström et al. 1970; Baldwin and Embleton 1974; Coggin et al. 1974; Hammarström et al. 1977). It is beyond the scope of this paper to attempt a comprehensive review of the immunology of human cancer. The interested reader is therefore referred to other literature for information on immunological aspects of human tumors outside the oral cavity (Immunology of malignancy 1973; International Conference on Immunobiology of Cancer 1976; Perlmann et al. 1977; Baldwin and Embleton 1978).

2:2 ORAL ASPECTS

Only a limited literature deals with immunological studies relevant to oral premalignancy and malignancy (Lehner 1970; Dabelsteen and Pindborg 1973; Roed-Petersen et al. 1973; Lehner et al. 1973a, 1973b; Cannell 1973, 1974; Dabelsteen et al. 1975). It appears from these studies that, although no attempts have been made to identify tumor associated antigens in oral carcinomas and premalignant lesions, some indirect evidences suggest that antigen changes have taken place in these lesions.

2:3 CELL MEMBRANE CHANGES

As already mentioned, the initiation of an immunological reaction against a tumor requires that the tumor cell membranes are different from those of normal cells. In the oral mucosa it has been shown that blood group substances A and B may be expressed at the cell membranes in the spinous cell layer of the epithelium (Brandtzaeg 1965; Dabelsteen and Fejerskov 1974). The expression in normal oral mucosa varies from person to person and is also dependent on the secretor status of the patient (Dabelsteen

1972). However, a partial or complete loss of blood group substances A and B respectively have been found in most oral carcinomas developing from epithelium in which these substances are normally present (Prendergast et al. 1968, Kovarik et al. 1968; Dabelsteen and Pindborg 1973; Lui et al. 1974; George 1977). (See Figure 1.) The blood group substances A and B associated with epithelial cell membranes are carbohydrates believed to be attached to either lipids or proteins in the cell membrane. The significance of the decreased expression of blood group substances in oral carcinomas is unknown, but it indicates a molecular change of the cell membranes associated with malignant transformation.

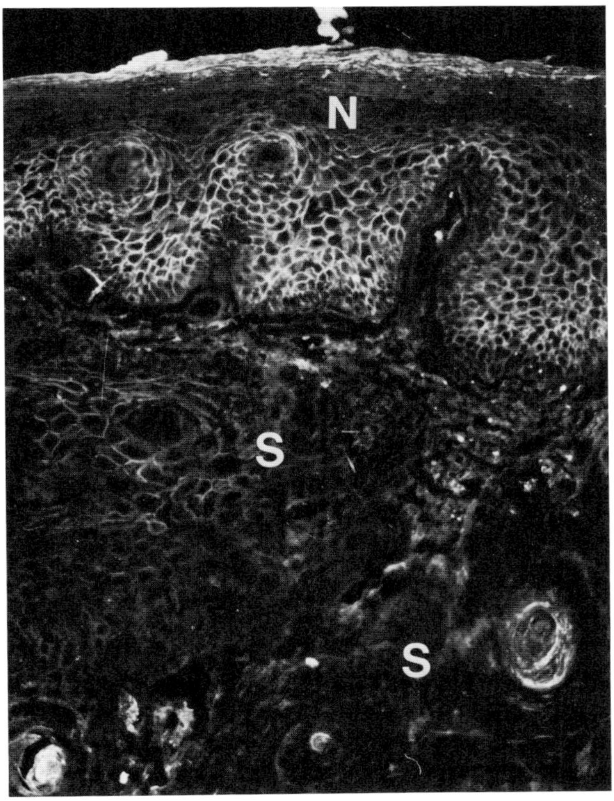

FIGURE 1. Normal mucosa (N) and squamous cell carcinoma (S). Immunofluorescent staining. Bright intercellular spaces in the spinous cell layer indicate the presence of blood group antigen A in normal epithelium. In the carcinoma, blood group antigens are absent except for one area. X 100.

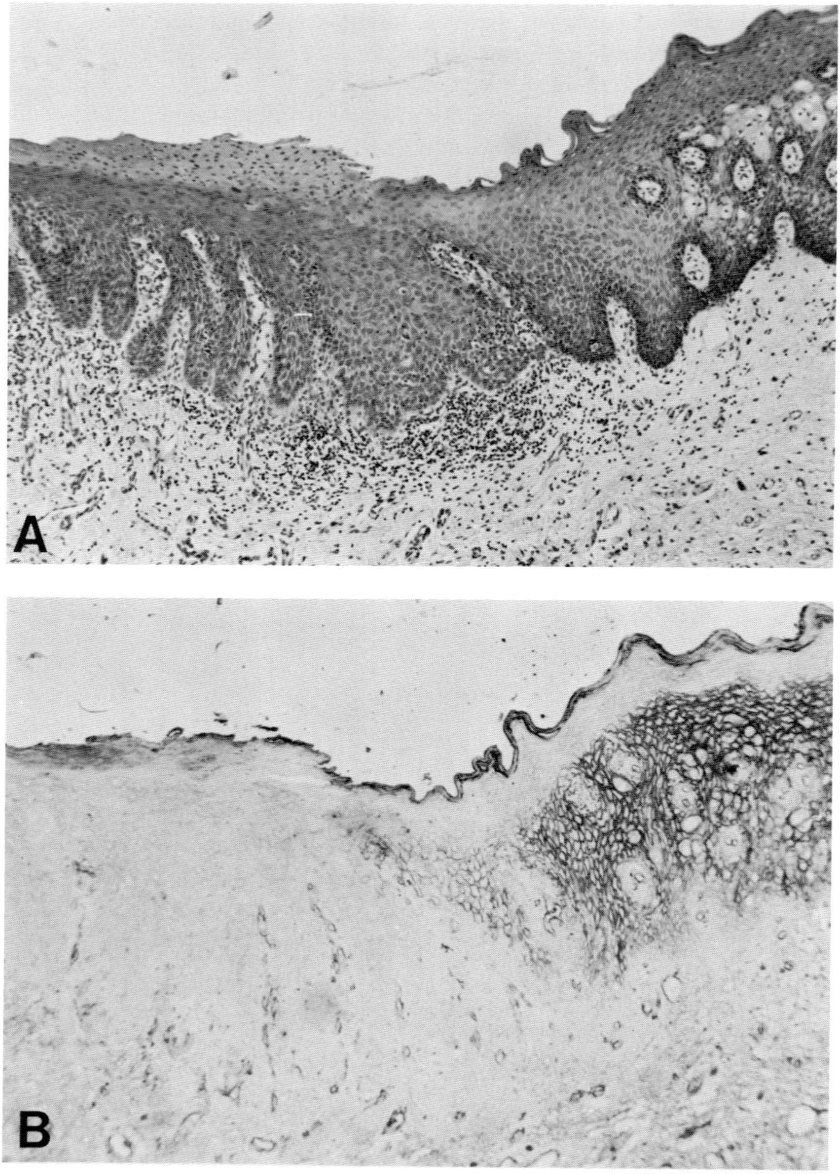

FIGURE 2. Borderline between normal and dysplastic epithelium. A. Hematoxylin and eosin staining, normal epithelium to the right. B. Immunoperoxidose staining of neighboring section. Black intercellular spaces indicate the presence of blood group antigen A.; these are only present in normal epithelium. X 100.

The distribution of blood group antigens has also been investigated in oral leukoplakias as well. Dabelsteen et al. (1975) found that all lesions with epithelial dysplasia and 20% of the lesions without epithelial dysplasia showed loss or decreased reactivity for blood group antigen A or B (Fig. 2). These findings are of interest when one considers the experimental work which has demonstrated that the antigen properties of preneoplastic cell populations are carried over into the resulting tumor (Lappé 1979; Halpin et al. 1972). The findings of decreased reactivity for blood group antigens A and B in oral premalignant and malignant lesions are in agreement with studies of similar lesions in the uterine cervix, and it has been suggested that the lesions with decreased blood group antigen activity are the ones most likely to become malignant (Davidsohn et al. 1969; Davidsohn 1972).

Loss of other cellular antigens during malignant transformation has previously been described in animal experiments as well as in other human tumors (Moragas et al. 1970; Seigler et al. 1971; Muller and Sutherland 1971; Baldwin and Glaves 1972; Burtin et al. 1972). Burtin et al. (1972) studied premalignant lesions of the colon. He investigated undifferentiated noninvasive polyps for three different antigens and concluded that, from an immunological viewpoint, polyps behave like cancer. Furthermore, Burtin et al. (1971) claimed that the loss of a normal intracytoplasmic antigen in colon carcinomas was accompanied by the appearance of an oncofetal antigen.

It has yet to be determined whether the loss of blood group antigens in oral premalignant and malignant lesions is accompanied by the appearance of tumor antigens against which there may be immunity.

As recent studies have shown loss of blood group antigen activity in the epithelium adjacent to healing wounds, it has been suggested that the change is related to cell movement rather than malignancy (Dabelsteen and Fejerskov 1974; Mackenzie et al. 1977). However, experimental studies of wound healing, and unpublished studies of oral carcinomas, suggest that a difference exists between blood group antigen expression in neoplastic and regenerating oral epithelial cells (Dabelsteen and Mackenzie 1976; Dabelsteen 1977). The studies suggest that the tumors exhibit wider changes in their cell membranes, with loss of what is believed to be glycoprotein as well as glycolipid-bound antigens, whereas only changes in glycoprotein-bound antigens are seen in wound healing.

The association between cell membrane changes in tumors and in regenerating oral epithelium may be a human example of what has been described in an experimental study of liver regeneration in mice. Hellström et al. (1975) have shown that lymphocytes from mice which have undergone partial hepatectomy, followed by liver regeneration, are cytotoxic to cultivated neoplastic cells but not to normal cells. These findings suggest that a normal tissue repair process may lead to a detectable immunological reaction against antigens present on neoplastic cells. There is evidence suggesting that fetal antigens are shared not only by normal embryonic cells and tumor cells but also by regenerating cells. It is therefore tempting to speculate whether the change in blood group antigens seen in oral carcinoma and wound healing is associated with the expression of embryonic antigens.

Other cell membrane changes in oral carcinomas have been demonstrated by use of lectins which, when conjugated with fluorescein, act as stains with specific properties for certain saccharide moities. Ricinus communis fraction$_{120}$ (RCA_{120}) is a lectin which binds to the surface region of basal and spinous cells of normal oral epithelium. Binding of RCA_{120} to the cell surface could not be demonstrated for most invading malignant cells and was decreased for epithelial cells at the margin of healing wounds. No studies of premalignant lesions have yet been performed by use of lectins.

Under ideal conditions one would like to associate the cell membrane changes described above directly with the appearance of tumor antigens against which immunity can be detected. Unfortunately, no such attempts have been made yet.

2:4 CELLULAR IMMUNITY TO ORAL MALIGNANT AND PREMALIGNANT LESIONS

Different in vitro tests have been used to provide evidence for cell-mediated immune response against specific antigens in oral carcinomas and oral leukoplakias. By use of a microcytotoxicity assay, Cannell (1973, 1974) demonstrated that lymphocytes from patients with oral cancer were capable of killing cultured oral tumor cells. In his studies, Cannell compared the cytotoxic effect of the patient's lymphocytes with the mean percentage cytotoxicity of normal controls. However, recent studies show that there are donors who have lymphocytes cytotoxic to different tumor cells, but who do not have cancer. The documentation of this natural cytotoxicity of human blood lymphocytes towards a variety of tumor cells has raised doubts concerning the validity of the cytotoxic assay in human tumor immunology (Skurzak et al. 1973; Takasugi et al. 1973, 1974, 1975). As different donors have lymphocytes with different levels of natural cytotoxicity, the specific cytotoxic effect of a cancer patient's lymphocytes against the tumor tissue can theoretically only be estimated after the elimination of the cells responsible for the non-disease-related cytotoxicity (Bakács et al. 1977).

In agreement with this, Perlmann et al. (1977) stated that the cytotoxicity assay at present is of limited value for monitoring individual patients, but that it is possible to demonstrate disease-related reactions in groups of patients.

It is obvious from this that the specific cytotoxic effect of lymphocytes from patients with oral cancer cannot be estimated by comparing the single cancer patient's cytotoxic reactions to the mean percentage cytotoxicity of several normals as a control as done by Cannell (1974).

Lehner (1970) used the lymphocyte transformation test with autologous saline homogenates of leukoplakia to study immunologic reactions against these lesions. The basis of this test is that when lymphocytes meet their specific antigen they are stimulated and undergo division. The degree of lymphocyte stimulation can then be assayed either by determining the percentage of morphologically altered cells or by the amount of radioactive DNA analogue incorporated into newly synthesized DNA. The lymphocyte transformation technique is particularly well suited for quantitation, but it seems that both B-lymphocytes, which are plasma cell precursors, as well as T-lymphocytes are taking part in the response. This makes the technique unsuitable for the dissection of the response of a mixed population of cells such as, for example, peripheral blood lymphocytes (Bloom and David 1976). Lehner (1970) found that the lesions with less severe histological changes were associated with the highest rates of transformation. A progressive impairment of lymphocyte transformation was seen when histological gradings were more severe, and Lehner suggested that the onset of carcinoma was accompanied by a depression in "cell-mediated" immune responses.

It would of course be tempting to suggest that a tumor develops from a premalignant lesion because the immunological defense for some reason breaks down, thus allowing the tumor to grow. This suggestion has not been confirmed for oral cancer but is in agreement with experimental studies and studies of human tumors such as urinary bladder carcinomas, hypernephromas, and malignant melanomas (Lewis 1972; Plescia et al. 1976; Kjaer and Bendixen 1976; Perlmann et al. 1977). However, there is some evidence that the immunodepression of the host is secondary to the tumor growth and is caused by the tumor itself (Kjaer and Bendixen 1976; Plescia et al. 1976).

The leukocyte migration inhibition technique is another in vitro technique which has been used in the study of oral premalignant lesions. This technique is based on the production by immunologically activated lymphocytes of a factor inhibiting the active migration of leukocytes or macrophages. The T-lymphocytes were previously believed to generate these substances. However, recent studies seem to indicate that B-cells can also produce migration inhibition factor (Bloom and David 1976). Consequently, results obtained by this technique cannot be regarded as reflecting a solely cell-mediated immune response.

Roed-Petersen et al. (1973) studied soluble extracts of leukoplakia and homologous normal oral mucosa, with the leukocyte migration inhibition technique. They found that five of eleven patients showed inhibition of migration with leukoplakia tissue extracts, and they suggested cell-mediated immunity against antigenic compartments in leukoplakia. The results are difficult to interpret as it is uncertain which immunological parameter the test measures. As antigens are generally used in very high concentrations in the test, it may sometimes be difficult to distinguish toxic reactions from specific immunological reactions.

The above-mentioned studies of "cell"-mediated immune response to oral precancerous and cancerous lesions used peripheral blood lymphocytes in their tests. It is possible that other results would have been obtained if lymphocytes from the lesions themselves had been studied. Experimental animal studies and a few human studies have shown that the nature of the cell infiltrate in tumors varies from one tumor to another. Further, the effect of the infiltrate may or may not correlate with what is found with lymphocytes from blood (Haskill et al. 1976; Klein et al. 1976). Studies with tissue localized lymphocytes would help to clarify the functional characteristics of the inflammatory cells seen in leukoplakias and carcinomas and could help to clarify the prognostic value of such infiltrates.

2:5 OTHER IMMUNOLOGICAL REACTIONS IN PATIENTS WITH ORAL MALIGNANT AND PREMALIGNANT LESIONS

The author is not aware of any studies of antibodies to tumor antigens in oral premalignant and malignant lesions. However, studies have investigated serum antibodies as well as cell-mediated immune reactions to herpesvirus hominis Type 1 (HSV-1) related antigens in patients with oral leukoplakia and oral carcinoma (Aurelian et al. 1973; Lehner 1973a, 1973b; Tarro and Sabin 1973; Smith et al. 1976).

The interest in antibodies to herpesvirus arises from studies of premalignant and malignant lesions in the uterine cervix. Essentially, patients with cervical carcinoma and its precursors have significantly higher titers of antibodies to herpesvirus Type 2 (HSV-2) than do control populations (Royston and Aurelian 1970; Hollinshead and Lee 1973). HSV-2 antigens have been demonstrated in cervical carcinoma, and in vitro studies have demonstrated that HSV-2 has oncogenic properties (Duff and Rapp 1971; Rapp and Reed 1977). Furthermore, some but not all studies have been able to demonstrate antibodies to a HSV-2 induced cell surface antigen in serum from patients with cervical precancerous and cancerous lesions (Aurelian et al. 1973; Sabin 1974; Christensen and

Espmark 1976). In two recent studies, Aurelian et al. (1977) found that the prevalence of antibodies to a HSV-2 induced cell surface antigen was significantly higher in patients with cervical precancerous and cancerous lesions, that the appearance of these antibodies reflects the progression of the neoplastic lesion, and that the antigen could be extracted from most biopsies of cervical squamous carcinomas, but not from other cervical tumors or from normal tissue. Consequently, the association between HSV-2 and carcinoma of the cervix has led to the proposal of HSV-2 as an etiologic agent of cervical neoplasia (Thiry 1976; Aurelian et al. 1977).

HSV-1 is the most commonly found virus in the mouth. In order to investigate whether a relationship exists between HSV-1 and oral carcinoma and leukoplakia, Lehner (1973a, 1973b) studied the cellular and humoral immune response to HSV-1 in patients with leukoplakia and carcinoma. Complement fixing antibodies to HSV-1 failed to show a significant change in titer in any group of subjects tested. By use of the lymphocyte transformation test and the macrophage migration inhibition test, Lehner et al. (1973a) demonstrated increasing values of stimulation and inhibition indices to HSV-1 in patients with epithelial dysplasia, but not in cancer patients and in patients with leukoplakia without epithelial dysplasia. The authors regarded this as an increase in cell-mediated immunity to HSV-1 in leukoplakia with epithelial dysplasia, and regarded this as being in favor of a possible participation of HSV-1 in the transformation of some leukoplakias into carcinomas. On the other hand, an increase in both lymphocyte transformation and macrophage migration inhibition to HSV-1 in patients with epithelial dysplasia may suggest that infection with virus follows the development of premalignant lesions. This concept is supported by the observation that herpesvirus grows better in actively replicating cells (Aurelian 1969).

HSV-1-induced antigen is a "non-virion" cell surface antigen present on HSV-1-infected cells. Smith et al. (1976) found in a recent study that antibodies to HSV-1 antigen were present in greater amounts in sera from patients with squamous cell carcinomas of the head and neck than in normal controls. These results are preliminary but promising as they seem to correspond to the above referred findings of Aurelian et al. (1973, 1977).

The studies of the relationship between oral cancer and HSV-1 virus are preliminary. The studies of the relationship between cervical cancer and HSV-2 virus seem promising, and although several differences between HSV-1 and HSV-2 have been pointed out, there is at present no reason to think that studies of oral cancer and HSV-1 should be less promising (Dowdle et al. 1967; Perol 1973).

3. CONCLUSION

Premalignant lesions in the oral cavity usually persist over a long period before developing malignancy (Einhorn and Wersäll 1966; Pindborg et al. 1968; Mincer et al. 1972; Bánóczy and Csiba 1976). It is possible that a prolonged period of malignant transformation, as in animal experiments, results in tumors with little immunogenicity. However, it is also possible that the leukoplakias have tumor antigens against which the host responds and that the long period of premalignancy partly is due to a successful host defense mechanism.

Thus, there is some, although not very strong, evidence suggesting that immunity plays a role in the biology of oral premalignant and malignant lesions. It seems well established that oral carcinomas and some oral leukoplakias have cell membrane changes seen as antigen simplification. On the other hand there is less evidence that new antigens, against which the host reacts, are present to a great extent. With the growing understanding of the heterogenecity of the lymphocyte population and the complexity of the immune reactions, future work should concentrate on reaching a better understanding of the mechanisms underlying the different immunological tests. Further there seems to be a great need for work dealing with the identification and isolation of antigens in normal mucosa, leukoplakias, and oral carcinomas. Finally, it seems unlikely that there will be any important progress in tumor immunology before a greater knowledge of the mechanism of self-tolerance and regulation of the immune response is gained.

REFERENCES

Alexander, P. 1972. Foetal "antigens" in cancer. *Nature* **235**, 137–140.

Alexander, P. 1974. Proceedings: Escape from immune destruction by the host through shedding of surface antigens: Is this a characteristic shared by malignant and embryonic cells. *Cancer Res.* **34**, 2077–2082.

Andersen, V., Bjerrum, O., Bendixen, G., Schiødt, T., and Dissing, I. 1970. Effect of autologous mammary tumour extracts on human leukocyte migration in vitro. *Int. J. Cancer* **5**, 357–363.

Aurelian, L. 1969. Factors affecting the growth of canine herpesvirus in dog kidney cells. *Appl. Microbiol.* **17**, 179–181.

Aurelian, L. Davis, J. H., and Julian, C. G. 1973. Herpesvirus type 2-induced, tumor-specific antigen in cervical carcinoma. *Am. J. Epidemiol.* **98**, 1–9.

Aurelian, L. Strnad, B. C., and Smith, M. F. 1977. Immunodiagnostic potential of a virus-coded, tumor-associated antigen (AG-4) in cervical cancer. *Cancer* **39**, 1834–1849.

Bakács, T., Gergely, P., Cornain, S., and Klein, E. 1977. Characterization of human lymphocyte subpopulations for cytotoxicity against tumor-derived monolayer cultures. *Int. J. Cancer* **19**, 441–449.

Baldwin, R. W. 1973. Immunological aspects of chemical carcinogenesis. In: *Advances in Cancer Research.* (Edited by Klein, G., and Weinhouse, S.), Vol. 18, pp. 1–75. Academic Press, New York.

Baldwin, R. W., and Embleton, M. J. 1974. Neoantigens on spontaneous and carcinogen-induced rat tumors defined by in vitro lymphocytotoxicity assays. *Int. J. Cancer* **13**, 433–443.

Baldwin, R. W., and Embleton, M. J. 1977. Assessment of cell-mediated immunity to human tumor-associated antigens. *Int. Rev. Exp. Pathol.* **17**, 49–95.

Baldwin, R. W., and Glaves, D. 1972. Deletion of liver-cell surface membrane components from aminoazo-dye-induced rat hepatomas. *Int. J. Cancer* **9**, 76–85.

Baldwin, R. W., and Robins, R. A. 1976. Factors interfering with immunological rejection of tumours. *Br. Med. Bull.* **32**, 118–123.

Bánóczy, J., and Csiba, A. 1976. Occurrence of epithelial dysplasia in oral leukoplakia. Analysis and follow-up study of 12 cases. *Oral Surg.* **42**, 766–774.

Berg, J. W. 1959. Inflammation and prognosis in breast cancer. A search for host resistance. *Cancer* **12**, 714–720.

Black, M. M., Cutler, S. J., and Barclary, T. H. 1972. Post biopsy breast carcinoma: A natural experiment in cancer immunology. *Cancer* **29**, 61–65.

Black, M. M., Leis, H. P., Shore, B., and Zachrau, R. E. 1974. Cellular hypersensitivity to breast cancer. *Cancer* **33**, 952–958.

Black, M. M., and Speer, F. D. 1958. Sinus histiocytosis of lymph nodes in cancer. *Surg. Gynec. Obstet.* **106**, 163–175.

Bloom, E. T., and David, J. R., eds. 1976. *In Vitro Methods in Cell-Mediated and Tumor Immunity.* Academic Press, New York.

Brandtzaeg, P. 1965. Localization of blood-group substances A and B in alcohol-fixed human gingivae by direct immunofluorescence technique. *Acta Odont. Scand.* **23**, 335–345.

Burtin, P., Kleist, S. von and Sabine, M. C. 1971. Loss of a normal colonic membrane antigen in human cancers of the colon. *Cancer Res.* **31**, 1038–1041.

Burtin, P., Martin, E., Sabine, M. C., and Kleist, S. von. 1972. Immunological study of polyps of the colon. *J. Natl. Cancer Inst.* **48**, 25–29.

Cannell, H. 1973. Oral cancer and immunity. *Br. J. Oral Surg.* **11**, 171–176.

Cannell, H. 1974. Cell-mediated and humoral immune responses to primary oral cancers. *J. Maxillofac. Surg.* **2**, 108–113.

Christenson, B., and Espmark, A. 1976. Long-term follow-up studies on herpes simplex antibodies in the course of cervical cancer. II. Antibodies to surface antigen of herpes simplex virus infected cells. *Int. J. Cancer* **17**, 318–325.

Coggin, J. H., Jr., Ambrose, K. R., Dierlam, P. J., and Anderson, N. G. 1974. Proceedings: Proposed mechanisms by which autochthonous neoplasms escape immune rejection. *Cancer Res.* **34**, 2092–2101.

Coggin, J. H., Jr., and Anderson, N. G. 1974. Cancer, differentiation and embryonic antigens: Some central problems. *Adv. Cancer Res.* **19**, 105–165.

Dabelsteen, E. 1972. Quantitative determination of blood group substances A of oral epithelial cells by immunofluorescence and immunoperoxidase methods. *Acta Pathol. Microbiol. Scand. (A)* **80**, 847–853.

Dabelsteen, E. 1977. Unpublished observations.

Dabelsteen, E., and Pindborg, J. J. 1973. Loss of epithelial blood group substances A in oral carcinomas. *Acta Pathol. Microbiol. Scand. (A)* **81**, 435–444.

Dabelsteen, E., and Fejerskov, O. 1974. Distribution of blood group antigen A in human oral epithelium. *Scand. J. Dent. Res.* **82**, 206–211.

Dabelsteen, E., Roed-Petersen, B., and Pindborg, J. J. 1975. Loss of epithelial blood group antigens A and B in oral premalignant lesions. *Acta Pathol. Microbiol. Scand. (A)* **83**, 292–300.

Dabelsteen, E., and Mackenzie, I. C. 1976. Selective loss of blood group antigens during wound healing. *Acta Pathol. Microbiol. Scand. (A)* **84**, 445–450.

Dabelsteen, E., and Mackenzie, I. C. 1978. Expression of Ricinus communis receptors on epithelial cells in oral carcinomas and oral wounds. *Cancer Res.* **38**, 4676–4680.

Davidsohn, I. 1972. Early immunologic diagnosis and prognosis of carcinoma. Phillip Levine Award Address. *Am. J. Clin. Pathol.* **57**, 715–730.

Davidsohn, I., Kovarik, S., and Ni, L. Y. 1969. Isoantigens A, B, and H in benign and malignant lesions of the cervix. *Arch. Pathol.* **87**, 306–314.

Dean, J. H., Silva, J. S., McCoy, J. L., Leonard, C. M., Middleton, M., Cannon, G. B., and Herberman, R. B. 1975. Lymphocyte blastogenesis induced by potassium chloride extracts of allogeneic breast carcinoma and lymphoid cells. *J. Natl. Cancer Inst.* **54**, 1295–1298.

Dowdle, W. R., Nahmias, A. J., Harwell, R. W., and Pauls, F. P. 1967. Association of antigenic type of herpesvirus hominis with site of viral recovery. *J. Immunol.* **99**, 974–980.

Duff, R., and Rapp, F. 1971. Oncogenic transformation of hamster cells after exposure to herpes simplex virus type 2. *Nature (New Biol.)* **233**, 48–50.

Einhorn, J., and Wersäll, J. 1966. Oral carcinoma in cases of leukoplakia of the oral mucosa. *Acta Otolaryngol.* (Suppl.) **224**, 20–22.

Evans, R. 1973. Macrophages and the tumour bearing host. *Br. J. Cancer* **28**, 19–25.

Foley, E. J. 1953. Antigenic properties of methyl cholanthrene-induced tumors in mice of the strain of origin. *Cancer Res.* **13**, 835–837.

George, D. 1977. Reactive properties of oral lesions to the specific red cell adherence test. Abstract. *J. Dent. Res.* **56**, A44.

Halliday, W. J., Maluish, A. E., Little, J. H., and Davis, N. C. 1975. Leukocyte adherence inhibition and specific immunoreactivity in malignant melanoma. *Int. J. Cancer* **16**, 645–658.

Halpin, Z. T., Vaage, J., and Blair, P. H. 1972. Lack of antigenicity of mammary tumors induced by carcinogens in a nonantigenic preneoplastic lesion. *Cancer Res.* **32**, 2197–2200.

Hammarström, S., Troye, M., Wahlund, G., Svenberg, T., and Perlmann, P. 1977. K cell mediated lysis of cultured colon carcinoma and urinary bladder carcinoma cells induced by monospecific antisera against carcino-embryonic antigen (CEA) and two CEA-related normal glycoproteins. *Int. J. Cancer* **19**, 756–766.

Haskill, J. S., Yamamura, Y., Radov, L., and Parthenais, E. 1976. Discussion paper: Are peripheral and in situ tumor immunity related? *Ann. N.Y. Acad. Sci.* **276**, 373–380.

Hellström, I. 1967. A colony inhibition (CI) technique for demonstration of tumor cell destruction by lymphoid cells in vitro. *Int. J. Cancer* **2**, 65–68.

Hellström, K. E., and Hellström, I. 1974. Lymphocyte-mediated cytotoxicity and blocking serum activity to tumor antigens. *Adv. Immunol.* **18**, 209–277.

Hellström, I., Hellström, K. E., and Nishioka, M. 1975. Reactivity to tumour-associated antigens detected in mice undergoing liver regeneration. *Nature* **253**, 744–746.

Hellström, I., Hellström, K. E., and Shepard, T. H. 1970. Cell-mediated immunity against antigens common to human colonic carcinomas and fetal gut epithelium. *Int. J. Cancer* **6**, 346–351.

Hellström, I., Hellström, K. E., Sjögren, H. O., and Warner, G. A. 1971. Demonstration of cell-mediated immunity to human neoplasms of various histological types. *Int. J. Cancer* **7**, 1–16.

Herberman, R. B. 1974. Cell mediated immunity to tumor cells. *Adv. Cancer Res.* **19**, 207–263.

Herberman, R. B., Aoki, T., Nunn, M., Lavrin, D. H., Soares, N., Gazclar, A., Holden, H., and Chang, K. S. 1974. Specificity of ^{51}Cr-release cytotoxicity of lymphocytes immune to murine sarcoma virus. *J. Natl. Cancer Inst.* **53**, 1103–1111.

Hewitt, H. B., Blake, E. R., and Walder, A. S. 1976. A critique of the evidence for active host defense against cancer based on personal studies of 27 murine tumors of spontaneous origin. *Br. J. Cancer* **33**, 241–259.

Hollinshead, A. C., Lee, O., Chretien, P. B., Tarpley, J. L., Rawls, W. E., and Adam, E. 1973. Antibodies to herpesvirus non-viron antigens in squamous carcinomas. *Science* **182**, 713–715.

Immunology of malignancy. 1973. Charles Salt Research Centre Symposium, fifth. *Br. J. Cancer Supplement No. I.* H. K. Lewis and Co., Ltd., London.

International conference on immunobiology of cancer. 1976. *Ann. N.Y. Acad. Sci.*, Vol. 276.

Kellen, J. A., and Anderson, K. M. 1971. The antigenicity of rat mammary tumours, induced by 7, 12-dimethylbenz (alpha) anthracene. *Oncology* **25**, 49–54.

Kirkwood, J. M., and Gershon, R. K. 1974. A role for suppressor T cells in immunological enhancement of tumor growth. *Prog. Exp. Tumor Res.* **19**, 157–164.

Kjaer, M., and Bendixen, G. 1976. Discussion paper: Tumor-directed cellular hypersensitivity detected by leucocyte migration in patients with renal carcinoma. *Ann. N.Y. Acad. Sci.* **276**, 260–271.

Klein, E., Becher, S., Svedmyr, E., Jondal, M., and Vánky, F. 1976. Tumor infiltrating lymphocytes. *Ann. N.Y. Acad. Sci.* **276**, 207–216.

Klein, G., Sjögren, H. O., Kelin, E., and Hellström, K. E. 1960. Demonstration of resistance against methylcholanthrene-induced sarcoma in the primary autochthonous host. *Cancer Res.* **20**, 1561–1572.

Kovarik, S., Davidsohn, I., and Stejskal, R. 1968. ABO antigens in cancer. Detection with the mixed cell agglutination reaction. *Arch. Pathol.* **86**, 12–21.

Lá, M. A. 1969. Tumour specific transplantation antigens: Possible origin in premalignant lesions. *Nature* **223**, 82–84.

Lehner, T. 1970. Immunopathology of oral leukoplakia. *Br. J. Cancer* **24**, 442–446.

Lehner, T., Shillitoe, E. J., Wilton, J. M., and Ivanyi, L. 1973a. Cell mediated immunity to herpesvirus Type 1 in carcinoma and pre-cancerous lesions. *Br. J. Cancer* **28**, 128–134.

Lehner, T., Wilton, J. M., Shillitoe, E. J., and Ivanyi, L. 1973b. Cell-mediated immunity and antibodies to herpesvirus Type 1 in oral leukoplakia and carcinoma. *Br. J. Cancer* **27**, 351–361.

Lewis, M. G. 1972. Immunology of human malignant melanoma. In: *Immunological Aspects of Neoplasia II.* (Edited by Anderson, Vagn), Vol. 5, No. 5, pp. 44–65. Munksgaard, Copenhagen.

Lui, P. I., McGregor, D. H., Liu, J. G., Dunlap, C. L., Jinks, W. L., Lin, F., Przybylski, C., and Miller, L. A. 1974. Carcinoma of the oral cavity evaluated by specific red cell adherence test. *Oral Surg.* **38**, 56–64.

Lund, C., Søgaard, H. Elbrønd, O., Jørgensen, K., and Andersen, A. P. 1975. Epidermoid carcinoma of the lip. Histologic grading in the clinical evaluation. *Acta Radiol.* **14**, 465–474.

Mackenzie, I. C., Dabelsteen, E., and Zimmerman, K. 1977. The relationship between expression of epithelial B-like blood group antigen, cell movement and cell proliferation. *Acta Pathol. Microbiol. Scand. (A)* **85**, 49–56.

Mincer, H. H., Coleman, S. A., and Hopkins, K. P. 1972. Observations on the clinical characteristics of oral lesions showing histologic epithelial dysplasia. *Oral Surg.* **33**, 389–399.

Moragas, J. M. de, Winkelmann, R. K., and Jordon, R. E. 1970. Immunofluorescence of epithelial skin tumours. I. Patterns of intercellular substance. *Cancer* **25**, 1399–1403.

Muller, H. K., and Sutherland, R. C. 1971. Epidermal antigens in cutaneous dysplasia and neoplasia. *Nature* **230**, 384–385.

Nathan, C. F., Karnovsky, M. L., and David, J. R. 1971. Alterations of macrophage functions by mediators from lymphocytes. *J. Exp. Med.* **133**, 1356–1376.

Old, L. J., and Boyse, E. A. 1964. Immunology of experimental tumors. *Ann. Rev. Med.* **15**, 167–186.

Perlmann, P., Perlmann, H., and Wigzell, H. 1972. Lymphocyte mediated cytotoxicity in vitro—induction and inhibition by humoral antibody and nature of effector cells. *Transplant. Rev.* **13**, 91–114.

Perlmann, P., O'Toole, C., and Ungsgaard, B. 1973. Lymphocyte-mediated tumor cell destruction in vitro. Some general principles and reactivities in human urinary bladder carcinoma. In: *Conference on Immunology of Carcinogenesis. National Cancer Institute Monograph No. 35*, pp. 223–230. U.S. Dept. of Health, Education, and Welfare.

Perlmann, P., Troye, M., and Pape, G. R. 1977. Cell-mediated immune reactions to human tumors. *Cancer* **40**, 448–457.

Perol, Y. 1973. Viroses et cavité buccale. *Rev. Stomatol. Chir. Maxillofac.* **74**, 37–78.

Pindborg, J. J., Jølst, O., Renstrup, G., and Roed-Petersen, B. 1968. Studies in oral leukoplakia: A preliminary report on the period prevalence of malignant transformation in leukoplakia based on a follow-up study of 248 patients. *J. Am. Dent. Ass.* **76**, 767–771.

Plescia, O. J., Grinwich, K., and Plescia, A. M. 1976. Subversive activity of syngeneic tumor cells as an escape mechanism from immune surveillance and the role of prostaglandins. *Ann. N.Y. Acad. Sci.* **276**, 455–465.

Prehn, R. T., and Main, J. M. 1957. Immunity to methyl-cholanthrene-induced sarcomas. *J. Natl. Cancer Inst.* **18**, 769–778.

Prehn, R. T. 1975. Relationship of tumor immunogenicity to concentration of the oncogen. *J. Natl. Cancer Inst.* **55**, 189–190.

Prehn, R. T., and Prehn, L. M. 1975. Pathobiology of neoplasia. A teaching monograph. *Am. J. Pathol.* **80**, 529–550.

Prendergast, R. C., Toto, P. D., and Gargiulo, A. W. 1968. Reactivity of blood group substances of neoplastic oral epithelium. *J. Dent. Res.* **47**, 306–310.

Rapp, F., and Reed, C. 1977. The viral etiology of cancer. A realistic approach. *Cancer* **40**, 419–429.

Roed-Petersen, B., Roed-Petersen, J., and Bendixen, G. 1973. Cell-mediated immunity to human oral leukoplakia demonstrated by the leukocyte migration test. *Int. J. Cancer* **12**, 66–72.

Royston, I., and Aurelian, L. 1970. The association of genital herpesvirus with cervical atypia and carcinoma in situ. *Am. J. Epidemiol.* **91**, 531–538.

Sabin, A. B. 1974. Herpes simplex-genitalis virus nonviron antigens and their implication in certain human cancers: Unconfirmed. *Proc. Natl. Acad. Sci. USA* **71**, 3248–3252.

Seigler, H. F., Kremer, W. B., Metzgar, R. S., Ward, F. E., Haung, A. T., and Amos, D. B. 1971. HL-A antigenic loss in malignant transformation. *J. Natl. Cancer Inst.* **46**, 577–584.

Skurzak, H., Steiner, L., Klein, E., and Lamon, E. 1973. Cytotoxicity of human peripheral lymphocytes for glioma, osteosarcoma and glia cell lines. In: *Conference and Workshop on Cellular Immune Reactions to Human Tumor-Associated Antigens. National Cancer Institute Monograph No. 37*, pp. 93–102. U.S. Dept. of Health, Education, and Welfare.

Sjögren, H. O., Hellström, I., and Klein, G. 1961. Resistance of polyoma virus immunized mice to transplantation of established polyoma tumors. *Exp. Cell Res.* **23**, 204–208.

Smith, H. G., Chretien, P. B., Henson, D. E., Silverman, N. A., and Alexander, J. C. 1976. Viral-specific humoral immunity to herpes simplex-induced antigens in patients with squamous carcinoma of the head and neck. *Am. J. Surg.* **132**, 541–548.

Steele, G., and Sjögren, H. O. 1974. Cross-reacting tumor-associated antigen(s) among chemically induced rat colon carcinomas. *Cancer Res.* **34**, 1801–1807.

Takasugi, M., and Klein, E. 1970. A microassay for cell-mediated immunity. *Transplantation* **9**, 219–227.

Takasugi, M., Mickey, M. R., and Terasaki, P. I. 1973. Reactivity of lymphocytes from normal persons on cultured tumor cells. *Cancer Res.* **33**, 2898–2902.

Takasugi, M., Mickey, M. R., and Terasaki, P. I. 1974. Studies on specificity of cell-mediated immunity to human tumors. *J. Natl. Cancer Inst.* **53**, 1527–1538.

Takasugi, M., Akira, D., and Kinoshita, K. 1975. Granulocytes as effectors in cell-mediated cytotoxicity of adherent target cells. *Cancer Res.* **35**, 2169–2176.

Taranger, L. A., Chapman, W. H., Hellström, I., and Hellström, K. E. 1972. Immunological studies on urinary bladder tumors of rats and mice. *Science* **176**, 1337–1340.

Tarro, G., and Sabin, A. B. 1973. Non-viron antigens produced by herpes simplex viruses 1 and 2. *Proc. Natl. Acad. Sci. USA* **70**, 1032–1036.

Thiry, L. 1976. Herpes simplex virus and carcinoma of the cervix. *Eur. J. Cancer* **12**, 851–858.

Troye, M., Perlmann, P., Larsson, A., Blomgren, H., and Johansson, B. 1977. Cellular cytotoxicity in vitro in transitional cell carcinoma of the human urinary bladder: ^{51}cr-release assay. *Int. J. Cancer* **20**, 188–198.

Vánky, F., Klein, E., Stjernswärd, J., and Nilsonne, U. 1974. Cellular immunity against tumor-associated antigens in humans: Lymphocyte stimulation and skin reaction. *Int. J. Cancer* **14**, 277–288.

Vánky, F., Klein, E., Stjernswärd J., and Nilsonne, U. 1974. Cellular immunity against tumor-associated antigens in humans: Lymphocyte stimulation and skin reaction. *Int. J. Cancer* **14**, 277–288.

Wood, W. C., and Morton, D. L. 1970. Microcytotoxicity test: Detection in sarcoma patients of antibody cytotoxic to human sarcoma cells. *Science* **170**, 1318–1320.

Discussion

Dr. Van Scott asked Dr. Mackenzie whether he had looked for any pattern of organization in the connective tissue which corresponded to the pattern of units in the overlying epidermis. Was there, for example, any vascular pattern related to the cell columns? Dr. Mackenzie replied that no dermal pattern had been identified; no regular position of connective tissue cells had been observed and larger patterns of dermal architecture such as the vascular network and dermal papillae are too large to be related to individual epidermal cell columns. Ultrastructurally, small indentations of the basal lamina were occasionally observed which appeared to be pierced by cellular processes, possibly of a neural nature, and these seem to be placed beneath and between the outer edges of the cell columns. A small unpublished study with Dr. Squier failed to demonstrate any statistically reliable evidence for a regular position of such structures.

Dr. Slavkin referred to experiments which had shown that embryonic skin mesoderm was capable of giving rise to pattern formation in an alien epidermis (see review by Kollar 1972). For example, feather formation in embryonic mouse skin epithelium, which would normally have formed hair, could be induced by chick skin mesenchyme. He asked why an intraepithelial mechanism of pattern formation was therefore suggested when such evidence unequivocally indicated the responsibility of mesenchyme for the spatial organization of the epithelium (see review by Slavkin et al. 1977). Dr. Mackenzie replied that it seemed most likely that the observed structure of an adult epithelium is primarily the result of the pattern of differentiation acquired during embryonic development. Continuing modulation of that pattern by the subepithelial connective tissue is also of importance. In that sense, it is clear that the mesenchyme determines the epithelial structure. However, once a particular pattern of epithelial organization is so regionally specified, for example columnar epidermis or papillary tongue epithelium, the actual assembly of epithelial cells in the spatially organized unit appears to take place as a result of interactions between the epithelial cells themselves. The mechanism of this intermediary stage appears to be worth studying, for an alteration in some aspect of the mechanism which implemented the mesenchymal instructions might be responsible for the grossly altered patterns of organization seen in pathologically involved epithelium.

Dr. Wilbanks pointed out that quantitative analysis had been used in evaluating cervical smears over 15 years ago, but the approach had not proved worthwhile. He asked Dr. Franklin whether the application of stereology to oral premalignancy was not merely inventing the wheel again? Dr. Franklin said he was aware of the type of quantification which had been undertaken on cervical epithelial cells obtained by exfoliative cytology. However, the methods used, such as planimetry, were very slow and laborious and examined only a small surface sample for simple parameters. Furthermore, no attempts had been made to put these methods to diagnostic use.

Dr. Slavkin asked about the application of devices such as the Zeiss double beam ultramicrospectrophotometer for obtaining quantitative data and whether it could be programmed to recognize a tumor histologically in terms of transmission of light at a given wavelength. Dr. Franklin replied that difficulties arose in determining what structures should be measured in this way, because of the unreliability of tinctorial properties; for example, hyperchromatism is evident in a range of conditions from benign to severe. However, Professor Kramer pointed out that one area where this approach has been useful is in determining ultraviolet absorption by DNA.

Dr. Outzen raised the problem of sampling of involved and uninvolved tissue during progression of a lesion towards malignancy. As a greater volume of tissue becomes involved then, even though the areas for measurement are selected, there are fewer differences evident in the remaining tissue; eventually it seems possible that no differences at all are discernible. Dr. Franklin agreed that there are, of course, problems with sampling any pathological material. During the final stages of carcinogenesis, for example, some of the data from two pathological stages tend to converge; this supported, in a numerical way, the subjective impression that the severe dysplasia progressed to malignancy.

Dr. Waldron asked Dr. Outzen's opinion of the significance of the large number of studies which indicate that the development or progression of carcinomas is associated with a deficient immunologic state of the host. There is, for example, evidence for an increasing depression of T-cell function with progression to metastases of carcinoma. Tests of cell-mediated immunity, such as patch testing early carcinoma patients with dinitrochlorobenzene, indicate a much lower rate of survival in those with a negative response. Dr. Outzen commented that the significance of such nonspecific tests is difficult to interpret because when people are very ill, irrespective of the cause of the illness, they frequently become anergic. Patients with tumors are usually very sick and depresssion of the immune response might not therefore be directly related to the tumor. Dr. Johnson stated that he had semiquantitatively examined patient survival in relation to a number of the histological features in a series of 100 oral squamous cell carcinomas. Some fairly obvious associations were found, such as lymph node involvement and depth of tumor infiltration, but there was little else of statistical significance except that the extent of the inflammatory infiltrate was positively correlated with survival (Johnson 1976; 1977). He asked Dr. Outzen whether he would consider this also to be a reflection of the general systemic health of the patient rather than evidence of a tumor-specific immune response? Dr. Outzen commented that the association of oral cancer with heavy smoking suggested that the development of such tumors might be comparable to chemical carcinogenesis in animals and that such tumors might therefore be antigenic. An inflammatory response would not therefore be surprising, but from observations of such a general nature as inflammation, it is not possible to make specific statements about the patient's immune status.

Dr. Smith asked Dr. Dabelsteen why basal epithelial cells did not display blood group antigens on their surfaces? Was this related to the age and degree of maturation of the cells? Dr. Dabelsteen said that he thought it probably was. Erythrocytes only express blood group antigens at a certain state of maturation. Dr. Slavkin asked whether there is evidence for immunologically-detectable cell surface molecules specifically related to epithelial cells. Dr. Dabelsteen replied that sera could be raised against epithelial cells which, when absorbed with connective tissue cells or purified biochemically, did not cross-react with nonepithelial tissues. Dr. Outzen said that there was considerable evidence from transplantation experiments that carcinogen-induced skin papillomas appear to be individually unique in terms of their antigens. Some studies had found some cross-reactivity after passage of such cells in culture, but under these conditions antigenicity resulting from viral contamination may lead to cross-reactivity. At present, it is difficult to make any firm statements of the validity and sensitivity of various in vitro and in vivo techniques, and the correlation found by examining the same material using different methods is often poor. For example, it has been shown that bladder tumors induced with a chemical carcinogen appeared to be individually unique in vivo, but these same tumors all cross-reacted in vitro (Wahl et al. 1974; Harmon et al. 1977).

Dr. Dabelsteen commented that although there has been work with in vitro tests using lymphocytes for cytotoxic assays, etc., there has been little work on the actual identification of cell membrane antigens in normal and malignant cells. In his opinion, this is primarily a problem of finding methods for isolation of the epithelial cell membranes. Dr. Slavkin commented that in trying to prepare cell surface markers for embryological studies, it has been found that plasma membrane preparations or intact cell preparations often fail to give an immunogenic response (see recent discussion by Moscona and Hausman 1977). Recently, it has been found that the immunogenic factor has to be unmasked, for example, by using an EDTA wash or a very light pronase or trypsin treatment to expose certain cell surface molecules. Sensitization then produced antisera with high specificity against many types of embryonic cells in a way that was not possible before these partial stripping techniques had been applied.

Dr. Slavkin asked whether it might be possible to obtain antibodies to, for example, leukoplakias, by raising sera which were absorbed with normal tissue. Dr. Outzen said that time and time again the results of animal experimentation and examination of human material have shown that most "spontaneous" lesions have little if any immunogenicity, and if they have no immunogenicity, they cannot be used to raise an antiserum. If all spontaneous tumors are nonantigenic or nonimmunogenic, then the whole concept of tumor immunology, even of immune stimulation, would become somewhat irrelevant. However, viral tumors and tumors induced by carcinogens are antigenic and perhaps many of the human tumors that were thought of as being spontaneous are not truly so, but occur in groups of genetically-susceptible individuals who are exposed to a common environmental carcinogen. If this were the case, such tumors may, in essence, be carcinogen-induced and highly antigenic. An extrapolation from animal work would suggest that these tumors would be individually specific and not cross-react, but if they were antigenic, there is at least a potential for immunotherapy.

Dr. Mackenzie said that there appears to be an enormous diversity of antigenic molecules exposed to the cell surface, and asked Dr. Outzen in what way each of these differing molecules is conceived to be functional. Dr. Outzen replied that there was indeed a large number of cell surface antigens, some being expressed early in development and then lost during differentiation when others were gained. Some, such as the H_2 and the T locus, have been extensively studied and these, and probably most of the antigenic cell surface molecules, function as receptors of some sort. Dr. Slavkin commented that the cell surface has species-specific information, tissue-specific information, spatial information, and information about the phase of the cell-cycle and pattern of cell differentiation (see Bennett et al. 1972). Given a projection of thousands of bits of information of this sort, an enormous diversity of receptors was perhaps not surprising. Dr. Mackenzie asked whether, as a tumor cell appeared to display a loss of normal function, a loss rather than a gain of specific antigen might not be expected. Dr. Dabelsteen replied that an alteration in the molecular configuration of a receptor might lead to a loss of physiological function, but that this loss of function might well be associated with a new antigenicity because of the altered molecule.

Dr. Dabelsteen asked Dr. Outzen whether immunostimulation of a lesion is viewed as a process specifically associated with a particular antigen, for example, could the immune response resulting from infection of a leukoplakia with Candida act as a nonspecific immune stimulation which leads to a tumor. Dr. Outzen replied that he did not see why this was not possible; an antigen common to both the tumor and the Candida could lead to stimulation. On the other hand, stimulation might not need to be so specific and perhaps just the presence of active lymphocytes in the local area is all that is necessary.

Dr. Slavkin asked about the role of proteases in the early stages of neoplasia. Are they normally present at the cell surface and when unmasked, for example by transformation, could this lead to the cell surface becoming enzymatically active? Dr. Smith replied that proteolytic enzymes have been located at the actively growing edges of tumors. However, whether the origin of this activity is from the tumor cells or the associated macrophages is uncertain and the techniques so far used do not provide adequate specificity or resolution. This might be provided by the new immunohistochemical techniques which are being developed.

REFERENCES

Bennett, D., Boyse, E. A., and Old, L. J. 1972. Cell surface immunogenetics in the study of morphogenesis. In: *Cell Interactions.* Lepetit Colloquium, 3d, London, 1971, Proceedings. (Edited by Silvestri, L. G.), pp. 247–263. Elsevier/North Holland, Amsterdam.

Harmon, R. E., Clark, E. A., Reddy, A. L., Hildemann, W. H., and Mullen, I. 1977. Immunity to MCA-induced rat sarcomas: Analysis of *in vivo* and *in vitro* results. *Int. J. Cancer* **20**, 748–758.

Johnson, N. W. 1976. The role of histopathology in diagnosis and prognosis of oral squamous cell carcinoma. *Proc. R. Soc. Med.* **69**, 740–747.

Johnson, N. W. 1977. Histological and histochemical studies of oral cancer. *Int. Dent. J.* **27**, 25–34.

Kollar, E. 1972. Histogenetic aspects of dermal-epidermal interactions. In: *Developmental Aspects of Oral Biology.* (Edited by Slavkin, H. C., and Bavetta, L. A.), pp. 125–149. Academic Press, New York.

Moscona, A. A., and Hausman, R. E. 1977. Biological and biochemical studies on embryonic cell-cell recognition. In: *Cell and Tissue Interactions.* (Edited by Lash, J. W., and Burger, M. N.), pp. 173–185. Raven Press, New York.

Slavkin, H. C., Trump, G. N., Brownell, A., and Sorgente, N. 1977. Epithelial-mesenchymal interactions: Mesenchymal specificity. In: *Cell and Tissue Interactions.* (Edited by Lash, J. W., and Burger, M. N.), pp. 29-46. Raven Press, New York.

PART FIVE
DIAGNOSIS AND PROGNOSIS

18

Clinical Features of Oral Malignancy in Relation to Prognosis

A. MASHBERG

Oral Surgery Section, Veterans Administration Hospital, East Orange, New Jersey

1. INTRODUCTION

Although oral squamous cancer in the United States accounts for approximately 5% of malignancies in males and 2% in females (Seidman et al. 1976), instruction about oral cancer within qualified institutions is frequently fragmented and departmentalized—especially in the area of diagnosis. The oral mucosa is easily accessible for visual examination and squamous carcinoma is easily discernible in its early asymptomatic stages, long before ulceration, bleeding, induration, and lymphadenopathy are present; yet at least 60% of intraoral lesions are well advanced (Stage III; American Joint Committee for Cancer Staging 1976) at the time of discovery (Batsakis 1974). The greatest concern of therapists is with the treatment of the *symptomatic lesion* which has been brought to their attention by the patient or by referral. Information disseminated to students and practitioners is usually related to surgical, radiotherapeutic, and chemotherapeutic management of comparatively large lesions, frequently with metastasis; a considerable interest remains in ablative techniques.

Misconceptions are common; etiology is obscure with a multiplicity of factors being indicated without scientific corroboration; natural history is unclear. New criteria for evaluating and diagnosing lesions are disseminated slowly. Diagnostic techniques other than biopsy are not wholly adequate. Morbidity and mortality continue to be high with 5 year survival rates of approximately 30 to 50%.

In recent years, numerous attempts have been made to increase the number of comparatively small *asymptomatic* carcinomas diagnosed and thereby reduce mortality and morbidity. There has been an increasing trend to establish cancer detection programs. Unfortunately, this positive approach has resulted in a limited yield which may be, in part, due to a scientific lag. This failure to effectively increase recognition rates of oral cancer in its early *asymptomatic* stages, and thereby increase survival rates—hopefully approaching that of the 80 to 95% which exists for lip and skin carcinomas—appears related to the dissemination of inadequate and ambiguous criteria for recognition of this disease. Cancer screening clinics are commendable; however, if the criteria utilized by the "screeners" are not adequate, then of necessity the yield will be low.

2. LEUKOPLAKIA[1]

The ubiquitous "leukoplakia"—white lesion—has been indicted as the most common "precancerous" lesion of the oral cavity (see chapters 1 and 2; Bhaskar 1965; MacComb 1960; MacComb et al. 1967). Although previous studies (Hobaek 1946) indicated the percent of leukoplakia which developed into cancer ranged from 10 to 100% with 25% as a generally cited figure, more recent studies by Einhorn and Wersall (1967) and Pindborg (1976; and chapter 1, this volume), indicated that about 4% of leukoplakias developed into cancer over a prolonged period. Malaowalla et al. (1976), in a study in India where leukoplakia abounds, indicated that of 11,610 leukoplakias, 0.13% became malignant in 2 years—a low rate of transformation for a select group at high risk.

There have been warnings on the overemphasis of the malignant potential of leukoplakia (Burket 1965; Lattes 1967; Robinson 1957), but generally this concept prevails in the literature and teaching institutions. The tendency to describe any mucosal aberration with keratotic components or white "slough" as a white lesion or leukoplakia, with disregard for other components of the lesion, still exists, as many clinicians are still reacting to historical concepts regarding their appearance.

3. ERYTHROPLASIA

Since 1961, in about 500 mucosal biopsies, the author has observed that the overwhelming number of asymptomatic white (keratotic) lesions were histologically benign with minimal or no cellular atypia. Less than 2% of these lesions have been diagnosed as carcinoma or carcinoma in situ; whereas asymptomatic lesions with *erythroplastic* (red) components often revealed malignant changes.

Pindborg (1963), in his studies, indicated that some leukoplakic lesions which were associated with epithelial dysplasia[2] or carcinoma had a speckled appearance—"white patches on an erythematous background." Shafer and Waldron (1975) in their most recent study on leukoplakia,

[1] All references to leukoplakia, white lesions, and keratotic lesions in this paper are related to clinical appearances only.

[2] The term epithelial dysplasia is used to describe alterations in the relationship of cells and the shape, size, and staining characteristics of the nucleus. Although all the criteria for malignancy may not be present microscopically, these cells individually resemble neoplastic cells.

indicate that lesions with mixed white and red components were included, and that prior to 1961, when the concept of "oral erythroplakia" was not well defined, lesions which were purely red were also included in their studies of leukoplakia. Sandler (1964) revealed that 50% of all cancers detected by his cytological screening technique were red; unfortunately, his emphasis was on the screening technique and not on the observation that the so-called "innocuous" red lesion was not, in reality, innocuous, but the earliest sign of oral cancer.

A direct relationship between these red, velvety, erythroplastic changes and oral cancer had not been suggested until the observations of Pindborg (1963), Shedd (1971), Mashberg et al. (1973), and Mashberg and Meyers (1976), were published. Pindborg indicated that of 35 lesions with white, nodular patches intermingled with erythematous areas, 51% were associated with epithelial dysplasia, and 14% with carcinoma. Studies by Shear (1972) and Shafer and Waldron (1975) indicate a growing interest in these lesions. In the study by Mashberg and Meyers (1976) of the location of 207 (excluding lip cancers) intraoral malignant lesions (color not indicated in published report), 69 (33.3%) were entirely erythematous, 124 (60%) were mixed (red and white), and only 10 (4.9%) were all white. Our studies of patients at high risk (heavy smokers and drinkers) have revealed that in the natural history of oral cancer, the red velvety lesion is the earliest visible mucosal alteration, signaling the presence of malignancy long before the appearance of ulceration, bleeding, induration, dysfunction, pain, or lymphadenopathy.

4. THE ERYTHROPLASTIC LESION

There are two distinct types of erythroplastic lesions that suggest the presence of carcinoma. The first is a granular, red, velvety lesion with either stippled or patchy areas of white (keratin) within or peripheral to the lesion (Fig. 1). These white areas appear to be lying on an inflamed mucosal surface that looks distinctly red. In describing these lesions, I frequently use the analogy that they appear as an area of worn velvet on which granules of farina have been spilled. The other is a smooth, nongranular lesion, primarily red, with minimal or no white areas (Fig. 2). The area once again looks like an inflammation. The mucosal surface, however, is not similar to that of a nonspecific inflammatory lesion, in that it seems atrophic and "worn."

These alterations in the mucosal surface may not have well defined boundaries. Many are irregular, with a blending of redness and normal mucosa. Some contain islands of entrapped normal mucosa, which have been created by the development and coalescence of a few malignant erythroplastic areas—field cancerization. Although these islands appear white or gray, they are not truly keratotic. Palpation is not revealing and only 20% are elevated above 1 mm.

Histologic studies of our specimens show 80% of these lesions to be invasive carcinomas. The erythematous character of the lesion appears to be related to an inflammatory barrier infiltrate present beneath the tumor (Fig. 3).

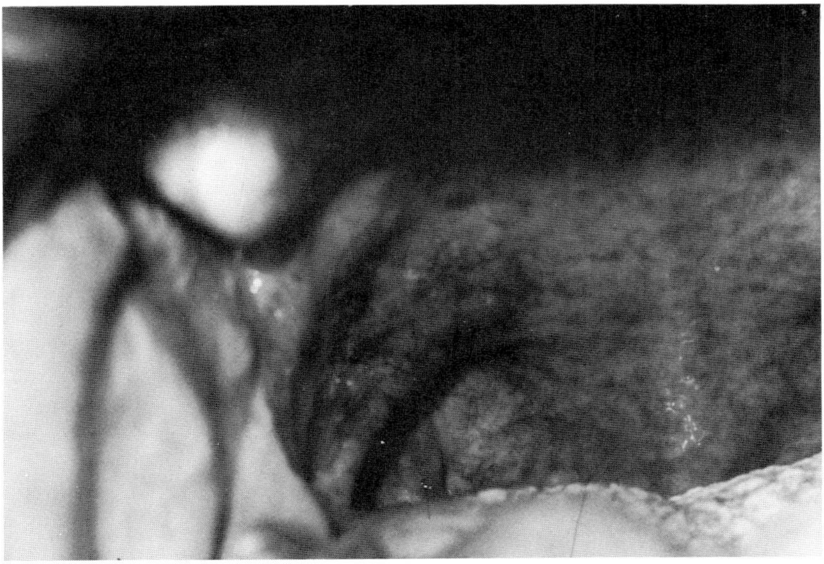

FIGURE 1. Reprinted by permission from Mashberg and Meyers 1976.

5. HIGH RISK SITES

The specific anatomical regions within the oral cavity have been defined by the American Joint Committee for Cancer Staging (Smith et al. 1968). We have further subdivided some of these sites in our studies of the distribution of carcinomas in the oral cavity (Mashberg et al. 1973).

In the past, the lips, hard palate, buccal mucosa, and gingiva, in addition to the floor of the mouth, soft palate, and tongue were all considered to harbor significant numbers of squamous carcinomas. However, in recent years this attitude has been altered. Based on the various studies by Moore and Catlin (1967), Mashberg et al. (1973), and others, the floor of the mouth, ventral tongue, and soft palate complex (i.e., soft palate proper, anterior pillar, and lingual aspect of retromolar trigone) have assumed much greater significance as sites predisposed to develop squamous carcinoma. The author has suggested that these sites be designated as *high*

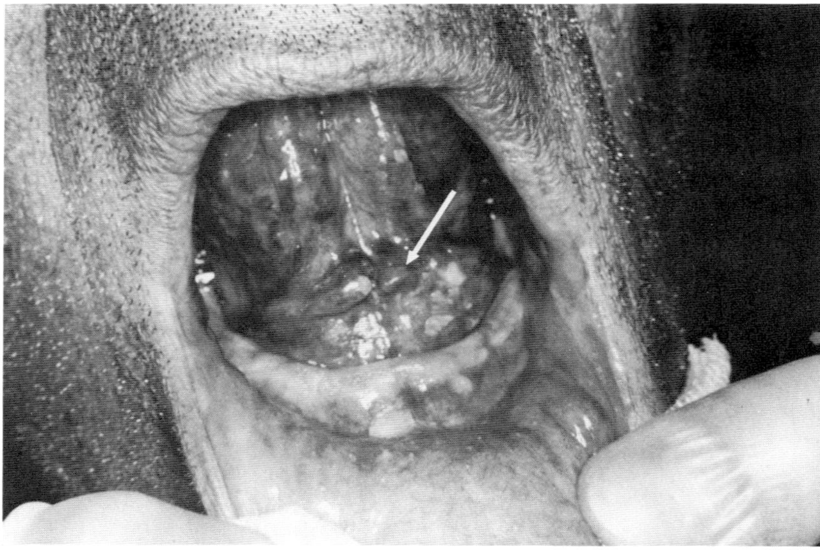

FIGURE 2. Reprinted by permission from Mashberg et al. 1973.

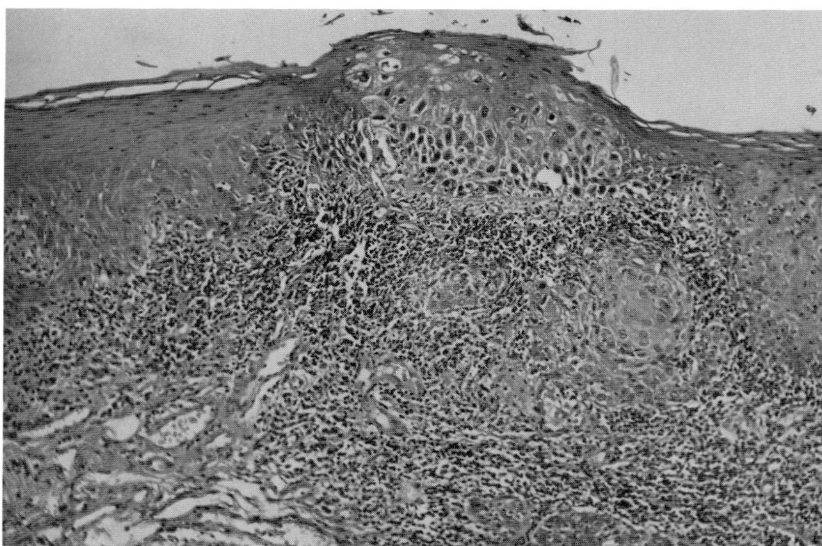

FIGURE 3. Reprinted by permission from Mashberg et al. 1973.

risk areas. Our previously noted prospective study of 222 asymptomatic, primarily erythroplastic squamous cell carcinomas of the oral mucosa in 161 patients (heavy smokers and drinkers), revealed that 201 (90.6%) lesions were found in three locations: floor of the mouth (101), ventral or lateral tongue (36), and soft palate complex (64). Significantly, only 6 were found distributed between the hard palate (1), alveolar gingiva (3), and buccal mucosa (2). Fifteen occurred on the lip. Of the 101 in the floor of the mouth, 73 occurred in the anterior portion, with 33 involving the papilla at the exit of Wharton's Duct (submaxillary gland).

The small number of asymptomatic hard palate, buccal, and alveolar lesions suggested that the site description of symptomatic lesions in the literature may be points of termination or extension rather than the site, or origin, e.g., a symptomatic lesion (at least 2–4 cm.) in the floor of the mouth may extend to and invade the alveolus, so that on clinical appearance and X-ray evidence, it may be documented as a gingival or alveolar lesion. A large soft palate lesion which has extended to the hard palate, necessitating a maxillectomy, may have been described as a hard palate malignancy. With the new clinical criteria developed for intraoral malignancies there seems to be a decrease in the relative number of lesions classified as lip lesions.

It may be of interest to note that there is great histological similarity in the tissues of the high risk areas. They are lined by a thin layer of epithelium which is devoid of keratin and a loose submucosa which contains fat and glands in contrast to the other areas which are either keratinized or highly specialized as is the dorsum of the tongue. Possibly high risk areas unprotected by keratin are more subject to the effect of carcinogenic agents (see chapter 9).

6. RECENT FINDINGS

6:1 COLOR OF LESIONS

In our most recent prospective study from 1973 to the present, documenting the color of persistent oral lesions, patients with *asymptomatic* and nonspecific oral lesions found during routine oral examination (which is mandatory for all inpatients in our institution) were reappointed for a second evaluation from 7 to 14 days later. If possible, in the interval, all known sources of irritation were withdrawn and all infections treated, if indicated. Upon re-examination, those persistent *asymptomatic* lesions in any portion of the oral cavity which clinically showed suspicion of invasive carcinoma, carcinoma in situ, or epithelial dysplasia as defined by our previous criteria, or those changes which did not correspond to visual criteria but were found in *high risk sites,* were carefully documented. Alterations considered clinically suspicious were recorded as epithelial dysplasia, carcinoma in situ, or invasive carcinoma; whereas lesions considered benign were diagnosed as keratoses, inflammation, or other. After biopsy, a final pathological diagnosis was recorded.

In evaluating the appearance of 169 intraoral lesions entered into the study (Table 1), we found red lesions to be more frequently carcinoma than white lesions. Of 90 lesions, appearing as red only (45) or red predominating with white (45), there were 62 (68.9%) with carcinoma, whereas of 75 lesions appearing white only (53) or white predominating with red (22), only 12 (16%) were carcinoma. Only 4 of 53 (7.5%) solely white lesions were cancer. Significantly, only 31.1% of the red or predominantly red lesions were benign. Table 2 indicates that of the 75 asymptomatic cancers in this group of 169 lesions, 82.7% were red or primarily red with some white component. Table 3, combining the 240 lesions in our study since 1961, reveals a similar pattern.

If one compares the accuracy of clinical impression with the final pathological diagnosis (Table 4), then the significance of erythroplasia is reinforced since the author's clinical impressions were guided primarily by the premise that erythroplasia in high risk areas without apparent etiology suggests the presence of early carcinoma. Note the false negative rate (underdiagnosis) of 5.3% (4/75) and a false positive (overdiagnosis) of 22.4% (22/98). Although not shown on these charts, epithelial dysplasias were evenly distributed among the red and the white lesions.

It is notable that of the 64 cancer patients with the 75 cancers, only 3 had lymphadenopathy. In 2 of these, the adenopathy was believed to be related to a primary tumor in the oropharynx. In the third patient, the cervical nodes were mobile, and since the patient received radiation therapy a determination could not be made relative to tumor involvement of the nodes.

6:2 HIGH RISK SITES

The anatomical distribution of 72 of 75 (96%) oral carcinomas again continues to support the premise that early carcinoma occurs primarily at the *high risk sites,* rather than being randomly distributed throughout the oral cavity (Table 5).

If we examine our cumulative statistics since 1961, of 240 intraoral lesions, 97.5% (234) were found in the high risk sites. Only 6 were distributed among the hard palate (1), buccal mucosa (2), and alveolar ridge (3) (Fig. 4). Additionally the number of early cancers (75) as compared to the number of benign lesions (94) is much greater than one would expect.

FIGURE 4.

ANATOMICAL DISTRIBUTION OF 240 ASYMPTOMATIC ORAL SQUAMOUS CELL CARCINOMAS

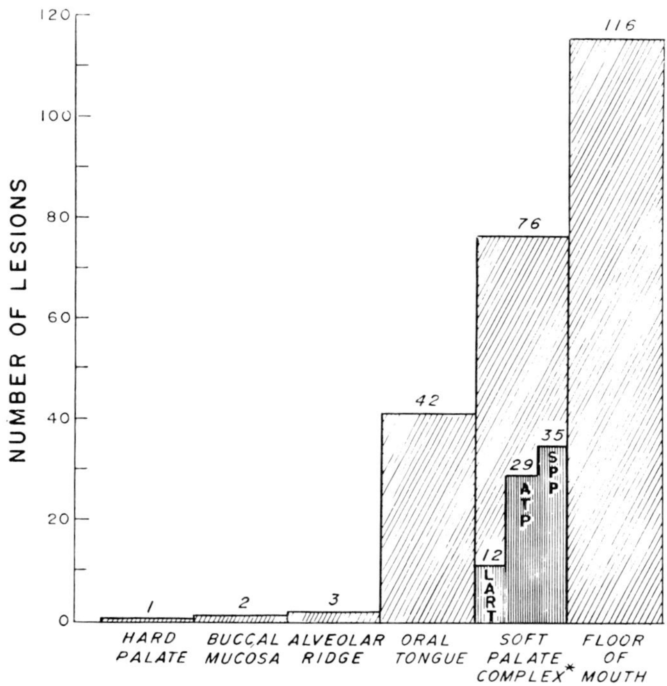

*SOFT PALATE COMPLEX INCLUDES THE LINGUAL ASPECT OF THE RETROMOLAR TONGUE, THE ANTERIOR TONSILLAR PILLAR AND THE SOFT PALATE PROPER

TABLE 1

Color Component for 169 Oral lesions
In High Risk Sites

Color	*Lesions*	*Carcinomas*	
Red only	45	29	64.4%
Red predominant with white	45	33	73.3%
White predominant with red	22	8	36.4%
White only	53	4	7.5%
Yellow-brown	2	1	–
Other and not stated	2	–	–
Total	169	75	

TABLE 2

Color Component for 75
Asymptomatic Oral Squamous-Cell Carcinomas

Red only	29	(38.7%)	
Red predominant with white	33	(44.0%)	54.7
White predominant with red	8	(10.7%)	
White only	4	(5.3%)	
Yellow-brown	1	(1.3%)	
Total	75	(100%)	

TABLE 3

Color Component of 240
Asymptomatic Oral Squamous Cell Carcinomas

Red only	81	(33.8%)
Red with white	145	(60.4%)
White only	11	(4.6%)
Yellow-brown	1	(0.4%)
Other or not stated	2	(0.8%)
Total	240	(100%)

TABLE 4

Asymptomatic Oral Squamous Cell Carcinoma
Clinical Suspicion vs Pathological Diagnosis

PATHOLOGIC DX		*Clinically Suspicious** *Yes*	*No*
Invasive carcinoma	(62)	59	3
Carcinoma in situ	(13)	12	1
Atypia	(9)	5	4
Benign	(85)	22	63
Total	169	98	71

False Negatives 4/75=5.3%
False Positives 22/98=22.4%
*A clinical diagnosis of Ca, Ca in situ or atypia indicates clinical suspicion.

TABLE 5

Anatomical Distribution of 75
Asymptomatic Oral Squamous Cell Carcinomas

Buccal mucosa	2	2.7%	
Lingual gingiva	1	1.3%	
Floor of mouth	39	52.0%	
Oral tongue	12	16.0%	
Hard palate	–	–	
Soft palate	9	12.0%	28.0%*
Anterior tonsillar pillar	10	13.3%	
Lingual aspect of retromolar trigone	2	2.7%	
Total	75	100.0%	

*72/75 lesions occurred in the floor of the mouth, ventrolateral tongue and soft palate complex.

7. MORBIDITY AND SURVIVAL

Since the etiology of oral cancer is obscure (although alcohol and tobacco appear to be related (see chapter 2)), and a definitive cure is still not within our grasp, early visual detection of oral cancer still remains the best available method to increase survival rates and decrease attendant morbidity.

In 1961, before the erythroplastic lesion in high risk sites was defined, two to three asymptomatic cancers per year were being diagnosed at this institution. Using the new criteria, we are finding approximately 25 asymptomatic squamous cell carcinomas in 5,000 patient examinations per year: that is, one oral cancer for every 200 routine oral examinations, or 500 cancers per 100,000 examinations as compared to 10 per 100,000 in the general population and 40 per 100,000 in the general population age group 60–64 (L. Garfinkel 1977, personal communication). However, these lesions are in male patients at high risk (i.e., heavy smokers and drinkers in the fifth, sixth, and seventh decades).

It has been firmly established that stage (Sandler 1970; Batsakis 1974), more than any other parameter, influences the survival rate of patients with squamous cell carcinoma. Moore (1966) stated, "... no lethal disease is easier to cure than oral cancer less than 1 cm in diameter." As more than 80% of these asymptomatic cancers are 2 cm or less, and 40% are 1 cm or less in diameter, treatment results are excellent; postoperative surgical morbidity and deformity are minimal since lesions are excised locally, with minimal soft tissue and bone loss. Few, if any, require extensive ablative procedures resulting in loss of bone continuity and gross soft tissue, scarring, and deformity. Radiotherapy is necessary only for broad diffuse lesions. External cosmetic defects are nonexistent and function is rated at least adequate.

Comparative survival rates for our patients at this time are difficult to assess since we are dealing with a hospital population at high risk, who are primarily admitted for a variety of chronic medical and surgical diseases, with an expected low survival rate. Ten percent of these patients had attendant bleeding, ulceration, induration, or a combination of these signs, and only one had lymphadenopathy related to the oral cancer. These findings in themselves suggest a more favorable prognosis since the presence of nodes reduces survival rate by 50% and certainly increases surgical and radiotherapeutic morbidity. Fewer than 10% of these patients with early asymptomatic carcinoma are not heavy drinkers and smokers; many are cirrhotic. Perhaps recurrence rates may be more easily assessed in determining the importance of utilizing these new criteria in early diagnosis to decrease morbidity and mortality. Although our data is still being analyzed, it is my impression that the recurrence rates for these small asymptomatic invasive cancers documented from 1961 to the present, is about 5%.

8. CONCLUSIONS

(1) Persistent erythroplastic asymptomatic lesions in high risk patients (smokers and drinkers) are suspect. In contrast to most leukoplakias, the erythroplastic lesion usually shows severe histologic changes. At the present stage of these studies, the evidence indicates that *red velvety lesions with or without white components in high risk sites of the oral cavity should be considered at the very least carcinoma in situ or invasive carcinoma—unless proven otherwise.*

(2) The recognition and treatment of asymptomatic lesions at this stage of development results in decreased morbidity, minimal recurrence, and, hopefully, an increased survival rate.

Portions of this paper are reprinted by permission from Mashberg, A. 1977. Erythroplasia vs. leukoplakia in the diagnosis of early asymptomatic oral squamous carcinoma. *N. Engl. J. Med.* **297**, 109–110; and Mashberg, A. 1978. Erythroplasia: The earliest sign of oral cancer. *J. Am. Dent. Assoc.* **96**, 615–620.

REFERENCES

American Joint Committee for Cancer Staging and End Results Reporting. 1976. *Classification and Staging of Cancer by Site: A Preliminary Handbook*. Chicago.

Batsakis, J. 1974. *Tumors of the Head and Neck: Clinical and Pathological Considerations*, pp. 86–100. Williams and Wilkins, Baltimore.

Bhaskar, S. N. 1965. *Synopsis of Oral Pathology*. 2d ed. C. V. Mosby, St. Louis.

Burket, L. W. 1965. *Oral Medicine*. 5th ed. J. B. Lippincott, Philadelphia.

Einhorn, J., and Wersäll, J. 1967. Incidence of oral carcinoma in patients with leukoplakia of the oral mucosa. *Cancer* **20**, 2189–2193.

Hobaek, A. 1946. Leukoplakia oris. *Acta Odontol. Scand.* **7**, 61–91.

Lattes, R. 1967. Precancerous lesions of the oral cavity and larynx. In: *The International Workshop on Cancer of the Head and Neck*. (Edited by Conley, John), pp. 33–40. Butterworth, Washington, D.C.

MacComb, W. S. 1960. Leukoplakia of the intraoral cavity. *Postgrad. Med.* **27**, 349–355.

MacComb, W. S., Fletcher, G. H., and Healey, J. E. 1967. Intra-oral cavity. In: *Cancer of the Head and Neck*. (Edited by MacComb, W. S., and Fletcher, G. H.), pp. 89–151. Williams and Wilkins, Baltimore.

Malaowalla, A. M., Silverman, S., Mani, N. J., Mani, B. D., Bilimoria, B. D., and Smith, L. W. 1976. Oral cancer in 57,518 industrial workers of Gujarat, India: A prevalence and follow-up study. *Cancer* **37**, 1882–1886.

Mashberg, A., Morrissey, J. B., and Garfinkel, L. 1973. A study of the appearance of early asymptomatic squamous cell carcinoma. *Cancer* **32**, 1436–1445.

Mashberg, A., and Meyers, H. 1976. Anatomical site and size of 222 early asymptomatic oral squamous cell carcinomas: A continuing prospective study of oral cancer. II. *Cancer* **37**, 2149–2157.

Moore, C. 1966. Education and oral cancer. In: *Oral Cancer, Interprofessional Symposium: Papers Presented at Interprofessional Symposium, Jan. 22–23, 1966*. (Sponsored by the Cancer Control Program, Health Services and Mental Health Administration), p. 89. U. S. Government Printing Office, Washington, D.C.

Moore, C., and Catlin, D. 1967. Anatomic origins and locations of oral cancer. *Am. J. Surg.* **114**, 510–513.

Pindborg, J. J., Renstrup, G., Poulsen, H. E., and Silverman, S. 1963. Studies in oral leukoplakias. V. Clinical and histologic signs of malignancy. *Acta Odontol. Scand.* **21**, 407–414.

Pindborg, J. J. 1976. Current concepts of oral precancerous lesions. Paper read at Greater New York Dental Meeting, Nov. 28–Dec. 2, 1976, New York City.

Robinson, H. B., ed. 1957. *Symposium on Tumors of the Oral Regions*. W. B. Saunders, Philadelphia.

Sandler, H. C. 1964. *Oral Exfoliative Cytology: Veterans Administration Cooperative Study*. U.S. Government Printing Office, Washington, D.C.

Sandler, H. C. 1970. A retrospective study of a head and neck cancer control program. *Cancer* **25**, 1153–1161.

Seidman, H., Silverberg, E., and Holleb, A. I. 1976. Cancer statistics, 1976: A comparison of white and black populations. *CA* **26**, 2–30.

Shafer, W. G., and Waldron, C. A. 1975. Erythroplakia of the oral cavity. *Cancer* **36**, 1021–1028.

Shear, M. 1972. Erythroplakia of the mouth. *Int. Dent. J.* **22**, 460–473.

Shedd, D. P. 1971. Clinical characteristics of early oral cancer. *JAMA* **215**, 955–956.

Smith, R. R., Bullock, W. K., Friedman, M., MacComb, W. S., Schulz, M. D., and Tollefsen, H. R. 1968. *Clinical Staging System for Carcinoma of the Oral Cavity*. Vol. 9, pp. 1–12. American Joint Committee for Cancer Staging and End Results Reporting, Chicago.

19

Prognosis from Features Observable by Conventional Histopathological Examination

I. R. H. KRAMER

Department of Oral Pathology, Institute of Dental Surgery
Eastman Dental Hospital, University of London, London, England

When assessing the prognosis in supposedly precancerous lesions of the oral mucosa, the histopathologist is attempting to do two things. Firstly, he is trying to judge in which particular patients the malignant change is most likely to occur, and secondly, he would like to put a time scale to the sequence of events. Furthermore, the histopathologist is inevitably (and rightly) influenced in his opinion not only by the microscopic features but also by the clinical data. From the histopathologic point of view, the principal guide to prognosis is epithelial dysplasia, so it is on this complex of changes that most emphasis must be placed in the present discussion.

There are four main ways in which an attempt is made to assess the prognosis from an assessment of epithelial dysplasia. The first of these is the traditional and essentially subjective method. This involves examining the biopsy and using, in a mainly subconscious way, the criteria discussed in chapter 3, deciding whether serious changes are impending or whether there is nothing that is cause for immediate concern.

Secondly, an attempt can be made to reduce or eliminate the subjective element by counting and measuring: i.e., by the application of morphometric methods (see chapter 15). Unfortunately, at present, such measurements cannot be fully automated, and consequently the process is immensely tedious and time-consuming. Furthermore, once everything has been measured, there is still the problem of deciding on the significance of the values obtained, in terms of the risk of malignant change and the time scale on which it may occur. These are still, therefore, research procedures, rather than procedures that can be used in routine diagnostic work.

Thirdly, and more practically, the pathologist can attempt some method of standardization of his assessment, using for example, photomicrographs such as those provided by Smith and Pindborg (1969). If he uses such semistandardized criteria, he may go further and attempt to express the degree of epithelial dysplasia in quantitative terms. Smith and Pindborg suggested a scoring method that might be applied, some components of epithelial dysplasia carrying a heavier numerical weighting than others, and each component being scored on its own scale according to the severity of that particular change. However, the numerical weighting they placed on each component of epithelial dysplasia was determined subjectively, on the basis of experience. This does not mean that it is wrong, but it is nevertheless subjective. For example, they suggested that the presence of mitoses in the upper half of the epithelium should score 10 points, whilst a marked increase in the nucleocytoplasmic ratio should score only 6, and that a marked disturbance in polarity should also score 6 points. It is likely that any pathologist could take the same list of components but produce a different scoring system.

The fourth approach that may be employed is the one explored by Kramer and his coworkers (Kramer 1969; Kramer et al. 1970a, 1970b; Kramer et al. 1974) involving the application of computer-aided analyses in an attempt to reduce the subjective element. These analyses are still at a primitive stage, and the methods contain many defects, but they may point the way to a method that has much promise for the future. These computer-aided studies have had three main objectives: to aid in the differential diagnosis of oral mucosal lesions, to aid in assessing the prognosis, and to give us a better insight into the workings of the traditional subjective methods.

Although diagnosis and prognosis are sometimes considered as two different things, they are essentially parts of of the same process, and this is a process of classification. It would be very convenient if each different disease had a single unique and easily recognizable feature from which it could be classified—in other words, from which the diagnosis could be made—and similarly it would be ideal if there were a single and easily recognizable or measurable feature from which the prognosis could be determined. Such ideal conditions do not exist. Instead, for each diagnosis or prognosis there is a large number of variables to be considered, no one of which, taken alone, acts as an absolute discriminator between one condition and another.

In his *Principles of Geology,* Lyell (1832) wrote: "The greater abundance of natural objects assembled together, the more do we discover proofs that everything passes by insensible shades into something else, that even the more remarkable differences are evanescent, and that Nature has, for the most part, left us nothing at our disposal for establishing distinctions, save trifling and, in some respects, puerile particularities." That comment applies as well to our own problems of histopathological diagnosis as to the problems of classification in geology, yet the interests of our patients demand that we must do what we can with the "trifling and, in some respects, puerile particularities."

Thus, in order to classify for diagnostic or prognostic purposes, it is necessary to base judgments on a considerable number of variables, each having its particular degree of relevance to the solution of the problem. If an attempt is made to separate a number of different entities by measuring only one variable, as in unidirectional chromotography, a very imperfect separation may be achieved: the different molecules may not be moved into well-separated patches or clusters. The addition of another variable, as in two-dimensional chromatography, may improve the separation. The measurement of a third variable, in a third dimension, may produce a better result still, but there are now no further dimensions available. However, the computer is not limited by these three dimensions. The computer can simultaneously explore how cases would group themselves in relation to almost any number of variables, for the computer can work in multidimensional space or "hyperspace," and it is this attribute of the computer that has been employed in one of the approaches to the differential diagnosis and prognosis of oral mucosal lesions (Kramer et al. 1970a).

If it were possible to link the computer to the microscope itself, and measure all of the variables in each biopsy, this would to a large extent eliminate the human element, and the element of subjectivity. Unfortunately, this is not possible: a section of a biopsy presents too complex an image for present computer-aided optical scanning to analyze. Therefore, it was necessary to interpose a human observer between the section and the computer. However, there was an attempt to reduce the human element to a minimum by training the observer simply to record what could be seen, under a large number of fairly clearly-defined headings and, above all, the observer was to make no attempt at interpretation or diagnosis. The data about what could be seen down the microscope were then fed into the computer, which was programmed to analyze all of the cases about which it had this information and place them into groups or clusters—very like the patches on the chromatogram, but in this instance the computer was working in 41 dimensions simultaneously. When fed with information on 41 variables on each of 248 cases (representing, according to conventional diagnostic methods, leukoplakia, lichen planus, and carcinomas), the computer separated out many of these cases into clusters that seemed to correspond to our diagnostic categories. Table 1 shows how the 248 cases were grouped by the computer when the program specified the formation of 7 clusters. Cluster 3 is almost wholly made up of cases that had been diagnosed by conventional methods as lichen planus, and cluster 2 consists almost entirely of cases diagnosed as "leukoplakia." At the time when these cases had been routinely diagnosed, a distinction was made between the milder forms of leukoplakia, termed "keratosis," and the more severe forms termed "leukoplakia," although they appear under one heading in Table 1.

TABLE 1

		Seven Clusters						
	No.	*1*	*2*	*3*	*4*	*5*	*6*	*7*
Carcinoma	13	11	–	–	–	–	–	2
"Leukoplakia"	187	9	101	1	21	27	12	16
Lichen planus	48	–	1	33	–	7	3	4

Seven cluster analysis of 248 cases in which the computer was provided with histological data. Each cluster formed by the computer has been analyzed to see what diagnoses were made for these cases by conventional methods.

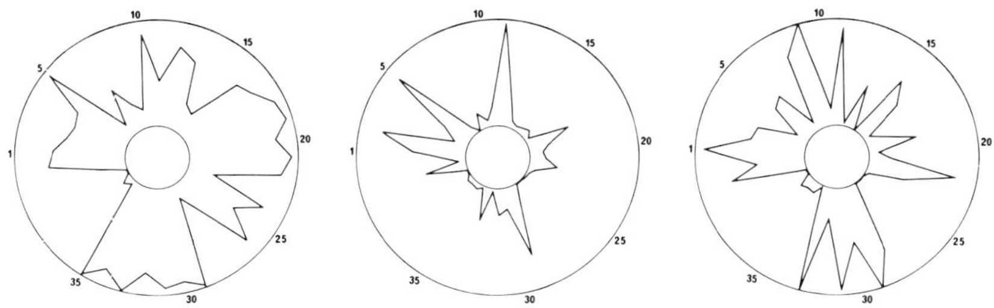

FIGURE 1. Polar vector diagrams depicting the histological characteristics of computer-selected clusters of cases representing:
left: carcinomas and more severe "leukoplakias."
middle: leukoplakias showing less severe changes (cases originally classified as "keratosis").
right: lichen planus.
(Reprinted by permission from Kramer et al., 1974).

Suppose that the 33 lichen planus cases placed together by the computer in cluster 3 represent histologically the most typical and characteristic lichen planus, and the 101 cases the computer has placed in cluster 2 represent histologically typical "keratosis" and "leukoplakia." It is now possible to program the computer to express in quantitative terms the histological characteristics that define the properties of each cluster.

The computer-calculated characteristics of each cluster were represented graphically in the form of polar vector diagrams (Kramer et al. 1974) which are simply based on graphs that are circular rather than having the x and y axes at right angles (Fig. 1). Each of 41 radii represents one variable, and the distance of the point from the inner circle represents the importance of that variable in defining the characteristics of that group or cluster of cases. When the points are joined to produce a closed figure, the difference between one of these diagrams and another can readily be seen.

In effect, each diagram represents the histological "fingerprint" of cases (selected and grouped together by the computer) that correspond to a conventional diagnostic category. As an example, the polar vector diagram depicting the histological characteristics of the computer-selected cases of lichen planus is compared in Fig. 1 with the diagram for the computer-selected cases of "keratosis" (the term we were using at that time for the milder forms of leukoplakia) and with the histological fingerprint of the group that contained the more severe leukoplakias. For any new case, it is now possible to determine mathematically the group to which it most closely corresponds, and this can be done in a relatively objective and quantitative way.

In these computer-aided studies, one of our principal aims was to see whether we could improve our ability to identify those cases with the greatest risk of malignant change. In the original cluster analyses, histological data on 13 cases of carcinoma were included (without telling the computer that there was invasion). These carcinomas acted as "markers" to see how the computer would group them in relation to the leukoplakias. In the cluster analysis shown in Table 2, the computer put 12 out of the 13 carcinomas in one cluster, but, out of the original 187 cases of keratosis and leukoplakia, it selected 11 and placed them in the same cluster as the carcinomas. As this was a retrospective survey, it was known that of the leukoplakia cases on which data had been fed to the computer, 4.8% subsequently developed carcinoma. But, of the leukoplakias that the computer split off from the main group and clustered with the carcinomas, 36% went malignant. In other words, the computer has tended to identify those leukoplakias that would subsequently develop carcinoma, and therefore, is tending to indicate the prognosis.

In the original cluster analyses, each histological variable was treated as being of equal importance to all of the other variables, but experience and common sense suggest that this is not so. For example, most pathologists would be more influenced by seeing abnormal mitoses than by seeing hyperorthokeratosis.

It is now possible to use a different type of analysis, in order to maximize the distinction between the clusters: this is the type of calculation that is termed discriminant analysis (Kramer et al. 1970b). In one of the discriminant analyses, the computer was given the histological data on two groups of cases; the leukoplakias that proceeded to carcinoma, and the leukoplakias that did not. It was then programmed to calculate a "weighting" or points value for each histological feature, and to do this in such a way that the separation of these two groups of cases was maximized.

The eight most important histological features distinguishing the leukoplakias that went malignant are listed in Table 3. Seven of these eight features or discriminators could probably have been predicted by any pathologist experienced in this field: one of them, the presence of Russell bodies, came as a complete surprise, although, in fact, Russell's original paper (Russell 1890) on these structures suggested that they were specially associated with cancer.

TABLE 2

		Six Clusters					
	No.	*1*	*2*	*3*	*4*	*5*	*6*
Carcinoma	13	12	–	–	1	–	–
"Leukoplakia"	187	11	110	6	20	28	12
Lichen planus	48	–	2	34	2	7	3

Six cluster computer-aided analysis of the cases shown in Table 1. In this analysis, note that, in cluster 1, the computer has placed most of the "marker" cases of carcinoma, together with 11 of the 187 cases of "leukoplakia." Whilst 4.8% of the 187 leukoplakia cases subsequently developed carcinoma, of the 11 leukoplakias placed by the computer in cluster 1, 36% developed carcinoma.

TABLE 3

Abnormal mitoses in the stratum spinosum
Disturbance of polarity of basal cells
Abnormal mitoses in the stratum basale
Nuclear hyperchromatism
Russell bodies in the lamina propria
Enlarged nucleoli
Pleomorphism
Intraepithelial keratinization

In the discriminant analysis to maximize the separation of leukoplakias that subsequently developed carcinoma from those that did not, these were the eight histological features calculated by the computer to be most important.

Thus by providing the computer with information about the histological features of a series of cases, the basis is established for a computer-aided classification of the cases by means of cluster analysis, and potentially this sort of cluster analysis or diagnosis could be more accurate than our subjective diagnosis methods. The computer can also calculate the histological characteristics—the histological "fingerprint"—of each cluster. The computer can then be instructed, by means of discriminant analysis, to give a numerical value to each histological feature in such a way that one group of cases is separated from another group with maximal efficiency, so that fewer cases fall into the overlap areas—the areas of diagnostic uncertainty.

Using the same type of discriminant analysis, it has also been shown that the computer can calculate the points value of each component of epithelial dysplasia and, indeed of all of the other histological features, for the specific purpose of helping to separate the cases that will become malignant from those that will not; in other words, the computer can help in assessing the prognosis. At this point it should be remembered that whilst a subjectively-devised "atypia index" will allocate points or weighting values to the features that the author believes to be important, this is only one side of the balance sheet. Although it does not have to do so, almost inevitably it will leave out what one might term "negative values" or points to be subtracted because of histological features that *reduce* the overall assessment of the seriousness of the lesion. In the computer-based calculations, numerical values are readily calculated for such features. It seems likely that, if an atlas of photographic standards of the type devised by Smith and Pindborg could be combined with a computer-calculated points system rather than a subjectively devised points system, then it might be possible to move a little closer to greater accuracy and uniformity in the prognosis of precancerous lesions of the mouth. Nevertheless the computer can only analyze the data that we provide; if certain histological variables that are of importance are omitted, or included in the wrong way, the help that the computer can provide will remain limited. Furthermore, the method is based on the assumption that adequate discriminators or prognostic features can actually be seen using the light microscope. In the present state of the art and until electron microscopists, or immunologists, or other workers provide a better way of assessing the prognosis, this assumption has to remain even though it may not be wholly true.

Certainly there is a correlation between the degree of epithelial dysplasia and the likelihood of invasive change, but this correlation is far from perfect. It is well established that, in the cervix, not all histological carcinoma in situ becomes invasive. There is evidence to support the view that apparently similar epithelial dysplasias in different sites (such as the cervix, the larynx, the conjunctiva, and the mouth) carry differing risks of proceeding to invasion. In some situations (such as the floor of the mouth) it is known that histologically "innocent" lesions carry a greater risk of malignant change than histologically innocent lesions in other sites (see chapter 18; Kramer et al. 1978). It is also known that certain factors (such as candidal infection) may produce dysplasia that seems to be reversible—although speckled leukoplakia, in which there is often a candidal infection, is more likely to become malignant than homogenous leukoplakia (see chapter 5).

Despite all of this evidence, some people still tend to think of epithelial dysplasia as a single complex of changes, always carrying the same meaning. However, we are forced to the conclusion that as a mirror of the underlying biological changes that lead to malignancy, epithelial dysplasia is a very imperfect mirror.

REFERENCES

Kramer, I. R. H. 1969. Precancerous conditions of the oral mucosa. A computer-aided study. *Ann. R. Coll. Surg. Engl.* **45**, 340–356.

Kramer, I. R. H., El-Labban, N. G., and Lee, K. W. 1978. The clinical features and risk of malignant transformation in sublingual keratosis. *Br. Dent. J.* **144**, 171–180.

Kramer, I. R. H., El-Labban, N. G., and Sonkodi, S. 1974. Further studies on lesions of the oral mucosa using computer-aided analyses of histological features. *Br. J. Cancer* **29**, 223–231.

Kramer, I. R. H., Lucas, R. B., El-Labban, N., and Lister, L. 1970a. A computer-aided study on the tissue changes in oral keratoses and lichen planus, and an analysis of case groupings by subjective and objective criteria. *Br. J. Cancer* **24**, 407–426.

Kramer, I. R. H., Lucas, R. B., El-Labban, N., and Lister, L. 1970b. The use of discriminant analysis for examining the histological features of oral keratoses and lichen planus. *Br. J. Cancer* **24**, 673–683.

Lyell, C. 1832. *Principles of Geology*, Vol. 2, p. 4. John Murray, London.

Russell, W. 1890. An address on a characteristic organism of cancer. *Br. Med. J.* **2**, 1356–1360.

Smith, C., and Pindborg, J. J. 1969. *Histological Grading of Oral Epithelial Atypia by the Use of Photographic Standards.* Copenhagen.

20

Biochemical and Histochemical Changes in Oral Premalignancy

N. W. JOHNSON,[1] A. W. EVANS,[1,2] P. R. MORGAN,[1] R. G. BUTCHER[2]

1. Department of Oral Pathology, London Hospital Medical College, London, England
2. The Midhurst Medical Research Institute, Midhurst, Sussex, England

1. INTRODUCTION

There are well documented differences in the metabolic activities of malignant cells when compared to their normal counterparts in the tissue of origin. These confer certain biological advantages on the cancer cell, and a recognizable pattern of enzymatic imbalance may be linked with the degree of malignancy (Weber 1977). An understanding of these processes has potential practical value in:

(a) Early detection of truly premalignant changes and of malignant transformation in the range of potentially malignant lesions, with a correspondingly increased chance of cure.

(b) The detection of sensitive enzymes or pathways amenable to chemotherapy.

It is important to realize, however, that the metabolic alterations involved may be substantially different in each of these applications and may thus require quite different research approaches (Potter 1962).

The development of a spectrum of tumors derived from rat liver and having different growth rates (Morris 1965; Morris and Wagner 1968) has made possible a detailed examination of the biochemical changes associated with different degrees of malignancy.

An extensive study of these tumors has been made by Weber and his associates (Weber et al. 1964; Weber 1966, 1972; Weber and Lea 1966, 1967). From his results has come the concept that the regulation of the rate and the direction of opposing and competing synthetic and catabolic pathways is achieved through the control of certain "key enzymes." These key enzymes may be of one of two types: transformation-linked discriminants, the activities of which are increased or decreased in all tumors; and progression-linked discriminants, the activities of which alter in parallel with the degree of malignancy. Other enzymes are not key enzymes—these are characterized by the following properties: they govern reversible equilibrium reactions, are shared by both synthetic and catabolic pathways, exhibit high activities, and are present in excess. In carbohydrate catabolism, these latter enzymes include aldolase and lactate dehydrogenase. A number of key enzymes from many pathways of intermediary metabolism have now been identified (Weber 1977). The changes observed in these enzymes, assayed under optimal biochemical conditions, have formed the basis of the "Molecular Correlation Concept" (Weber 1966, 1972, 1977; Weber and Lea 1966, 1967). According to this theory, the key enzymes of each metabolic pathway are governed by separate genetic units whose coordinated activity regulates the overall balance in tissues.

Apart from the quantitative differences described, there are qualitative changes in the nature of certain enzymes which exist in different molecular forms called isozymes or isoenzymes (for reviews see Criss 1971; Weinhouse 1971). In relation to the diagnosis of human neoplasms, isoenzymes of lactate dehydrogenase and of alkaline phosphatase have been most extensively investigated. They are usually studied in body fluids and may be of value in detecting deep-seated solid tumors. However, their application to small mucosal lesions would require histochemical approaches which are not yet adequately developed, although immunohistochemical methods show promise in this regard (Miyayama et al. 1976).

2. PROBLEMS IN THE APPLICATION OF METABOLIC STUDIES TO ORAL PREMALIGNANT LESIONS

Many studies of tissues from oral as well as other sites do not set out to test a stated hypothesis, but merely scan a tissue for activities of a range of enzymes which are not necessarily significant in the neoplastic process. The choice of enzyme studied is often based primarily on the existence of a convenient technique for demonstrating its presence. Unless an enzyme is known to be one of the "key" or "rate limiting" enzymes of a particular biochemical pathway, its activity need not bear any relation to the flux through that pathway. Further, if these key enzymes are under genetic control, they must be studied under optimal reaction conditions so that the activities detected truly reflect the enzyme content of the cell; this indicates the metabolic potential of the tissue in vivo though not necessarily the activity under physiological conditions. Similarly, unless key enzymes are chosen, the study of multiple enzymes within the same pathway provides empty information which only serves to confuse.

A major problem in interpreting data on enzyme activities in oral lesions is the paucity of information on the metabolism of normal oral mucosa in man and of the variations between lining, masticatory, and specialized mucosa in different sites (Squier et al. 1976). Questions of the validity of the animal models of oral carcinogenesis referred to earlier in chapter 7 also arise, for it cannot be taken for granted that the premalignant stages of, say, a carcinogen-treated hamster cheek pouch result in the same alterations as exist in a potentially malignant human mucosa. Faced with these unavoidable difficulties, most workers have chosen to relate the potentially new diagnostic feature under study to the degree of cellular atypia detectable by histological methods. Therein lies a major logical trap, however, for we are unable to differentiate those kinds or degrees of cellular atypia and epithelial dysplasia which really indicate pre- or early malignant change from those which do not (see chapter 19).

Perhaps most important of all, it cannot be assumed that the alterations seen are specific to neoplastic transformation unless they can be shown to be absent in other situations involving increased cell proliferation and cell movement, such as in wound healing and benign hyperplasia.

3. METHODS USED FOR STUDYING METABOLIC CHANGES IN PREMALIGNANT AND MALIGNANT EPITHELIA

The methods which have been most extensively applied to such studies can be gathered into three groups, namely standard biochemical techniques, stain histochemical techniques and quantitative microchemical techniques; this last can be further subdivided into ultramicrochemical methods based on the reaction in the test tube of minute pieces of tissue whose site and structure have been first identified by microscopy, and quantitative histochemical methods.

Standard biochemical methods have the advantages of permitting a wide range of techniques to be applied so that many enzymes and metabolic pathways can be studied. They are usually very sensitive, so that small changes in activity can be detected, and they are quantitatively accurate. Based on the rate of disappearance of substrate and/or rate of appearance of a product of a key enzyme-catalyzed reaction, the flux through the pathway involved can be determined. Biochemical methods have the major disadvantage however of requiring homogenates of tissue. This means that mean values are obtained and we are unable to distinguish the contribution from tumor parenchyma, from stromal cells, or from any inflammatory infiltrate present. As an example of the latter, much of the proteolytic activity detected in tumor homogenates may be derived from the macrophages and polymorphonuclear leucocytes which are so often present. Similarly it is impossible to isolate metabolic changes to individual cells or clones of cells, a requirement of prime importance in searching for pre- or early malignant changes in a tissue.

Stain histochemical methods depend upon the deposition of a colored reaction product at the site of enzyme activity, so that localization to cell and tissue type is possible. Diffusion artifact is, however, common. In order to overcome problems, many workers, for example Anderson and Hoyer (1974), have reduced the concentrations of the reagents to such an extent that the rate-limiting step becomes the final capture reaction. This is an artificial situation and no conclusions as to enzyme activity or enzyme content can be drawn from it. Furthermore, reactions which result in colored end products are limited in number so that the range of enzymes amenable to histochemical study is also limited. Finally, the small sample taken for histochemistry may be unrepresentative of the tissue as a whole, although this is a problem common to all microscopic methods.

Ultramicrochemical methods involve microdissection of thin slices of tissues or of freeze-dried frozen sections (see review by Gerson and Meyer 1970) into fragments which are weighed and incubated with substrate, after which the reaction products are estimated by standard measuring techniques. They thus provide better localization than routine biochemical methods, but the dissection techniques are difficult and slow, and they require especially sensitive detection reactions. However, they are quantitative and accurate and could with benefit be much more widely applied.

Quantitative histochemistry involves measurement of light absorbed by a given volume of the tissue section using a photometer or densitometer built into a microscope (Deely 1955). The application of this technique to enzyme histochemistry (Butcher 1972; Chayen et al. 1973), combined with the greater understanding of the physiochemical characteristics of the colored reaction products (Altman and Butcher 1973; Butcher and Altman 1973; Altman 1976), now permits precise measurements of the biochemical activity to be made at the cellular level.

A combination of methods is thus desirable in arriving at an understanding of the metabolism of neoplastic tissues, quantitative methods being likely to prove of particular value.

4. CARBOHYDRATE METABOLISM AND ENERGY PRODUCTION IN MALIGNANT EPITHELIUM WITH SPECIAL REFERENCE TO ORAL EPITHELIUM

Because tumor growth is accompanied by increased energy requirements of the neoplastic cells, an examination of the enzymes involved in cellular energy production may be of assistance in the early diagnosis of the premalignant lesion.

Cellular energy is mainly produced by the metabolism of carbohydrates so that Warburg's postulation (1930, 1956) that a high rate of glycolysis and a lack of its inhibition in the presence of oxygen were essential characteristics of neoplasms, has stimulated much interest in the enzymes of carbohydrate metabolism.

Glycolysis is opposed by the synthetic pathway of glucose production, gluconeogenesis. Weber has proposed that the site and direction of these opposing pathways are controlled by the amounts and activities of three key glycolytic enzymes and four key gluconeogenic enzymes (Weber et al. 1965). The key glycolytic enzymes are hexokinase, phosphofructokinase, and pyruvate kinase; those of gluconeogenesis are glucose-6-phosphatase, fructose-1, 6-diphosphatase, phosphoenolpyruvate carboxykinase, and pyruvate carboxylase. All of these enzymes are progression-linked in the experimental hepatoma system, i.e., they increase or decrease with the degree of tumor differentiation. Other changes of carbohydrate metabolism are said to occur throughout the range of hepatomas and are thus transformation-linked changes. These changes include a decrease in glycogen storage, a decrease in the conversion of glucose to fatty acids, and a decrease in fructose uptake when compared to normal liver.

4:1 GLYCOLYSIS (THE EMBDEN-MEYERHOF PATHWAY)

Glycolysis is an important energy-producing pathway of the epithelial cell. A useful aid in early diagnosis may be the relatively high glycolytic metabolism of malignant tissue which helps to distinguish it from its tissue of origin.

Hexokinase, catalysing the conversion of glucose to glucose-6-phosphate, is the only key enzyme of glycolysis which has been shown to alter in oral premalignant lesions. Scott et al. (1960, 1962) assayed this enzyme biochemically at intervals during chemically induced carcinogenesis of the hamster cheek pouch and found that, after an initial fall in activity, the level of this enzyme rose during the period of hyperplasia and tumor formation until, in the malignant lesion, the level of hexokinase was 1.5 to 5.5 times the level of the control.

Another key enzyme in the glycolytic pathway is phosphofructokinase. Shonk et al. (1965) studied the activities of glycolytic enzymes in carcinomas of the rectum and colon. In these lesions they found phosphofructokinase to be the rate-limiting enzyme, which limited the extent of increased glycolytic capacity of the tumors. Changes in the activity of this enzyme could therefore markedly influence the glycolytic rate and assays of this enzyme in the development of oral neoplasms may well prove to be of diagnostic aid. However the histochemical demonstration of phosphofructokinase is difficult.

The first step of the second stage of glycolysis is catalyzed by glyceraldehyde-3-phosphate dehydrogenase. This enzyme is a good indicator of the potential of the glycolytic pathway, as it functions under both aerobic and anaerobic conditions. Although it is not a rate-limiting enzyme, ultramicrochemical methods have been used to assay this enzyme in normal oral epithelium and in nondysplastic hyperkeratinized epithelium ("leukoplakia"). Glyceraldehyde-3-phosphate dehydrogenase activity was slightly higher in "leukoplakic" tissue, suggesting a higher potential for the operation of the Embden-Meyerhof pathway in the heavily keratinized epithelium (Gerson and Silverman 1973). Henderson (1976) has recently published a technique for measuring the activity of this enzyme histochemically.

Pyruvic kinase catalyzes the transfer of phosphate from phosphoenol pyruvate to ADP to yield ATP and pyruvic acid. This is another key enzyme of glycolysis and according to Weber (1977) is progression-linked in the rat hepatoma system, alterations in the level of this enzyme occurring in parallel with the rise in the growth rate of the neoplasm. Knowledge of its activity in oral lesions might yield valuable information, though Hammar and Alvares (1974) were unable to find differences between "leukoplakic" and noninvolved epithelium in this regard. However, if it is also a progression-linked enzyme in oral epithelium, changes in its activity may only be evident at a late stage.

Lactate dehydrogenase is probably the enzyme most commonly used as an indicator of the level of glycolysis. It catalyses the interconversion of pyruvic acid and lactic acid. Biochemical and histochemical analysis of lesions in experimentally induced carcinogenesis of the hamster cheek pouch and of human leukoplakia and carcinomatous oral tissue have confirmed the increased activity of lactate dehydrogenase in these tissues (Alvares et al. 1972; Mori et al. 1962; Mori 1968; Shklar 1965, 1966; Oka 1969). However, Weber (1977) states that, as this is not a key enzyme, it exhibits random alterations in neoplastic tissue and its usefulness in the early diagnosis of malignancy must be considered doubtful.

The development of "leukoplakia" is also associated with a shift in lactate dehydrogenase isoenzymes towards the fetal pattern; this enzyme modification is similar to that seen in tumor tissue (Langvad and Roed-Petersen 1970).

Thus, in studies on the glycolytic pathway in oral neoplasms, all the results indicate an increase in activity of the enzymes involved in the pathway.

4:2 THE TRICARBOXYLIC ACID (TCA) CYCLE

It might be expected that, since a cyclic series of reactions occur, the pattern of enzyme changes in the TCA cycle would follow a common course, i.e., would either all increase or all decrease. In studies on oral premalignant and malignant lesions, the change in the pattern of enzyme activity from normal tissue in relation to this cycle is extremely confused. The picture is further complicated by an increase in keratin formation in many premalignant and some malignant lesions.

The primary control point of the TCA cycle in most tissues occurs when acetyl CoA reacts with oxaloacetic acid to produce citric acid. The reaction is catalyzed by citrate synthase, but little work has been carried out on the activity of this enzyme in oral neoplasms.

Nicotinamide adenine dinucleotide (NAD) -dependent isocitrate dehydrogenase catalyzes the conversion of isocitric acid to α-ketoglutaric acid and acts as a secondary regulatory control point of the cycle. Using ultramicrochemical techniques, this enzyme has been found to have a higher activity in "leukoplakic" oral epithelium than in normal tissue, and Gerson and Silverman (1973) suggest that this indicates a higher potential in the keratotic tissue for operation of the TCA cycle. Experimental results are, however, conflicting as Hammar and Alvares (1974) found reduced activities of this enzyme in hyperorthokeratinized mucosa, consistent with their observation that mitochondria were reduced in number. Each author's definition of "leukoplakia" is crucial to interpretation of such studies.

It seems to be generally accepted that the activity of succinate dehydrogenase (SDH) in potentially malignant, premalignant, and malignant oral lesions is reduced from that of normal tissue (Shklar 1965, 1966; Cabrini 1973; Itoiz et al. 1974). Itoiz et al. (1974) and Cabrini (1973) suggested that reduced SDH activity may be related to depresson of the tricarboxylic acid cycle in order to utilize the pentose phosphate shunt, since glucose-6-phosphate dehydrogenase activity is correspondingly increased.

Another indicator of TCA cycle activity is malate dehydrogenase which is involved in the conversion of malic to oxaloacetic acid. In a histochemical study of oral epidermoid carcinomas, Mori (1968) found that malate dehydrogenase was highly active in neoplastic epithelium in relation to keratin pearls. Oka (1969) found many intensely reactive cells in papillomas and carcinomas of hamster cheek pouch. However Alvares et al. (1972) found that malate dehydrogenase activity was reduced by 32% in hyperorthokeratinized and hyperparakeratinized oral leukoplakia in a biochemical analysis; the observed reduction may, however, have been affected by the large amount of keratin present, which tends to exaggerate results expressed on a dry weight or protein basis.

4:3 CYTOCHROME OXIDASE

Cytochrome oxidase is a major respiratory enzyme, being the terminal electron acceptor in the electron transport chain. Tissue with a high metabolic activity normally exhibits high cytochrome oxidase activity (Burstone 1961).

Decreased levels have been found in a number of tumors (Burstone 1959). Unfortunately there do not appear to be any definitive studies of cytochrome oxidase in oral neoplasms.

4:4 THE PENTOSE PHOSPHATE PATHWAY

Another route for the metabolism of glucose is the pentose phosphate pathway (or shunt) which is a major source of reduced nicotinamide adenine dinucleotide phosphate (NADPH). This pathway also provides ribose for the synthesis of RNA and DNA and thus for protein synthesis and nucleic acid replication (Butcher 1975). The activity of this shunt would be expected to increase considerably in malignancy, and Weber (1977) claims that glucose-6-phosphate dehydrogenase (G6PD), the key enzyme of this pathway, is a transformation-linked discriminant in the hepatoma model. This is borne out by reports of markedly increased activity of the enzyme in carcinomas from many different sites in man (see review by Livni and Laufer 1975). Bronchial carcinomas have strikingly high G6PD activity, in marked contrast to normal bronchial epithelium (Butcher 1975; Johnson 1977).

The findings of different research workers in respect of oral carcinomas are however conflicting. Increase in the activity of G6PD has been reported in both hamster cheek pouch and in human oral squamous cell carcinoma in biochemical and histochemical studies (Scott et al. 1960, 1962; Mori 1968; Oka 1969). In quantitative histochemical studies, Cabrini (1973) and Itoiz et al. (1974) confirmed these results. They suggest that similar changes in lichen planus and irradiated epithelium meant that these variations in enzymatic activity were associated with common metabolic variations of the oxidative system and that, in part, higher G6PD activity corresponded to increased keratinization of the tissue. In contrast, in an ultramicrochemical analysis of human oral leukoplakic epithelium, Gerson and Silverman (1973) found that G6PD was approximately one third lower than in normal nonkeratinized oral epithelium.

A recent major advance in dehydrogenase histochemistry has been the introduction of phenazine methosulphate (PMS) into the incubation medium. Dickens and McIlwain (1938) first used it as an artificial hydrogen carrier in biological systems and Farber and Bueding (1956), using PMS in dehydrogenase histochemistry, showed that it could in turn reduce tetrazolium salts quantitatively. As PMS reacts directly with reduced flavoproteins and reduced coenzymes and then nonenzymatically with tetrazolium salts, it completely bypasses the endogenous diaphorase system in the tissue, and the localization and quantitation of the dehydrogenase is improved (Altman 1972).

Heyden (1974) histochemically examined potentially malignant and malignant oral epithelium for G6PD activity in rat and human tissue using PMS and the oxygen-insensitive tetra nitro-blue tetrazolium salt in the incubation medium. By carefully modifying the conditions of incubation, he was able to identify activity only in malignant cells and groups of cells in potentially malignant lesions, and thus to detect "atypia of oxidative metabolism" before morphological signs of cellular atypia were present. By controlling his incubation conditions in this way, however, it is possible only to observe variations in enzyme activity in a given specimen without reference to standard values in either normal or overtly malignant tissue. There is, therefore, the need to assess by means of quantitative histochemical techniques, the activity of G6PD using PMS in the incubation medium. Our own recent studies (Figs. 1 and 2, Table 1), using these techniques in dimethyl benzanthracene-induced carcinomas of hamster cheek pouch, showed reduced G6PD activity in malignant lesions (Fig. 2c). In the earlier stages of neoplastic transformations, however, there are areas of high G6PD activity adjacent to areas of decreased activity (Fig. 2b), and it is uncertain whether it is the areas of high or low activity that are more likely to become malignant. It is interesting to note, from Table 1, that the mean activity at 14 weeks is the same as in control tissue, in spite of the marked regional variations, so that had biochemical methods been used no differences would have been detected. Preliminary studies suggest that at all stages the lactate dehydrogenase activity remains constant and uniform throughout the tissue, as might be expected from a nonrate-limiting enzyme, and that there is a fall in succinate dehydrogenase activity. These results suggest, therefore, that the irregular distribution of groups of cells with abnormal G6PD activity may be of particular importance in detecting neoplastic transformation, particularly as they do not occur in benign hyperplastic lesions produced in the hamster cheek pouch by topical application of turpentine (Evans, unpublished). However, the difficulties of determining which areas of tissue are truly premalignant remain and cause considerable difficulties in the interpretation of results.

5. PROTEIN AND NUCLEIC ACID METABOLISM

In the hepatoma model, the incorporation of amino acids such as alanine, aspartate, glycine, serine, and valine into protein increases as tumor differentiation decreases and there is a corresponding increase in the activity of the postmicrosomal protein synthesizing system. In contrast, the enzymes of amino acid catabolism decrease with loss of differentiation.

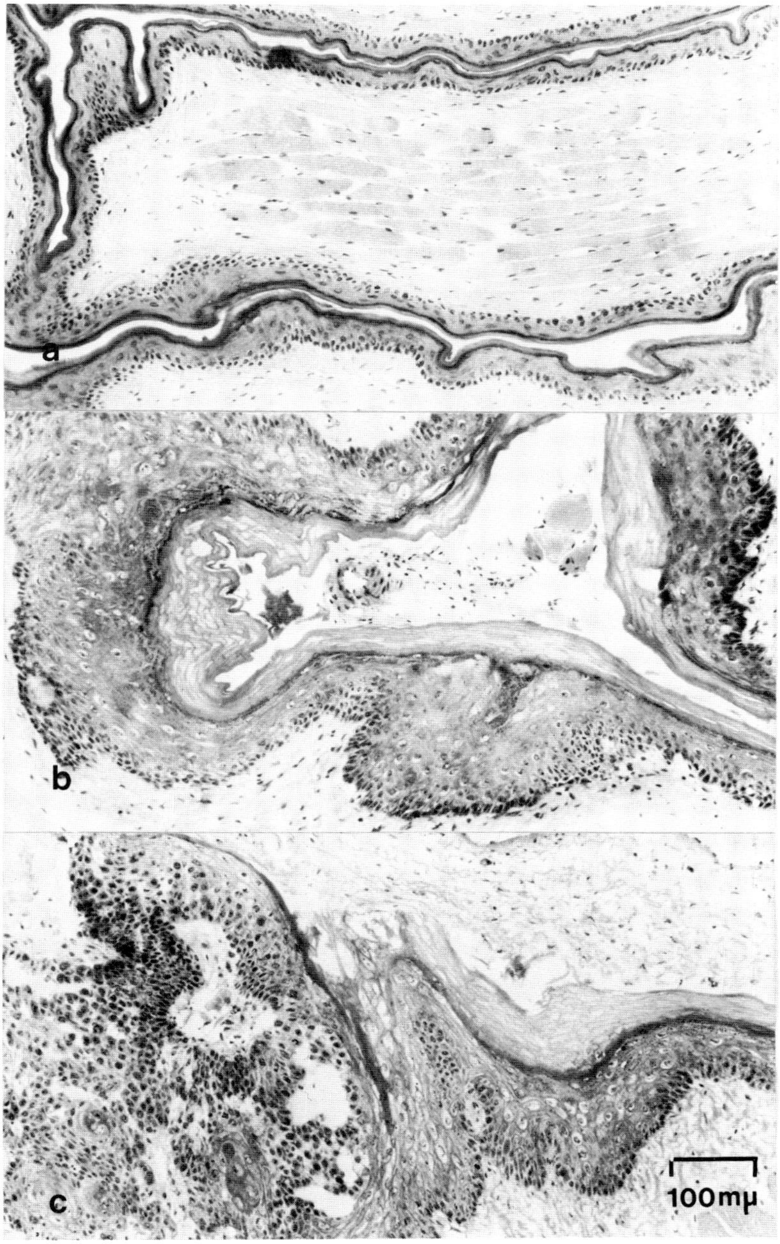

FIGURE 1. 10μm cryostat sections of hamster cheek pouch: (a) No DMBA, (b) 6 weeks painting with DMBA, and (c) 14 weeks painting with DMBA. Hematoxylin and eosin. X 120. The tissue has been rolled before freezing to facilitate sectioning.

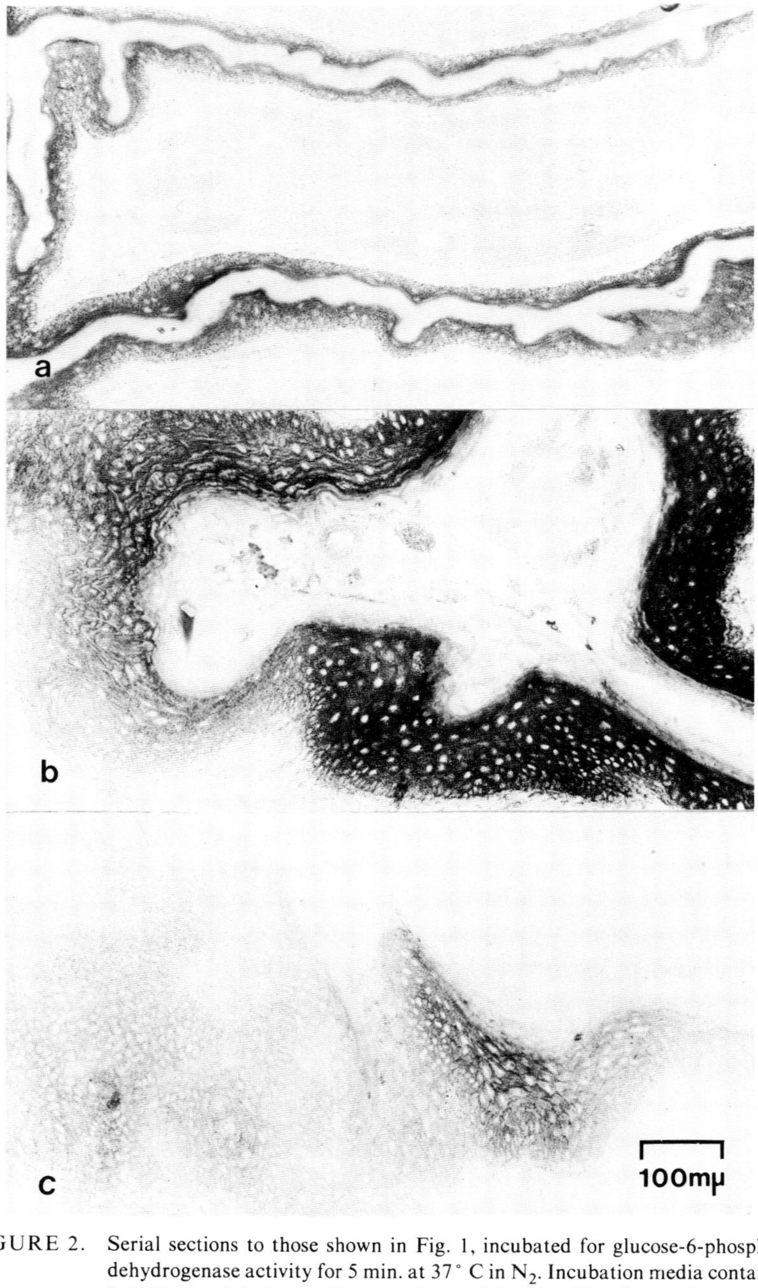

FIGURE 2. Serial sections to those shown in Fig. 1, incubated for glucose-6-phosphate dehydrogenase activity for 5 min. at 37° C in N_2. Incubation media contained 0.05M glycylglycine buffer containing 12% PVA (Grade G18/140); 0.5% (7.5mM) neotetrazolium chloride; 1mg/ml (1.3mM) NADP; 1mg/ml (3.3 mM) glucose-6-phosphate; and 0.2 mg/ml (0.65mM) phenazine methosyl-phate. Final pH 7.5.

TABLE 1 Glucose-6-phosphate dehydrogenase Activity (p moles H_2 cm^{-2} sec^{-1}) and its Variation in the Epithelium of the Hamster Cheek Pouch Treated with DMBA

	(a) From whole sample		*(b) From selected cells*	
Application of DMBA (weeks)	*Mean and SD*	*Range*	*Least Active Cells*	*Most Active Cells*
0	156.0 ± 36.4	110.6–206.4	142.5	195.6
6	249.7 ± 113.0	73.8–449.6	128.5	406.6
14	151.9 ± 79.8	33.6–395.2	79.6	210.1

DMBA = 0.5% 9,10-Dimethyl- 1,2-Bezanthracene in liquid paraffin applied three times per week.

Moreover, the normal control mechanisms of certain enzymes are modified; thus in normal liver, a high-protein diet induces an increase in the levels of the catabolic enzymes threonine dehydrase and serine dehydrase; in the hepatomas such a diet fails to alter the enzyme activities.

The relative rates of incorporation of thymidine into DNA, and of degradation of thymidine to carbon dioxide, correlate closely with the growth rates of the spectrum of transplantable hepatomas, and can thus be used as a measure of the malignancy of these neoplasms (Weber 1974; Ferdinandus et al. 1971). Many enzymes involved in the biosynthetic pathways of purine, pyrimidine, and DNA metabolism increase in the hepatomas. Moreover, this increase is greatest in those tumors furthest removed in characteristics from normal rat liver. In contrast, there is a progressive decrease in the activity of the enzymes of degradation of purines and pyrimidines with loss of differentiation of the tumor.

Little work, however, appears to have been done on the activities of these enzymes in oral tissues, apart from studies on the pentose-phosphate pathway referred to earlier. This pathway is relevant to a number of biosynthetic pathways, including synthesis of nucleic acids.

Measurement of the DNA content of nuclei of cells has been used in an attempt to distinguish normal, premalignant, and malignant oral epithelium. The procedure is discussed by Dabelsteen in chapter 21.

6. HYDROLYTIC ENZYMES

It has long been considered probable that cancer cells can liberate proteolytic enzymes, and that these may contribute to the invasiveness of a tumor (Carrel and Ebling 1928; Rifkin et al. 1974). To invade normal tissues, malignant epithelial cells must penetrate across the basement membrane, through connective tissue, and between host cells; it is possible that hydrolases released from tumor cells are required for this process, and these are most likely to be of lysosomal origin. The functions of lysosomes in cancer have been reviewed by Poole (1973) and Allison (1974).

6:1 LYSOSOMAL ACID HYDROLASES

Lysosomes are membrane-bounded cytoplasmic organelles, which contain hydrolytic enzymes with an acid pH optimum. There have been several biochemical studies showing higher levels of lysosomal enzyme activities in tumors than in the corresponding normal tissues. Elevated enzyme levels include acid phosphatase, cathepsin D, and β-glucuronidase in mouse skin tumors (Shamberger and Rudolph 1967); ribonuclease and deoxyribonuclease in human carcinoma of the cervix (Goldberg and Pitts 1966); and N-acetylglucosaminidase (Conchie and Levy 1957) and arylsulphatases in other human tumors (Boyland et al. 1955). Indeed, there is evidence that the invasiveness of a tumor is directly related to its lysosomal enzyme content. Thus, levels of cathepsin B1 (Blackwood et al. 1965) and β-glucuronidase (Watts and Goldberg 1969) correlated with the degree of invasiveness of tumors of the female genital tract.

Histochemical demonstrations of acid phosphatase activity, and that of other acid hydrolases, have been applied to a wide variety of neoplasms, and the intensity and location of the reaction product have been considered to indicate the degree and site of lysosomal activity (see chapter 15). However, there are several interpretative difficulties to be overcome before the results of such studies can be viewed in terms of tumor behavior.

Firstly, in common with most current histochemical techniques, it is rarely possible to establish whether the activity of hydrolases is at all indicative of the cell's own use of that metabolic pathway, particularly as the majority of histochemical substrates are grossly unphysiological. Secondly, criteria have been established for the unequivocal identification of lysosomes (De Duve 1963), which are rarely possible to adopt with heterogeneous tissue such as oral mucosa, although lysosome fragility tests represent a realistic compromise (Bitensky 1962, discussed by Smith 1972a). Thirdly, the several different histochemical techniques available for the demonstration of acid hydrolases may produce quite different results, so that comparison of different studies must be made with care. Finally, and in the present context most importantly, lysosomes have been implicated in so many functions of normal cells (Lloyd and Beck 1974) that independent corroboration from other investigative techniques is usually necessary before their altered state can be linked to a specific event in a disease process.

Nevertheless, the argument favoring a link between increased lysosomal activity and tumor invasion is attractive, particularly when presented together with ultrastructural evidence of simultaneous irregularity of the basal cell surface and loss of basal lamina (Smith 1972b). At least in the skin, however, a marked rise in acid hydrolase activity has been noted in a variety of other lesions such as Darier's disease and psoriasis (Mier and van den Hurk 1976). In addition, ultrastructural studies of several nonneoplastic skin diseases, including psoriasis again (Brody 1962) and lichen planus (Johnson and Fry 1967), have revealed deficiencies in the epidermal basal lamina. It should be stressed that no ultrastructural demonstration of the discharge of lysosomal contents into the connective tissue has so far been produced which might support the simple view that lysosomes carry the mediators of tumor invasion.

6:2 ACID PHOSPHATASE

Acid phosphatase activity in normal human and rodent oral epithelia is highest in the upper prickle cell layers, and has been demonstrated cytochemically to lie within lysosomes (Squier and Waterhouse 1967). As in normal skin (Lazarus et al. 1975), lysosomal activity in basal cells of oral epithelium is generally weak. Mori et al. (1962) and Santis et al. (1964) found raised acid phosphatase activity in experimentally induced dysplasia and carcinoma of the hamster cheek pouch, and this activity was located in the upper epithelial layers. They interpreted the rise as reflecting the increased keratin formation by their generally well-differentiated tumors. Using the same experimental model, Smith (1972a) accepted only particulate reaction product as evidence of lysosomal activity, and found a progressive increase confined to groups of basal cells and to subepithelial macrophages during carcinogenesis and in overt carcinomas. He found a similar distributon in human oral "leukoplakias" and carcinomas.

6:3 LEUCYL NAPHTHYLAMIDASE

In a series of studies on the mechanism of the leucyl naphthylamidase (sometimes more loosely termed leucine amino-peptidase) reaction, Sylvén and coworkers have demonstrated its localization to lysosomes, particularly "autophagosomes" (see Niemi and Sylvén 1969). Thus, they have presented the technique as a possible means of denoting early cellular injury. Previously, Sylvén and Malmgren (1957) had correlated naphthylamidase activity with the degree of invasiveness of experimental tumor transplants but, as numerous studies have shown (see Burstone 1962 for review), marked activity can be demonstrated in normal fibroblasts and in inflammatory infiltrates as well as in neoplastic epithelial cells themselves. Of particular relevance to tumor invasion is the suggestion that the reaction may be used selectively to demonstrate cathepsin B by means of inhibitors (Sylvén 1968). This group of enzymes, whether released from the tumor or as part of the host response, might be expected to aid invasive activity, particularly as there is some evidence that one of these enzymes, cathepsin B1, is able to degrade native collagen (Burleigh et al. 1974).

With regard to oral malignancy, Smith (1972a) found a patchy granular reaction product in basal cells in human oral squamous cell carcinoma and in his hamster cheek pouch model. In the latter, the increased activity during the period of carcinogenesis paralleled that of acid phosphatase and it, too, was prominent in the cytoplasm of subjacent macrophages.

6:4 OTHER ACID HYDROLASES

The activity of β-glucuronidase, which catalyses the hydrolysis of acid mucopolysaccharides, might be expected to be raised in malignant tumors—the destruction of ground substance thus aiding tumor spread. In oral malignancy, there is no evidence that β-glucuronidase alters the stroma. In both hamster cheek pouch carcinoma (Mori et al. 1962) and human oral carcinoma (Kawakatsu and Mori 1963; Mori 1968), the distribution and intensity of β-glucuronidase reaction product appear to be comparable to those of the normal epithelia.

The biochemistry of esterases, another group of lysosomal enzymes, is a controversial field. Problems stem from the difficulty in demonstrating specific esterases, a task requiring the rigorous use of inhibitors. Nonspecific esterase activity has been demonstrated cytochemically in human and rat oral epithelium, where it was localized to Golgi vesicles and lysosomes in the prickle and basal cell layers (Squier and Waterhouse 1970). Santis et al. (1964) described the presence of nonspecific esterase activity in the basal cells of normal hamster cheek pouch epithelium, but indicated that this was lost during stages towards carcinoma. A slight loss in activity was also shown by Mori (1968) and by Oka (1969) in human and hamster oral carcinomas. Willighagen et al. (1974) found that well-differentiated laryngeal carcinomas contained higher nonspecific esterase activity than did more poorly differentiated types.

In summary, although the histochemical demonstration of lysosomal enzyme activity has aided the identification of stages in the progression of experimental carcinogenesis, variations in activity in the epithelium and stroma in both malignant and nonneoplastic lesions at present precludes its use for the diagnosis of potential malignancy of man.

6:5 COLLAGENASES

In an electronmicroscopic study, Birbeck and Wheatley (1965) showed collagen degradation in basement membranes ahead of infiltrating ascites tumor cells. Similar observations in skin and mammary tumors have been made by Tarin (1969). Unfortunately, there is not yet a technique for the unquestionable histochemical demonstration of collagenases, enzymes which degrade native collagen, so studies on the turnover of collagen in relation to tumors must depend on biochemical techniques. Collagenases may be assayed either by the ability of tissue extracts to release from collagen detectable cleavage products or by the more recently introduced immunofluorescent techniques (Reed 1976). These techniques have been used with some precision. For example, Strauch (1972) has reviewed studies in which tissues have been sampled at varying distances from the center of the tumors. Measuring a profile of collagenase activity through the lesion, he found levels to be highest at the tumor margins, although it was not possible to locate the source of the enzyme. Moreover, there was some correlation between the collagenase activity and the degree of invasiveness of the tumor.

Human skin carcinoma has been shown to possess a significantly higher degree of collagenase activity than normal skin (Hashimoto et al. 1973), but the precise source of the activity again remains in doubt; inflammatory cells are bound to contribute. The collagen content of skin is known to fall during experimental carcinogenesis, and the activity of collagen peptidase rises, especially in the connective tissue (Rohrbach et al. 1970), so there is reason to suspect that similar changes take place in oral mucosa. In a series of oral and laryngeal squamous cell carcinomas, Abramson et al. (1975) have demonstrated a pronounced increase in collagenase production in vitro compared to normal tissue from comparable sites. Oral carcinomas were the more potent source of collagenase activity and although an attempt was made to correlate this activity with survival prognosis, the number of cases was too small to provide statistical support for the relationship.

Invasive oral carcinoma may destroy collagen as it enlarges, and the demonstration of collagenase activity may prove of value in the future for assessing degrees of invasiveness and thus prognosis. However, it is not yet established whether collagenases are a direct product of malignant epithelium, or whether they are activated as an indirect consequence of aggressive tumor behavior. If the latter, collagenase techniques would be unlikely to provide useful information on potentially malignant oral lesions.

6:6 ALKALINE PHOSPHATASE

Alkaline phosphatase is a collective term for a group of enzymes whose activities vary with the tissue and substrate (see Pearse 1968), but techniques for their demonstration have long been used in applied histochemistry. The enzymes are generally considered to be active in membrane transport and/or to help regulate the intracellular phosphate concentration.

Santis et al. (1964) described raised alkaline phosphatase activity both in human oral carcinomas and in those from the hamster cheek pouch. An increase has also been found in laryngeal squamous cell carcinoma, particularly the more poorly differentiated types (Willighagen et al. 1974). In contrast, Mori (1968) and Oka (1969) could detect no alkaline phosphatase activity in human oral carcinoma, in hamster cheek pouch carcinogenesis, or in comparable normal epithelium.

Rubin and Levij (1975) have shown that inducers of alkaline phosphatase activity suppress the induction by dimethyl benzanthracene (DMBA) of carcinoma in the hamster cheek pouch, whilst alkaline phosphatase inhibitors promote tumor formation. As yet it is not clear whether these dramatic effects on the carcinogenic process are mediated directly by alkaline phosphatase, but these findings would certainly seem to warrant further investigation.

6:7 5′-NUCLEOTIDASE

5′-nucleotidase cleaves the phosphate at the 5 carbon position of ribose and deoxyribose. Willighagen et al. (1974) found increased activity of 5′-nucleotidase (as well as alkaline phosphatase and lactate dehydrogenase) in the more poorly differentiated laryngeal carcinomas. On the other hand, Magnusson et al. (1974) studied the cytochemical localization of 5′-nucleotidase activity in rat palatal epithelium during early invasive stages of DMBA-induced carcinoma. They showed that the activity, which was localized to the plasma membrane of basal cells in the normal palate, was lacking on microinvasive cell processes in areas where the basal lamina was breached. Further controlled studies with 5′-nucleotidase are needed, however, if we are to learn how specific is the relationship between malignant transformation and loss of enzyme activity.

7. CONCLUSIONS

It has to be concluded that, at present, there are no reliable histochemical or biochemical methods for testing the malignant potential of human oral mucosa lesions.

Further study of animal models and further large scale prospective studies of human lesions are required, particularly in a search for transformation-linked changes in the metabolic acivities of the tissues. Such an approach is likely to prove more meaningful than the study of progression-linked changes in overtly malignant tissues, although the latter has potential prognostic value, both in terms of deciding how radical treatment should be and in the planning of rational chemotherapy.

We believe it is essential to use quantitative methods, and a combination of quantitative histochemistry and ultramicrobiochemistry is likely to be of most value. Immunohistochemical techniques are also bound to become increasingly important.

Enzyme studies should be carried out under optimum incubation conditions, and only key enzymes for the particular metabolic pathway under study should be chosen. Several key enzymes of the Embden-Myerhof pathway may require additional study, but further information on lactate dehydrogenase activities is of doubtful value.

So far as the Kreb's cycle is concerned, further study of succinate dehydrogenase is probably indicated because, although not a key enzyme, activity of this enzyme falls dramatically in the early stages of hamster cheek pouch carcinogenesis. The similar fall in cytochrome oxidase found in other sites suggests that studies of this enzyme in oral tissues may be of value.

More work is clearly needed on the pentose phosphate pathway, for the activity of its key enzyme, glucose-6-phosphate dehydrogenase, rises early in experimental cheek pouch carcinogenesis and then, intriguingly, can no longer be demonstrated in certain clones of cells. Concomitant study of nuclear DNA content in animal models would also be of value.

Finally, more work on hydrolytic enzymes, particularly in relation to stromal changes, is desirable, but the histochemical techniques employed need to be refined, particularly for the selection of cathepsins. Identification of the activity and source of specific collagenases would be even more valuable.

ACKNOWLEDGMENT

We are grateful for the support of the Medical Research Council to A.W.E.

REFERENCES

Abramson, M., Schilling, R. W., Huang, C. C., and Salome, R. G. 1975. Collagenase activity in epidermoid carcinoma of the oral cavity and larynx. *Ann. Otol. Rhinol. Lar.* **84**, 158–163.

Allison, A. C. 1974. Lysosomes in cancer cells. *J. Clin. Pathol.* (Supplement 1) **7**, 43–50.

Altman, F. P. 1972. Quantitative dehydrogenase histochemistry with special reference to the pentose shunt dehydrogenases. *Prog. Histochem. Cytochem.* **4**, 241–247.

Altman, F. P. 1976. Tetrazolium salts. A consumer's guide. *Histochem. J.* **8**, 471–485.

Altman, F. P., and Butcher, R. G. 1973. Studies on the reduction of tetrazolium salts. I. The isolation and characterisation of a half-formazan intermediate produced during the reduction of neotetrazolium chloride. *Histochemie* **37**, 333–350.

Alvares, O., Hammar, H., Pindborg, J., and Roed-Petersen, B. 1972. Lactate and malate dehydrogenase activities in normal oral mucosa and in homogeneous leukoplakia. *Acta Derm. Venereol.* **52**, 484–488.

Andersen, H., and Hoyer, P. E. 1974. Simplified control experiments in the histochemical study of coenzyme-linked dehydrogenases. *Histochemistry* **38**, 71–83.

Atkin, N. B. 1976. Prognostic significance of ploidy level in human tumours. II. Extra-uterine cancers and summary of data on 1171 tumours. *Cytobios* **15**, 233–237.

Birbeck, M. S., and Wheatley, D. N. 1965. An electron microscopic study of the invasion of ascites tumor cells into the abdominal wall. *Cancer Res.* **25**, 490–497.

Bitensky, L. 1962. The demonstration of lysosomes by the controlled temperature, freeze-sectioning method. *Quart. J. Micr. Sci.* **103**, 205–210.

Bitensky, L. 1967. Histochemistry of liver disease. In: *Symposium of the Colston Research Society, 19th, University of Bristol, 1967. The Liver.* (Edited by Read, A. E.), pp. 61–69. Butterworth, London.

Blackwood, C. E., Mendl, I., and Long, M. E. 1965. Proteolytic enzymes and their inhibitors in human gynecological tumors. *Am. J. Obstet. Gynecol.* **91**, 419–429.

Boyland, E., Wallace, D. M., and Williams, D. C. 1955. The activity of the enzymes sulphatase and β-glucuronidase in the urine, serum, and bladder tissue. *Br. J. Cancer* **9**, 62–79.

Brody, I. 1962. The ultrastructure of the epidermis in psoriasis vulgaris as revealed by electron microscopy. 1. The dermo-epidermal junction and the stratum basale in parakeratosis without keratohyalin. *J. Ultrastruct. Res.* **6**, 304–323.

Burleigh, M. C., Barret, A. J., and Lazarus, G. S. 1974. Cathepsin B1. A lysosomal enzyme that degrades native collagen. *Biochem. J.* **137**, 387–398.

Burstone, M. S. 1959. New histochemical techniques for the demonstration of tissue oxidase (cytochrome oxidase). *J. Histochem. Cytochem.* **7**, 112–122.

Burstone, M. S. 1961. Histochemistry of oral cancer. *J. Oral surg.* **19**, 290–295.

Burstone, M. S. 1962. *Enzyme Histochemistry, and its Application in the Study of Neoplasms.* Academic Press, New York.

Butcher, R. G. 1972. Precise cytochemical measurement of neotetrazolium formazan by scanning and integrating microdensitometry. *Histochemie* **32**, 171–190.

Butcher, R. G. 1975. Pentose shunt oxidation in bronchogenic carcinoma. (Abstract) Proceedings of Ninth Annual Meeting of European Society for Clinical Investigation **186**, 48–49.

Butcher, R. G., and Altman, F. P. 1973. Studies on the reduction of tetrazolium salts. II. The measurement of the half reduced and fully reduced formazans of neotetrazolium chloride in tissue sections. *Histochemie* **37**, 351–363.

Cabrini, R. L. 1973. Histochemistry of early oral cancer. *Int. Dent. J.* **23**, 100–107.

Carrell, A., and Ebling, A. A. 1928. The fundamental properties of the fibroblast and the macrophage. The malignant fibroblast of sarcoma 10 of the Crocker Foundation. *J. Exp. Med.* **48**, 105–123.

Chayen, J., Bitensky, L., and Butcher, R. G. 1973. *Practical Histochemistry.* John Wiley, London.

Conchie, J., and Levy, G. A. 1957. Comparison of different glycosidase activities in conditions of cancer. *Br. J. Cancer* **11**, 487–493.

Criss, W. E. 1971. A review of isozymes in cancer. *Cancer Res.* **31**, 1523–1542.

De Duve, C. 1963. The lysosome concept. In: *Ciba Foundation Symposium: Lysosomes.* (Edited by De Reuck, A. V., and Cameron, M. P.), pp. 1–31. Little, Brown, Boston.

Deeley, E. M. 1955. An integrating microdensitometer for biological cells. *J. Sc. Instr.* **32**, 263–267.

Dickens, F., and McIlwain, H. 1938. Phenazine compounds as carriers in the hexosemonophosphate system. *Biochem. J.* **32**, 1615–1625.

Farber, E., and Bueding, E. 1956. Histochemical localization of specific oxidative enzymes. V. The dissociation of succinic dehydrogenase from carriers by lipase and the specific histochemical localization of the dehydrogenase with phenazine methosulphate and tetrazolium salts. *J. Histochem. Cytochem.* **4**, 357–362.

Ferdinandus, J. A., Morris, H. P., and Weber, G. 1971. Behavior of opposing pathways of thymidine utilization in differentiating, regenerating, and neoplastic liver. *Cancer Res.* **31**, 550–556.

Gerson, S., and Silverman, S. 1973. Activity levels of some oxidoreductases of carbohydrate metabolism in leukoplakia and normal human buccal epithelium. *J. Oral Pathol.* **2**, 77–85.

Gerson, S., and Meyer, J. 1970. Biochemical assay of heterogeneous soft tissues of the oral cavity. *Advances Oral Biol.* **4**, 289–312.

Goldberg, D. M., and Pitts, J. F. 1966. Enzymes of the human cervix uteri. Comparison of nucleases and adenosine deaminase in malignant and non-malignant tissue samples. *Br. J. Cancer* **20**, 729–742.

Hammar, H., and Alvares, O. 1974. Activities of glycolytic and citric acid cycle enzymes in oral leukoplakia. *Scand. J. Dent. Res.* **82**, 85–92.

Hashimoto, K., Yamanishi, Y., Maeyens, E., Dabbous, M. K., and Kansaki, T. 1973. Collagenolytic activities of squamous cell carcinoma of the skin. *Cancer Res.* **33**, 2790–2801.

Henderson, B. 1976. Quantitative cytochemical measurement of glyceraldehyde 3-phosphate dehydrogenase activity. *Histochemistry* **48**, 191–204.

Heyden, G. 1974. Histochemical investigation of malignant cells. *Histochemistry* **39**, 327–334.

Itoiz, M. E., Trasch, A. C., Crivelli, M. E., and Barros, R. E. 1974. Microspectrophotometric study of succinic dehydrogenase and glucose-6-phosphate dehydrogenase in the hyperkeratinized epithelium of oral lesions in man. *Arch. Oral Biol.* **19**, 1101–1104.

Johnson, F. R., and Fry, L. 1967. Ultrastructural observations on lichen planus. *Arch. Dermatol.* **95**, 596–607.

Johnson, N. W. 1977. Histological and histochemical studies of oral cancer. *Int. Dent. J.* **27**, 25–34.

Kawakatsu, K., and Mori, M. 1963. Histochemical evaluation of enzymatic activities in human squamous cell cancer. *Cancer Res.* **23**, 539–545.

Langvad, E., and Roed-Petersen, B. 1970. Lactate dehydrogenase isoenzymes patterns in oral leukoplakias and in clinically uninvolved oral mucosa of the same persons. *Acta Pathol. Microbiol. Scand. A* **78**, 505–508.

Lazarus, G. S., Hatcher, V. B., and Levine, N. 1975. Lysosomes and the skin. *J. Invest. Dermatol.* **65** 259–271.

Livni, N., and Laufer, A. 1975. Histochemical studies of human breast tumors: Activity of alkaline phosphatase, acid phosphatase, and glucose 6-phosphate dehydrogenase. *Pathol. Microbiol.* **42**, 159–170.

Lloyd, J. B., and Beck, F. 1974. Lysosomes. In: *The Cell in Medical Science.* (Edited by Beck, F., and Lloyd, J. B.), Vol. 1, pp. 272–313. Academic Press, London and New York.

Magnusson, B. C., Heyden, G., and Svensson, S. E. 1974. Histochemical observations on 5′-nucleotidase activity in squamous cell carcinomas of the rat. *Histochemistry* **42**, 1–8.

Mier, P. D., and van den Hurk, J. J. 1976. Lysosomal hydrolases of the epidermis. 6. Changes in disease. *Br. J. Dermatol.* **95**, 271–274.

Miyayama, H. Doellgast, G. J., Memoli, V., Gandbhir, L., and Fishman, W. H. 1976. Direct immunoperoxidase staining for regan isoenzyme of alkaline phosphatase in human tumor tissues. *Cancer* **38**, 1237–1246.

Mori, M. 1968. Methods for early diagnosis of oral tumors: Histochemistry. *Int. Dent. J.* **18**, 724–738.

Mori, M., Miyaji, T., Murata, I., and Nagasuna, H. 1962. Histochemical observations on enzymatic processes of experimental carcinogenesis in hamster cheek pouch. *Cancer Res.* **22**, 1323–1326.

Morris, H. P. 1965. Studies on the development, biochemistry, and biology of experimental hepatomas. *Adv. Cancer Res.* **9**, 227–302.

Morris, H. P., and Wagner, B. P. 1968. Introduction and transplantation of rat hepatomas with different growth rate (including minimal deviation hepatomas). In: *Methods in Cancer Research.* (Edited by Busch, H.), Vol. 4, pp. 125–152. Academic Press, New York.

Niemi, M., and Sylvén, B. 1969. The naphthylamidase reactions as a diagnostic tool for the demonstration of cellular injury and autophagy. *Histochemie* **18**, 40–47.

Oka, R. 1969. Cytology and enzyme histochemistry of squamous carcinoma of the hamster cheek pouch and human oral mucosa. *Gann* **60**, 631–648.

Pearse, A. G. 1968. *Histochemistry: Theoretical and Applied.* 3d ed., Vol. 1. Little, Brown, Boston.

Poole, A. R. 1973. Tumour lysosomal enzymes and invasive growth. In: *Frontiers of Biology, Vol. 29. Lysosomes in Biology and Pathology.* (Edited by Dingle, J. T.), Vol. 3, pp. 303–337. Elsevier/North Holland, Amsterdam, American Elsevier, New York.

Potter, V. R. 1962. Enzyme studies on the deletion hypothesis of carcinogenesis. In: *The Molecular Basis of Neoplasia*, pp. 367–407. M. D. Anderson Hospital and Tumor Institute at Houston. University of Texas Press, Austin.

Reed, F. B. 1976. Collagenase assays. In: *The Methodology of Connective Tissue Research.* (Edited by Hall, D. A.), Chap. 29, pp. 275–282. Joynson-Bruvvers, Oxford.

Rifkin, D. B., Loeb, J. N., Moore, G., and Reich, E. 1974. Properties of plasminogen activators formed by neoplastic human cell cultures. *J. Exp. Med.* **139**, 1317–1328.

Rohrbach, R., Thomas, C., Rumpler, R., and Lau, M. 1970. Die kollagenas enaktivität und der Kollagengehalt der Haut wahrend der Carcinogenese. *Verh. Dtsch. Ges. Pathol.* **54**, 442–450.

Rubin, D., and Levij, I. S. 1975. Chemical carcinogenesis in the hamster cheek pouch. Influence of inhibitors and inducers of alkaline phosphatase. *Pathol. Microbiol.* **43**, 26–30.

Santis, H., Shklar, G., and Chauncey, H. H. 1964. Histochemistry of experimentally induced leukoplakia and carcinoma of the hamster buccal pouch. *Oral Surg.* **17**, 207–218.

Scott, D. B. McN., Morris, A. L., Reiskin, A. B., and Pakoskey, A. M. 1960. Changes in hexokinase and dehydrogenases for glucose-6-phosphate and 6-phosphoguconate during carcinogenesis in the hamster cheek pouch. (Abstract) *Fed. Proc.* **19**, 397.

Scott, D. B. McN., Morris, A. L., Reiskin, A. B., and Pakoskey, A. M. 1962. Carcinogenesis in the hamster cheek pouch. II. Changes in enzymes of glucose-6-phosphate oxidation. *Cancer Res.* **22**, 857–866.

Shamberger, R. J., and Rudolph, G. 1967. Increase of lysosomal enzymes in skin cancers. *Nature* **213**, 617–618.

Shklar, G. 1965. Metabolic characteristics of experimental hamster pouch carcinomas. *Oral Surg.* **20**, 336–339.

Shklar, G. 1966. Enzyme histochemistry of human oral carcinoma. *Oral Surg.* **21**, 764–769.

Shonk, C. E., Arison, R. N., Koven, B. J., Majima, H., and Boxer, G. E. 1965. Enzyme patterns in human tissues. III. Glycolytic enzymes in normal and malignant tissues of the colon and rectum. *Cancer Res.* **25**, 206–213.

Smith, C. J. 1972a. Variations in histochemical properties of hydrolytic enzymes in oral precancerous conditions. *J. Dent. Res.* **51**, 308–318.

Smith, C. J. 1972b. The epithelial-connective tissue junction in the pathogenesis of human and experimental oral cancer. In: *Tissue Interactions in Carcinogenesis.* (Edited by Tarin, D.), pp. 191–225. Academic Press, London and New York.

Squier, C. A., Johnson, N. W., and Hopps, R. M. 1976. *Human Oral Mucosa: Development, Structure, and Function.* Blackwell Scientific Publications, London.

Squier, C. A., and Waterhouse, J. P. 1967. Localization of acid phosphatase in oral epithelium. *Nature* **215**, 664–665.

Squier, C. A., and Waterhouse, J. P. 1970. Lysosomes in oral epithelium: The ultrastructural localization of acid phosphatase and non-specific esterase in keratinized oral epithelium in man and rat. *Arch. Oral Biol.* **15**, 153–168.

Strauch, L. 1972. The role of collagenases in tumour invasion. In: *Tissue Interactions in Carcinogenesis.* (Edited by Tarin, D.), pp. 399–433. Academic press, London and New York.

Sylvén, B. 1968. Studies on the histochemical 'leucine aminopeptidose' reaction. VI. The selective demonstration of cathepsin B activity by means of the naphthylamide reaction. *Histochemie* **15**, 150–159.

Sylvén, B. and Malmgren, H. 1957. The histological distribution of proteinase and peptidase activity in solid mouse tumor transplants. A histochemical study on the enzymic characteristics of different tumor cell types. *Acta Radiol.* Suppl. **154,** 1–24.

Tarin, D. 1969. Fine structure of murine mammary tumours: The relationship between epithelium and connective tissue in neoplasms induced by various agents. *Br. J. Cancer* **23**, 417–425.

Warburg, O. 1930. *Metabolism of Tumours.* R. R. Smith, New York.

Warburg, O. 1956. On the origin of cancer cells. *Science* **123**, 309–314.

Wattenberg, L. W. 1959. A histochemical study of five oxidative enzymes in carcinoma of the large intestine in man. *Am. J. Pathol.* **35**, 113–137.

Watts, C., and Goldberg, D. M. 1969. New observations on β-glucuronidase in human cervical cancer. *Eur. J. Cancer* **5**, 465–473.

Weber, G. 1961. Behavior of liver enzymes during hepatocarcinogenesis. *Adv. Cancer Res.* **6**, 403–494.

Weber, G. 1966. The molecular correlation concept: Studies on the metabolic pattern of hepatomas. In: *Biological and Biochemical Evaluation of Malignancy in Experimental Hepatomas. Gann Monogr. Cancer Res.*, Vol. 1, pp. 151–178. Japanese Cancer Association, Tokyo.

Weber, G. 1972. Molecular correlation concept: Ordered pattern of gene expression in neoplasia. In: *Isozymes and Enzyme Regulation in Cancer. Gann Monogr. Cancer Res.* (Edited by Weinhouse, S., and Ono, T.), Vol. 13, pp. 47–77. Japanese Cancer Association, Tokyo.

Weber, G. 1974. The molecular correlation concept: Recent advances and implications. *The Molecular Biology of Cancer.* (Edited by Busch, H.), Chap. 11, pp. 488–521. Academic Press, New York.

Weber, G. 1977. Enzymology of cancer cells. *N. Eng. J. Med.* **296**, 486–492 and 541–551.

Weber, G., Henry, M. C., Wagle, S. R., and Wagle, D. S. 1964. Correlation of enzyme activities and metabolic pathways with growth rate of hepatomas. *Adv. Enzyme Regul.* **2**, 335–346.

Weber, G., and Lea, M. A. 1966. The molecular correlation concept of neoplasia. *Adv. Enzyme Regul.* **4**, 115–145.

Weber, G., and Lea, M. A. 1967. The molecular correlation concept: An experimental and conceptual method in cancer research. *Meth. Cancer Res.* **2**, 523–578.

Weber, G., Singhal, R. L., and Srivastava, S. K. 1965. Action of glucocorticoid as inducer and insulin as suppressor of biosynthesis of hepatic gluconeogenic enzymes. *Adv. Enzyme Regul.* **3**, 43–75.

Weinhouse, S. 1971. Isoenzymes in cancer. *Cancer Res.* **31**, 1166–1167.

Weinhouse, S., Warburg, O., Burk, D., and Schade, H. L. 1956. On respiratory impairment in cancer cells. *Science* **124**, 267–272.

Willighagen, R. G., Kluyskens, P., and Thiery, M. 1974. Enzyme histochemistry of squamous cell carcinoma of the larynx. *Acta Otolaryngol.* **78**, 282–286.

Willighagen, R. G., and Planteydt, H. T. 1959. Aminopeptidase activity in cancer cells. *Nature* **183**, 263–264.

21

Cytological and Immunological Approaches to Prognosis of Oral Premalignant Lesions

E. DABELSTEEN

Departments of Oral Pathology and Oral Diagnosis, The Royal Dental College, Copenhagen, Denmark

1. INTRODUCTION

From epidemiological studies it appears that certain oral lesions are predisposed to oral carcinoma. However, it also appears that it is often a minority of patients with such premalignant lesions who subsequently develop carcinoma (Pindborg 1971). Consequently, it would be of great importance at an early stage to assess with accuracy the likelihood of malignant change in a particular patient.

Besides the clinical features, certain histological changes are known to be indicators of impending premalignancy. The term epithelial dysplasia of the oral mucosa is generally used to describe such histological changes (Pindborg et al. 1963; Kramer 1973; chapter 3). However, the significance of epithelial dysplasia and its relationship to invasive carcinoma is obscured by the fact that not all lesions diagnosed as dysplastic progress to an invasive carcinoma if left untreated (Brocheriou et al. 1973; Mincer et al. 1972; Pindborg and Roed-Petersen 1973).

The histological diagnosis of epithelial dysplasia is based on the presence of certain tissue changes which are also characteristics associated with carcinomas. In reaching a diagnosis, the pathologist registers changes or combinations of them, and usually also gives more weight to some features than to others (Smith and Pindborg 1970; chapter 19). This is a subjective process, and the reliance on a subjective interpretation of morphology is probably the most important factor accounting for the difficulties in predicting malignant development in a premalignant lesion (chapters 15 and 19; Ringsted et al. 1978).

It is therefore desirable to identify preinvasive lesions by means of criteria that are more objective than the traditional morphological features. This means seeking more definite and quantifiable characteristics of the lesion or the host which might indicate impending malignancy.

The period of premalignancy is often characterized by one or more early cell populations which may undergo apparent regression or differentiation, and by later populations which persist as immediate precursors for cancer (Farber 1973). Most studies of markers of initial malignancy rest on the unproved hypothesis that the cancer cell has only few biological variables associated with its malignant behavior, and that these can be characterized and used to identify populations of cells which are immediate precursors for cancer. However, as no studies have yet characterized the essential attributes of a population of cancer cells, the markers studied up to now have of necessity been tumor-associated rather than tumor-specific.

The present paper will discuss cytological and immunological changes which may be associated with malignant transformation in oral premalignant lesions.

1:1 FOLLOW-UP STUDIES

Before discussing tumor-associated markers in oral premalignant lesions, it should be recognized that the only way a marker can be evaluated is by means of follow-up studies. Such studies are, for several reasons, rare. There are obvious ethical problems involved in follow-up studies of patients with premalignant lesions; there are also technical problems because it is impossible to follow a lesion histologically without altering the lesion (Koss 1968; Richart 1966), and finally it is a very time-consuming task because only a few oral premalignant lesions actually develop malignancy every year, and lesions may thus persist for more than ten years before they become malignant (Dabelsteen et al. 1975; Bánóczy and Csiba 1976; Pindborg et al. 1968; Mincer et al. 1972; Einhorn and Wersäll 1966). Most studies of markers of malignant transformation in oral premalignant lesions have therefore concentrated on identifying tumor-associated changes in premalignant lesions. The hope has generally been to identify a tumor-associated factor, which when present in premalignant lesions considerably increases the likelihood of malignant development of these lesions.

2. EXFOLIATIVE CYTOLOGY

Exfoliative cytology, by which the superficial cell layers of the epithelium are removed, is an alternative way to get information on the histology of the lesion in question. The widespread acceptance of exfoliative cytology as a technique for detecting malignant and premalignant changes in the uterine cervix has been followed by its application to other sites (Papanicolaou 1954; Richart 1968). If cytodiagnosis is to be adopted as a procedure in cases of suspected oral premalignancy, its sensitivity must be high. Dabelsteen et al. (1971) found that 10 out of 16 leukoplakias with histological evidence of epithelial dysplasia had normal cytology, thus providing a false negative diagnosis. Almost identical results were obtained by Mehta et al. (1970), who studied oral leukoplakias and submucous fibrosis. It also appears from a study by Dabelsteen et al. (1971) that clinical criteria for selection of lesions which on subsequent biopsies showed epithelial dysplasia were far more successful than the exfoliative cytology. This is an important finding, as it is often suggested that exfoliative cytology gives useful information on where or when to biopsy (Selbach and Von Haam 1963; Shapiro et al. 1964; Sandler 1966; Folsom et al. 1972; Poswillo 1975).

Most oral premalignant lesions have a keratinized surface, and it is most probably this keratin which covers the dysplastic cells and is responsible for the high percentage of false negative smears (Bánóczy and Rigo 1976; Mehta et al. 1970; Dabelsteen et al. 1971). It seems that exfoliative cytology is not a useful marker for oral premalignancy, and at best only provides some of the information a conventional clinical and histological investigation of the lesion would have given.

3. DNA MEASUREMENTS

To the pathologist, nuclear abnormalities are common features of malignant and premalignant lesions. In an attempt to study these changes objectively, the nuclear DNA content has been measured by cytophotometry of tissues stained with specific DNA stains (Wied et al. 1966). By this method it has been shown that benign proliferative lesions have a diploid-to-tetraploid DNA distribution, whereas epithelial cancer precursors and cancer generally are aneuploid with an increase in nuclear DNA (Sandritter et al. 1966; Wilbanks et al. 1967; Ng and Atkin 1973; Wied et al. 1966; Atkin and Richards 1956; Nødskov-Petersen 1971; Izuo et al. 1971).

Although measurements of the DNA content of single cells have contributed valuable information on the understanding of the pathogenesis of cervical neoplasia, only limited work has been done on oral lesions (Wilbanks et al. 1967; Valeri et al. 1967; Sandritter et al. 1966).

In a preliminary report Doyle and Manhold (1975) estimated the DNA content of individual nuclei in biopsies of normal oral epithelium, hyperplastic epithelium, oral leukoplakias, and oral carcinomas. They found that normal and benign hyperplastic epithelium had DNA values in the diploid range. Four out of 6 leukoplakias with moderate to severe dysplasia, and 5 out of 10 carcinomas had increased DNA values, some of them with aneuploid stem lines. Among 10 leukoplakias without any signs of dysplasia, 8 cases demonstrated high DNA content. Unfortunately, there is no follow-up information on these leukoplakias. These preliminary findings are in agreement with studies of premalignant lesions in other human tissues (Cole and McKalen 1960; Stich et al. 1960; Sandritter and Seidel 1965; Levi et al. 1969; Goldfarb et al. 1971; Cabrini 1973; Pfitzer and Pape 1975). In studies of the uterine cervix it has been shown that even lesions with mild dysplasia are aneuploid with increased DNA values (Weid et al. 1964; Sandritter et al. 1966; Wilbanks 1976), and in a follow-up study of patients with cystic disease of the breast, it has been demonstrated that lesions with aneuploid DNA values are more likely to develop malignancy than lesions with a diploid DNA content (Izuo et al. 1971).

It would certainly be of interest to know whether changes in nuclear DNA in a leukoplakia indicate an early step in the malignant transformation of this lesion. However, it is important to realize that the reliance on cytophotometry for detection of DNA as a marker for early invasiveness would be dangerous as 50% of the carcinomas had diploid stem lines.

4. ELECTRON MICROSCOPY

Although the distinguishing characteristic of a malignant cell is not its structure, it may be useful to investigate the ultrastructure of premalignant cells in order to get more detailed information on cell changes during malignant transformation.

Studies with transmission microscopy of lesions from the uterine cervix have revealed that cells of lesions with histological evidence of beginning malignancy have an increase in microvilli and a decrease in the number of desmosomes (Shingleton et al. 1968; Shingleton and Wilbanks 1974). Similar changes have been found with the scanning electron microscope, the cells showing microvilli that were variable in size, shape, and distribution, instead of the orderly ridges seen on normal cells (Williams et al. 1973). Similar microvilli have been described in experimental premalignant lesions of the urinary bladder (Hicks and Wakefield 1976). These changes at the cell membranes are interesting, for one of the prominent features of cancer cells is the loss of contact inhibition of cell proliferation and movement; these are features which are probably controlled by cell membrane interactions (Abercrombie and Ambrose 1962; Edelman 1976). Data from experimental oral carcinogenesis suggests a marked loss of cell attachments in malignant tissue (MacDonald 1973; White and Squier 1974). However, there does not seem to be data available on the numbers of desmosomes and the presence of microvilli in oral premalignant lesions.

A fundamental feature of epidermal carcinogenesis appears to be the failure of the neoplastic epithelium to maintain a basal lamina at its interface with the underlying connective tissue. Electron microscopic studies of several different malignant tumors, including oral carcinoma, have shown protrusions of epithelial cells through the basal lamina into the connective tissue (Ashworth et al. 1961; Frei 1962; Listgarten et al. 1963; Tarin 1967). Similar pseudopodial formations have been seen in oral leukoplakias, with histological changes considered indicative of impending malignancy (Frithiof 1969; Woods and Smith 1969). Basal cell processes through a defective basement membrane are, however, also found in association with regenerating epithelium (Salpeter and Singer 1960) and in epithelium in organ culture (Hill, 1978). Although not specific for malignant development, the demonstration of epithelial cell protrusion into the connective tissue may offer a means of identifying those lesions which have the essential properties of invasive carcinoma within a group of premalignant lesions.

It is obvious that markers which are only detectable by transmission electron microscopy are not very useful in routine diagnosis. However, detection of cell membrane changes by use of scanning electron microscopy may in the future prove a useful marker for premalignant changes in oral lesions.

5. EPITHELIAL CELL KINETICS

When the pathologist evaluates a premalignant lesion, he looks for signs of altered epithelial behavior. One of these is increased numbers of mitoses which reflect changes in the cell kinetics of the lesion (see chapter 13). Quantitative studies of epithelial kinetics in oral premalignant lesions are limited and no studies have tried to correlate cell kinetics of oral premalignant lesions with the natural history of the lesion. Cell kinetics of premalignant lesions of the uterine cervix have been studied by incubating biopsies with tritiated thymidine, and subsequently preparing autoradiographs (Richart 1963; Rubio and Lagerlöf 1974). The general pattern seen in these studies has been that various grades of epithelial lesions show a linear increase when the amount of DNA synthesis is compared to the increase in the severity of the histological changes. Furthermore, it was shown that unlike normal epithelium, lesions diagnosed as severe dysplasia and carcinoma in vitro had labeled cells well above the basal layer (Rubio and Lagerlöf 1974; Chi et al. 1977).

Only a few studies describe the pattern of cell proliferation in oral leukoplakias (Alvares et al. 1972; MacDonald and Warnakulasuriya 1976). Alvares incubated biopsy specimens of six homogeneous leukoplakias and of normal buccal mucosa from the contralateral sites of the leukoplakia with tritiated thymidine. None of the leukoplakias showed histological signs of dysplasia. In the normal mucosa as well as in the leukoplakia, labeled cells were only found in the three layers closest to the basement membrane. In the leukoplakias, cell renewal and mitotic cycles were faster than in the normal epithelium. These data are preliminary; such studies should be extended to include leukoplakias showing various grades of dysplasia, and with follow-up cases before the use of in vitro labeling as a marker can be fully assessed.

6. CELL MEMBRANE CHANGES

Numerous molecular changes in cell membranes have been demonstrated in association with malignant transformation. Although none of these changes have been successfully correlated with the characteristic biological properties of the tumor cells, they may serve as markers of beginning malignancy (Hakomori 1973).

Studies have shown that blood group antigens A and B are present at cell membranes of normal oral epithelial cells but disappear in most oral carcinomas (Brandtzaeg 1965; Prendergast et al. 1968; Dabelsteen 1972; Dabelsteen and Pindborg 1973; Dabelsteen and Fejerskov 1974).

Dabelsteen et al. (1975) have recently studied tissue from 40 oral lesions for the presence of cell membrane-bound blood group antigens A and B. The material included 21 lesions with epithelial dysplasia and 18 lesions without histological evidence of impending malignancy. All lesions with dysplasia showed decreased reactivity for blood group antigen. Among the leukoplakias without signs of dysplasia, 4 cases demonstrated loss of antigen reactivity. None of 38 benign keratotic lesions showed any change in reactivity as compared to normal adjacent epithelium. Ten of the lesions with epithelial dysplasia had been followed histologically for periods from 6 months up to 10 years. During the follow-up period 3 cases developed from slight dysplasia into carcinoma. In all 3 cases a decreased blood group antigen activity had already been seen in the first biopsy. One lesion diagnosed clinically and histologically as lichen planus developed into a lesion with moderate dysplasia after 9 years. At the time dysplasia was diagnosed, a change from normal to loss of blood group antigen activity was apparent. Unfortunately, no follow-up exists of the leukoplakias with decreased antigen reactivity and a histology without signs of dysplasia. It would be important to see whether these cases are more likely to develop into dysplasia and cancer than the rest of the leukoplakias without severe epithelial changes. Similar results have been obtained by George (1977), who found loss of blood group antigens in oral carcinomas, and oral lesions with epithelial dysplasia, whereas tissue from lichen planus and oral ulcers reacted as normal epithelium.

It appears that oral epithelial dysplasia and oral carcinomas are associated with decreased blood group antigen activity at the epithelial cell membranes. However, the loss of blood group antigen in an oral lesion does not imply that this lesion is developing into cancer, nor does the normal expression of blood group antigen in a lesion exclude malignancy. This conclusion is reached from experimental studies of wound healing where loss of blood group antigens has been described in oral epithelium adjacent to a wound (Dabelsteen and Fejerskov 1974), from follow-up studies showing that not all lesions with epithelial dysplasia develop into cancer, although they show decreased blood group antigen activity (Brocheriou et al. 1973; Mincer et al. 1972; Dabelsteen et al. 1975), and from studies of oral carcinomas showing that few carcinomas express blood group antigens in the same way as normal epithelium (Dabelsteen and Pindborg 1973; Liu et al. 1974).

Recent studies seem to indicate that it is possible to distinguish between blood group antigen loss in wound healing and in malignancy (Dabelsteen and Mackenzie 1978). If blood group antigen patterns are investigated in unfixed frozen sections, antigen loss is seen in oral carcinomas and lesions with epithelial dysplasia, but not in the epithelial outgrowth from the wound margin. Where the wounded epithelium was treated with nonpolar solvents, antigen activity disappeared from the epithelial outgrowth, but not from normal epithelium. This finding may suggest that glycoprotein, but not glycolipid associated antigen, is lost from the surface of epithelial cells during wound healing, a pattern of selective loss which may reflect a difference between regenerative and neoplastic cells.

Dabelsteen et al. (1975) found that all lesions with diagnosed epithelial dysplasia had decreased blood group antigen activity. However, because of the lack of objective criteria, the diagnosis of epithelial dysplasia varies between different investigators. It is therefore reasonable to expect that some of the lesions Dabelsteen et al. (1975) classified as epithelial dysplasia, by other investigators would have been classified as nondysplastic. Likewise, the 5 lesions in the material which were not classified as epithelial dysplasias, but in which loss of blood group antigen was seen, may have been classified by others as dysplasia.

As the reactivity of blood group antigen in oral epithelium can be estimated with high reproducibility, measurements of blood group antigen activity in oral lesions may be a step closer to the establishment of objective criteria for the beginning epithelial malignancy (Dabelsteen 1972).

7. IMMUNOLOGY

The lymphocyte infiltrate seen in many tumors is usually thought to reflect the host's immunological defense mechanism towards the tumor.

It appears from studies of human cancer, and from a variety of animal tumor models, that there is a relationship between host immunocompetence and prognosis (Hersh et al. 1975). Thus, tumor-bearing individuals with good immunocompetence have a good prognosis, while individuals with poor immunocompetence have a poor prognosis. This relationship has been observed at every stage of disease, and thus holds true for individuals with metastatic malignancy (Hersh et al. 1975, 1976). A variety of in vivo as well as in vitro tests have been useful in evaluating immunocompetence in the cancer patient. These tests are all nontumor-specific and it is presumed that they indirectly reflect the host ability to mount an attack on his own tumor cells (Hersh et al. 1976). Lehner et al. (1973a, and 1973b) used the mitogenic response of lymphocytes to phytohemagglutinin to study the immunocompetence of patients with oral premalignant and malignant lesions. They found that patients with leukoplakias had a slight decrease in immunocompetence, whereas most patients with carcinoma had more severely depressed immunocompetence. In patients who became tumor free following treatment, the lymphocyte response to phytohemagglutinin returned to normal. In patients with recurrent tumors, the response fell but could recover if the patient again became tumor free after treatment (Lehner et al. 1973a, and 1973b). It was suggested on the basis of these studies that the lymphocyte transformation to phytohemagglutinin may serve as a marker in the prognosis and management of leukoplakia and carcinoma. However, as the material studied by Lehner et al. (1973a, and 1973b) was limited, it seems that a broader survey of immunological competence in patients with oral premalignant and malignant lesions is needed before immunological reactivity of a patient can be used as a marker.

Histological studies have shown a correlation between the intensity of lymphocyte infiltration and improved survival of the patients (Black and Speer 1958; Lund et al. 1975; Eneroth and Moberger 1973; Noone et al. 1974). Infiltrates of lymphocytes and plasma cells are usually also seen in the connective tissue in oral leukoplakias. An attempt to study the correlation between this infiltrate and the prognosis of the leukoplakia was made by Lehner in 1971. He assessed quantitatively the lymphocyte and plasma cell infiltrates in biopsy specimens of leukoplakias and correlated this data with the histological appearance of the lesions. Leukoplakias without dysplasia had very few lymphocytes and plasma cells, whereas there was an increase in these cells which paralleled the increase in severity of the histological changes.

However, recent studies show that only some lesions diagnosed as epithelial dysplasia actually develop into cancer, and that cancer may in some cases develop in a leukoplakia without any recognizable period of dysplasia (Brocheriou et al. 1973; Mincer et al. 1972; Pindborg and

Roed-Petersen 1973). Therefore, at present there is no obvious correlation between the intensity of the lymphocyte infiltrate in the leukoplakia and the prognosis of the lesion.

In recent years, it has become obvious that the patients' immunological reactions against their tumors are extremely complex, and it is therefore not surprising that differences between lymphocyte counts in leukoplakias are difficult to interpret (Klein et al. 1976; Haskill et al. 1976). However, functional analysis of lymphocytes from tumor-bearing patients have shown disease-related immunological responses, and it is generally considered that cell-mediated immune reactions are of prime importance for tumor development (Perlmann et al. 1977; Hellström and Hellström 1974; chapter 16).

Lehner (1970) assayed cell-mediated immunity to leukoplakia tissue in patients with oral leukoplakias. He used the lymphocyte transformation test. This is an in vitro test where the immune response of the patient is studied by measuring stimulation of DNA or induction of blast transformation in lymphocytes exposed to tumor extracts (Lehner 1970; Vänky et al. 1974). Lehner found the highest rate of lymphocyte transformation in lesions without dysplasia, and a decrease in transformation when the histological grading progressed towards carcinoma. He also compared the transformation rate with the plasma cell infiltrate and found that plasma cells were only seen in carcinomas and lesions with carcinoma in situ. It was finally suggested that depression of lymphocyte transformation and raised plasma cell count may signify a change from leukoplakia to carcinoma. These results appear to be similar to findings of reactions to tumors in other sites. In a study of hypernephromas, Kjaer and Bendixen (1976) found that small tumors which were locally dispersed, or showed early metastases, had a low antigenicity. Analogous to the above findings, Perlmann et al. (1977), in their studies of disease-related cytotoxicity in patients with transitional cell carcinoma of the urinary bladder, showed that the cytotoxicity was highest in patients with small tumor burden and reduced in patients with large tumors.

Cell-mediated immunity to leukoplakia tissue was also demonstrated by Roed-Petersen et al. (1973). They used the leukocyte migration inhibition technique where addition of antigenic extracts to the blood leukocytes from a sensitized individual inhibits their cell migration from capillary tubes. By this technique it was possible to demonstrate migration inhibition in 5 of 11 patients with leukoplakias. However, as there was only 1 lesion showing epithelial dysplasia, it was not possible to correlate the migration inhibition to premalignant or malignant changes.

Such studies seem promising and may, if reproducible, be used in future as prognostic and diagnostic tools for monitoring patients with premalignant lesions. However, it must be remembered that the in vitro tests for cell-mediated immunity to premalignant and malignant tissue frequently reflect the patients' response against a variety of antigens. While some of these antigens may be tumor-associated to tumor-specific, others are not and may give rise to responses in apparently healthy individuals (Perlmann et al. 1977). Until the molecular basis for these reactions is established, these tests do not seem to be useful markers of oral malignancy.

7:1 HERPES VIRUS

Several studies have indicated a relationship between herpes simplex virus type 2 (HSV-2) and carcinoma of the uterine cervix (see chapter 8). Of special interest for the present discussion is the recent finding that antibodies to a defined HSV-2 induced cell surface antigen were present in most patients with cervical precancerous and cancerous lesions, but not in normal controls. This finding raised the possibility that there might be an immunological marker for cervical neoplasia (Aurelian et al. 1977).

Although there are only a limited number of studies dealing with the association of herpes simplex type 1 (HSV-1) and oral cancer, it has been proposed that there exists a correlation between lip cancer and HSV-1 (Hollinshead and Tarro 1973; chapter 17). Most relevant for the present discussion are preliminary findings by Smith et al. (1976), which have shown antibodies to virus induced surface antigen on HSV-1 infected cells in a greater percentage of sera from patients with squamous cell carcinomas of the head and neck than in normal controls.

With the limited data yet available, it is impossible to interpret the findings of immunological reactions to HSV-1 induced antigens in patients with oral premalignant and malignant lesions. However, the studies of the relationship between cervical cancer and antibodies to HSV-2 induced antigens seem promising, and there is at present no reason to think that studies of oral cancer and HSV-1 should be less promising.

8. CONCLUSION

At present no specific markers of malignant transformation in oral premalignant lesions have been identified. Several markers are promising, but can at present not be used in routine diagnosis, because of lack of carefully controlled follow-up studies. Until highly specific markers are identified, it seems that the best evaluation of the lesions may come from examining a battery of well-defined and quantifiable characteristics of the premalignant lesion, or the host.

REFERENCES

Abercrombie, M., and Ambrose, E. J. 1962. The surface properties of cancer cells: A review. *Cancer Res.* **22,** 525–548.

Alvares, O., Skougaard, M. R., Pindborg, J. J., and Roed-Petersen, B. 1972. In vitro incorporation of tritiated thymidine in oral homogeneous leukoplakias. *Scand. J. Dent. Res.* **80**, 510–514.

Ashworth, C. T., Stembridge, V. A., and Luibel, F. J. 1961. Symposium on probable or possible malignant cervical lesions—carcinoma in situ. I. Histology of carcinoma in situ. A study of basement membranes of normal epithelium, carcinoma in situ and invasive carcinoma of the uterine cervix utilizing electron microscopy and histochemical methods. *Acta Cytol.* **5**, 369–384.

Atkin, N. B., and Richards, B. M. 1956. Deoxyribonucleic acid in human tumours as measured by microspectrophotometry of Feulgen stain: A comparison of tumours arising at different sites. *Br. J. Cancer* **10**, 769–786.

Aurelian, L., Schumann, B., Marcus, R., and Davis, H. 1973. Antibody to HSV-2 induced tumor specific antigens in serums from patients with cervical carcinoma. *Science* **181**, 161–164.

Aurelian, L., Strnad, B. C., and Smith, M. F. 1977. Immunodiagnostic potential of a virus-coded, tumor-associated antigen (AG-4) in cervical cancer. *Cancer* **39**, 1834–1849.

Bánóczy, J. 1969. Exfoliative cytologic changes in oral leukoplakia. *J. Dent. Res.* **48**, 17–21.

Bánóczy, J., and Csiba, A. 1976. Occurrence of epithelial dysplasia in oral leukoplakia. Analysis and follow-up study of 12 cases. *Oral Surg.* **42,** 766–774.

Bánóczy, J., and Rigo, O. 1976. Comparative cytologic and histologic studies in oral leukoplakia. *Acta Cytol.* **20**, 308–312.

Black, M. M., and Speer, F. D. 1958. Sinus histiocytosis of lymph nodes in cancer. *Surg. Gynecol. Obstet.* **106**, 163–175.

Brandtzaeg, P. 1965. Localization of blood-group substances A and B in alcohol-fixed human gingivae by indirect immunofluorescence technique. *Acta Odontol. Scand.* **23**, 335–345.

Brocherious, C., Chomette, G., Cernéa, P., Auriol, M. and Helenon, R. 1973. Cancer in situ et micro-invasif de law cavité buccale. *Pathol. Microbiol.* **39,** 214–221.

Cabrini, R. L. 1973. Histochemistry of early oral cancer. *Int. Dent. J.* **23**, 100–107.

Chi, C. H., Rubio, C. A., and Lagerlöf, B. 1977. The frequency and distribution of mitotic figures in dysplasia and carcinoma in situ. *Cancer* **39**, 1218–1223.

Christenson, B., and Espmark, A. 1976. Long-term follow-up studies on herpes simplex antibodies in the course of cervical cancer. II. Antibodies to surface antigen of herpes simplex virus infected cells. *Int. J. Cancer* **17**, 318–325.

Cole, J. W., and McKalen, A. 1960. Observations on the cytochemical composition of adenomas and carcinomas of the colon. *Ann. Surg.* **152**, 615–620.

Dabelsteen, E. 1972. Quantitative determination of blood group substances A of oral epithelial cells by immunofluorescence and immunoperoxidase methods. *Acta Pathol. Microbiol. Scand. (A)* **80**, 847–853.

Dabelsteen, E., and Fejerskov, O. 1974. Distribution of blood group antigen A in human oral epithelium. *Scand. J. Dent. Res.* **82**, 206–211.

Dabelsteen, E., and Mackenzie, I. C. 1978. Expression of Ricinus Communis receptor sites in normal human oral cancer and oral wounds. *Cancer Res.* **38**, 4676–4680.

Dabelsteen, E., and Pindborg, J. J. 1973. Loss of epithelial substance A in oral carcinomas. *Acta Pathol. Microbiol. Scand. (A)* **81**, 435–444.

Dabelsteen, E., Roed-Petersen, B., and Pindborg, J. J. 1975. Loss of epithelial blood group antigens A and B in oral premalignant lesions. *Acta Pathol. Microbiol. Scand (A)* **83**, 292–300.

Dabelsteen, E., Roed-Petersen, B., Smith, C. J., and Pindborg, J. J. 1971. The limitations of exfoliative cytology for the detection of epithelial atypia in oral leukoplakias. *Br. J. Cancer* **25**, 21–24.

Doyle, J. L., and Manhold, J. H. 1975. Feulgen microspectrophotometry of oral cancer and leukoplakia. *J. Dent. Res.* **54**, 1196–1199.

Duff, R., and Rapp, F. 1971. Oncogenic transformation of hamster cells after exposure to herpes simplex virus Type 2. *Nature (New Biol.)* **233**, 48–50.

Edelman, G. M. 1976. Surface modulation in cell recognition and cell growth. *Science* **192**, 218–226.

Einhorn, J., and Wersäll, J. 1966. Oral carcinoma in cases of leukoplakia of the oral mucosa. *Acta Otolaryngol. Suppl.* **224**, 20–22.

Eneroth, C. M., and Moberger, G. 1973. Histological malignancy grading of squamous cell carcinoma of the palate. *Acta Otolaryngol.* **75**, 293–295.

Farber, E. 1973. Carcinogenesis—cellular evolution as a unifying thread. Presidential address. *Cancer Res.* **33**, 2537–2550.

Folsom, T., White, C. P., Bromer, L., Canby, H. F., and Garrington, G. E. 1972. Oral exfoliative study. Review of the literature and report of a three-year study. *Oral Surg.* **33**, 61–74.

Frei, J. V. 1962. Fine structure of the basement membrane in epidermal tumors. *J. Cell Biol.* **15**, 332–342.

Frithiof, L. 1969. Ultrastructure of the basement membrane in normal and hyperplastic human oral epithelium compared with that in preinvasive and invasive carcinoma. *Acta Pathol. Microbiol. Scand. Suppl. 200.*

George, D. 1977. Reactive properties of oral lesions to the specific red cell adherence test. (Abstract) *J. Dent. Res.* **56**, A44.

Goldfarb, S., Richart, R. M., and Okagaki, T. 1971. A cytophotometric study of nuclear DNA content of cyto- and syncytiotrophoblast in trophoblastic disease. *Cancer* **27**, 83–92.

Hakomori, S. 1973. Glycolipids of tumor cell membrane. In: *Advances in Cancer Research.* (Edited by Klein, G., and Weinhouse, S.), No. 18, pp. 265–315. Academic Press, New York.

Haskill, J. S., Yamamura, Y., Radov, L., and Parthenais, W. 1976. Discussion paper: Are peripheral and in situ tumor immunity related? *Ann. N.Y. Acad. Sci.* **276**, 373–380.

Hellström, K. E., and Hellström, I. 1974. Lymphocyte-mediated cytotoxicity and blocking serum activity to tumor antigens *Adv. Immunol.* **18**, 209–277.

Hersh, E. M., Gutterman, J. U., and Mavligit, G. M. 1975. Cancer and host defense mechanisms. In: *Pathobiology Annual.* (Edited by Iachim, H. L.), Vol. 5, pp. 133–167. Academic Press, New York.

Hersh, E. M., Gutterman, J. U., Mavligit, G. M., Mountain, C. W., McBride, C. M., Burgess, M. A., Lurie, P. M., Zelen, M., Takita, H., and Vincent, R. G. 1976. Immunocompetence, immunodeficiency and prognosis in cancer. *Ann. N.Y. Acad. Sci.* **276**, 386–406.

Hicks, R. M., and Wakefield, J. J. 1976. Membrane changes during urothelial hyperplasia and neoplasia. *Cancer Res.* **36**, 2502–2507.

Hill, M. W. 1978. The ultrastructure of rat palatal mucosa maintained in organ culture. *J. Anat.* **127,** 475–490.

Hollinshead, A. C., Lee, O., Chretien, P. B., Tarpley, J. L., Rawls, W. E., and Adam, E. 1973. Antibodies to herpes-virus non-viron antigens in squamous carcinomas. *Science* **182,** 713–715.

Hollinshead, A. C., and Tarro, G. 1973. Soluble membrane antigens of lip and cervical carcinomas: Reactivity with antibody for herpesvirus non-virion antigens. *Science* **179,** 698–700.

Izuo, M., Okagaki, T., Richart, R. M., and Lattes, R. 1971. Nuclear DNA content in hyperplastic lesions of cystic disease of the breast with special reference to malignant alteration. *Cancer* **28,** 620–627.

Kjaer, M., and Bendixen, G. 1976. Discussion paper: Tumor directed cellular hypersensitivity detected by leukocyte migration in patients with renal carcinoma. *Ann. N.Y. Acad. Sci.* **276,** 260–271.

Koss, L. G. 1968. *Diagnostic Cytology and its Histopathologic Bases.* 2d ed. Lippincott, Philadelphia.

Klein, E., Becker, S., Svedmyr, E., Jondal, M., and Vánky, F. 1976. Tumor infiltrating lymphocytes. *Ann. N.Y. Acad. Sci.* **276,** 207–216.

Kramer, I. R. H. 1973. Carcinoma-in-situ of the oral mucosa. *Int. Dent. J.* **23,** 94–99.

Lehner, T. 1970. Immunopathology of oral leukoplakia. *Br. J. Cancer* **24,** 442–446.

Lehner, T. 1971. Quantitative assessment of lymphocytes and plasma cells in leukoplakia, candidiasis and lichen planus. *J. Dent. Res.* **50,** 1661–1665.

Lehner, T., Shillitoe, E. J., Wilton, J. M., and Ivanyi, L. 1973a. Cell mediated immunity to herpesvirus Type 1 in carcinoma and pre-cancerous lesions. In: *Immunology of Malignancy* (*Br. J. Cancer* **28,** Suppl. I.) (Edited by Moore, N., Nisbet, N. W., and Haigh, M. V.), pp. 128–134. Lewis, London.

Lehner, T., Wilton, J. M., Shillitoe, E. J., and Ivanyi, L. 1973b. Cell-mediated immunity and antibodies to herpesvirus hominis Type 1 in oral leukoplakia and carcinoma. *Br. J. Cancer* **27,** 351–361.

Levi, P. E., Cooper, E. H., Anderson, C. K., Path, M. C., and Williams, R. E. 1969. Analysis of DNA content, nuclear size and cell proliferation of transitional cell carcinoma in man. *Cancer* **23,** 1074–1085.

Listgarten, M. A., Albright, J. T., and Goldhaber, P. 1963. Ultrastructural alterations in hamster cheek pouch epithelium in response to a carcinogen. *Arch. Oral Biol.* **8,** 145–165.

Liu, P. I., McGregor, D. H., Liu, J. G., Dunlap, C. L., Jinks, W. L., Lin, F., Przybylski, C., and Miller, L. A. 1974. Carcinoma of the oral cavity evaluated by specific red cell adherence test. *Oral Surg.* **32,** 56–64.

Lund, C., Søgaard, H., Elbrond, O., Jorgensen, K., and Andersen, A. P. 1975. Epidermoid carcinoma of the lip. Histologic grading in the clinical evaluation. *Acta Radiol.* **14,** 465–474.

MacDonald, D. G. 1973. Experimental oral carcinogenesis. Ph.D. dissertation. University of Glasgow, Scotland.

MacDonald, D. G., and Warnakulasuriya, K. A. A. S. 1976. Epithelial cell kinetics in leukoplakia. (Abstract) *J. Dent. Res.* **55,** Special Issue D, D110.

Mehta, F. S., Daftary, D. K., and Sahiar, B. E. 1970. A correlative histocytological study of epithelial atypia in leukoplakic and submucous fibrosis lesions amongst Indian villagers in a mass screening programme. *Indian J. Cancer* **7,** 18–23.

Mincer, H. H., Coleman, S. A., and Hopkins, K. P. 1972. Observations on the clinical characteristics of oral lesions showing histological epithelial dysplasia. *Oral Surg.* **33**, 389–399.

Ng, A. B., and Atkin, N. B. 1973. Histological cell type and DNA value in the prognosis of squamous cell cancer of uterine cervix. *Br. J. Cancer* **28**, 322–331.

Noone, B. R., Bonner, H., Raymond, S., Brown, A. S., Graham, W. P., and Lehr, H. B. 1974. Lymph node metastases in oral carcinoma: A correlation of histopathology with survival. *Plast. Reconstr. Surg.* **53**, 158–166.

Nødskov-Pedersen, S. 1971. Degree of malignancy of cancer involving the cervix uteri, judged on the basis of clinical stage, histology, size of nuclei, and content of DNA. *Acta Pathol. Microbiol. Scand. (A.)* **79**, 617–628.

Papanicolaou, G. N. 1954. *Atlas of Exfoliative Cytology.* Harvard University Press, Cambridge, Mass.

Perlmann, P., Troye, M., and Pape, G. R. 1977. Cell-mediated immune reactions to human tumors. *Cancer* **40**, 448–457.

Pfitzer, P., and Pape, H. D. 1975. Investigation of DNA-content of leukoplakia cells of oral mucosa. *J. Maxillofac. Surg.* **3**, 119–124.

Pindborg, J. J. 1971. Oral leukoplakia. *Aust. Dent. J.* **16**, 83–93.

Pindborg, J. J., Renstrup, G., Poulsen, H. E., and Silverman, S. 1963. Studies in oral leukoplakias. V. Clinical and histologic signs of malignancy. *Acta Odontol. Scand.* **21**, 407–414.

Pindborg, J. J., Jølst, O., Renstrup, G., and Roed-Petersen, B. 1968. Studies in oral leukoplakia: A preliminary report on the period prevalence of malignant transformation in leukoplakia based on a follow-up study of 248 patients. *J. Am. Dent. Assoc.* **76**, 767–771.

Pindborg, J. J., and Roed-Petersen, B. 1973. Personal communication.

Poswillo, D. 1975. Evaluation, surveillance and treatment of panoral leukoplakia. *J. Maxillofac. Surg.* **3**, 205–211.

Prendergast, R. C., Toto, P. D., and Gargiulo, A. W. 1968. Reactivity of blood group substances of neoplastic oral epithelium. *J. Dent Res.* **47**, 306–310.

Rapp, F., and Reed, C. L. 1977. The viral etiology of cancer. A realistic approach. *Cancer* **40**, 419–429.

Richart, R. M. 1963. Radioautographic analysis of cellular proliferation in dysplasia and carcinoma in situ of the uterine cervix. *Am. J. Obstet. Gynecol.* **86**, 925–930.

Richart, R. M. 1966. Influence of diagnostic and therapeutic procedures on the distribution of cervical intraepithelial neoplasia. *Cancer* **19**, 1635–1638.

Richart, R. M. 1968. Natural history of cervical intraepithelial neoplasia. *Modern Treatment* **5**, 748–784.

Ringsted, J., Amtrup, F., Asklund, C., Baunsgaard, P., Christensen, H. E., Hansen, L., Jakobsen, C., Jensen, N. K., Moesner, J., Rasmussen, J., Reintoft, I., Rolschau, J., Starklint, H., Thommesen, and Vrang, J. 1978. Reliability of histo-pathological diagnosis of squamous epithelial changes of the uterine cervix. *Acta Pathol. Microbiol. Scand [A]* **86**, 273–278.

Roed-Petersen, B., Roed-Petersen, J., and Bendixen, G. 1973. Cell-mediated immunity to human oral leukoplakia demonstrated by leukocyte migration test. *Int. J. Cancer* **12**, 66–72.

Royston, I., and Aurelian, L. 1970. The association of genital herpesvirus with cervical atypia and carcinoma in situ. *Am. J. Epidemiol.* **91**, 531–538.

Rubio, C. A., and Lagerlöf, B. 1974. Autoradiographic studies of dysplasia and carcinoma in situ in cervical cones. *Acta Pathol. Microbiol. Scand. [A]* **82**, 411–418.

Sabin, A. B. 1974. Herpes simplex-genitalis virus nonvirion antigens and their implication in certain human cancers: Unconfirmed. *Proc. Natl. Acad. Sci. USA* **71**, 3248–3252.

Salpeter, M. M., and Singer, M. 1960. Differentiation of the submicroscopic epidermal membrane during limb regeneration in adult Triturus, including a note on the use of the term basement membrane. *Anat. Rec.* **136**, 27–39.

Sandler, H. C. 1966. Oral cytology. *CA* **16**, 97–101.

Sandritter, W., Seidel, A., Kleinhans, D., Paddags, I., and Dontenwill, W. 1965. Cytophotometrische Messungen des DNA-Gehaltes an menschlichen und tierenexperimentellen Bronchialepithelmetaplasien. *Z. Krebsforsch* **67**, 69–79.

Sandritter, W., Carl, M., and Ritter, W. 1966. Cytophotometric measurements of the DNA content of human malignant tumors by means of the Feulgen reaction. *Acta Cytol.* **10**, 26–30.

Selbach, G. J., and Von Haam, E. 1963. The clinical value of cytology. *Acta Cytol.* **7**, 337–345.

Shapiro, B. L., Gorlin, R. J., and Jordan, W. A. 1964. The role of exfoliative cytology in oral cancer detection. *Oral Surg.* **17**, 327–330.

Shingleton, H. M., Richart, R. M., Wiener, J., and Spiro, D. 1968. Human cervical intraepithelial neoplasia: Fine structure of dysplasia and carcinoma in situ. *Cancer Res.* **28**, 695–706.

Shingleton, H. M., and Wilbanks, G. D. 1974. Fine structure of human cervical intraepithelial neoplasia in vivo and in vitro. *Cancer* **33**, 981–989.

Smith, C., and Pindborg, J. J. 1969. *Histological Grading of Oral Epithelial Atypia by Use of Photographic Standards.* Copenhagen.

Smith, H. G., Chretien, P. B., Henson, D. E., Silverman, N. A., and Alexander, J. C. 1976. Viral-specific humoral immunity to herpes simplex induced antigens in patients with squamous carcinoma of the head and neck. *Am. J. Surg.* **132**, 541–548.

Stich, H. F., Florian, S. F., and Emson, H. E. 1960. The DNA content of tumor cells. I. Polyps and adenocarcinomas of the large intestine of man. *J. Natl. Cancer Inst.* **24**, 471–482.

Tarin, D. 1967. Sequential electron microscopical study of experimental skin carcinogenesis. *Int. J. Cancer* **2**, 195–211.

Thiry, L., Sprecher-Goldberger, S., Hannecart-Pokonni, E., Gould, I., and Bossens, M. 1977. Specific non-immunoglobulin G antibodies and cell-mediated response to herpes simplex virus antigens in women with cervical carcinoma. *Cancer Res.* **37**, 1301–1306.

Vánky, F., Klein, E., Stjernswärd, J., and Nilsone, M. 1974. Cellular immunity against tumor-associated antigens in humans: Lymphocyte stimulation and skin reaction. *Int. J. Cancer* **14**, 277–288.

Valeri, V., Cruz, A. R., Brandão, H. J., and Lison, L. 1967. Relationship between cell nuclear volume and deoxyribonucleic acid of cells of normal epithelium, of carcinoma in situ and of invasive carcinoma of the uterine cervix. *Acta Cytol.* **11**, 488–496.

White, F. H., and Squier, C. A. 1974. A quantitative study of the intercellular and basal attachment apparatus in hamster cheek pouch epithelium during carcinogenesis. (Abstract) *J. Dent. Res.* **53**, 1072.

Williams, A. E., Jordan, J. A., Allen, J. M., and Murphy, J. F. 1973. The surface ultrastructure of normal and metaplastic cervical epithelia and of carcinoma in situ. *Cancer Res.* **33**, 504–513.

Wied, G. L., Messina, A. M., and Rosenthal, E. 1966. Comparative quantitative DNA-measurements on Feulgen-stained cervical epithelial cells. *Acta Cytol.* **10**, 31–37.

Wilbanks, G. D., 1976. In vivo and in vitro "markers" of human cervical intraepithelial neoplasia. *Cancer Res.* **36**, 2485–2494.

Wilbanks, G. D., Richart, R. M., and Terner, J. Y. 1967. DNA content of cervical intraepithelial neoplasia studied by two-wavelength Feulgen cytophotometry. *Am. J. Obstet. Gynecol.* **98**, 792–799.

Woods, D. A., and Smith, C. J. 1969. Ultrastructure of the dermal-epidermal junction in experimentally induced tumors and human oral lesions. *J. Invest. Dermatol.* **52**, 259–263.

Discussion

Dr. Slavkin asked Dr. Mashberg whether there were noninvasive clinical methods which could be used to augment the diagnostic information obtained by visual examination. Dr. Mashberg replied that the use of toluidine blue might be considered helpful but gave a slightly higher rate of false negative signs than clinical impressions. Visual clinical signs are, in his opinion, still the most reliable to the experienced clinician. Professor Kramer commented to Dr. Slavkin that it is important to realize that the reliability of such clinical impressions depends on the expertise of highly trained observers. Unfortunately, the average clinician in a position to detect oral cancer does not possess this high degree of clinical diagnostic ability. He also believed that as far as the mouth in concerned, not too much emphasis should be placed on noninvasive techniques. The taking of a biopsy is still the most reliable diagnostic method and, as far as is known, is simple and safe.

Dr. Binnie asked Professor Kramer how his computer calculated weightings compared to the weightings previously developed by Professors Pindborg and Smith and whether he used his own weightings when routinely making diagnoses from histological preparations. Professor Kramer replied that the weightings he had developed were rather different from those of Smith and Pindborg; he attached more importance to some tissue changes than to others as a result of these studies but not in a precise and quantifiable way. Professor Smith asked whether Professor Kramer had thought of putting into his diagnostic scheme other factors, such as the position of a lesion in the floor of mouth, that are now emerging as important indicators of a lesion's potential for malignant transformation. Professor Kramer replied that attention had so far been concentrated on what could be seen microscopically. However, in making a diagnosis, one is influenced by all sorts of other factors, and there is no reason why such additional information should not be built into a system such as his. Professor Smith commented that the weighting system that Professor Pindborg and he had described was indeed subjective, and that it was time that it was revised, or at least varied. However, what had struck him about Professor Kramer's list was that these features also required to be interpreted subjectively, and the observer was asked to make value judgments about features such as abnormal mitoses, hyperchromatism, and pleomorphism, which are very difficult to recognize in a consistent fashion. Photographic standards, together with Professor Kramer's weighting of them, could be used for training observers, but perhaps a much better approach would be to look for new, quantifiable, parameters to put into the computer. Human error would then be removed. Professor Kramer said that he wholly accepted that, in studies of this type, the more the human component could be eliminated the better.

Dr. Waldron remarked that Dr. Mashberg's finding of a second or third primary tumor in over 20% of his oral cancer patients indicated a considerably higher association than previously reported figures. Was this because of a more intensive examination, or was it a reflection of the particular population group being studied? Dr. Mashberg replied that several reports indicated a general impression of a relationship with tumors of the upper aerodigestive tract (Marcheta et al. 1965; Moertel 1964; Wynder et al. 1969), but that his figures indicated that second primary tumors could be found at a rate two or three times higher than reported in other studies. He thought this was because of the high proportion of his population who are heavy smokers and drinkers, and was partly a reflection of the fact that he pressed for an intensive search for asymptomatic tumors at other sites once an oral lesion was demonstrated.

Dr. Mackenzie asked Professor Johnson what sort of work had been done to examine histochemically-detectable variation in epithelial enzyme patterns between species and between epithelia from one region and the next. He pointed out that Professor Johnson's slides had shown abrupt changes in glucose-6-phosphate dehydrogenase (G6PD) activity from one region of the premalignant cheek pouch to the next. Was this to be considered primarily as an epithelial change, for example a clone of cells with altered enzyme patterns, or was it secondary, perhaps, to some change in the connective tissue? Had the same sort of examination of epithelial enzyme patterns been undertaken following application of friction, or after wounding to produce epithelial hyperplasia? Professor Johnson replied that the cause of the observed change remained uncertain, but turpentine-induced hyperplasia of the cheek pouch produced no elevation of G6PD activity. There were in fact marked regional variations in epithelial enzyme activity; for example, activity for G6PD in the human bronchus is relatively low so that the distinction between a healthy bronchus and a neoplastic bronchus was readily made. Healthy oral epithelium, on the other hand, had an intrinsically higher G6PD activity, and the change in a potentially or fully malignant oral lesion was therefore less marked. Dr. Smith commented that data obtained by colleagues working in his laboratory, using electron microscopy, indicated a sequential reduction in the number of mitochondria per unit volume of epithelial cell cytoplasm, with transition from the normal, through hyperplastic and dysplastic stages, to malignant epithelium (Gohari 1977). This appeared to tie in very nicely with histochemical data about the distribution of succinic dehydrogenase.

Dr. Slavkin commented that the "housekeeping proteins," including enzymes associated with oxidative phosphorylation, appear to be essentially the same throughout vertebrate cells and that, even in the G_1, G_2, and S phases, and throughout circadian rhythms and normal shifts associated with hormones, there were only relatively small fluctuations. He expressed concern at the sort of basic scientific strategy that assumes that there might be something missing or dramatically reduced in the oxidative phosphorylation of an animal cell which could serve as a key toward the diagnosis of malignancy.

Dr. Mashberg referred to Dr. Dabelsteen's findings of altered blood group antigens in premalignant oral lesions without dysplasia. As such tissues develop carcinoma infrequently, would it be worthwhile to use such techniques to evaluate high risk areas of mucosa in high risk patients? In other words, would more definitive results be produced, for example, by examining mucosa from the floor of the mouth of smoking alcoholics than by examining recognizable premalignant lesions which may remain for 20 years before development of malignancy? Perhaps the mucosa of the type of patient that he was describing might have the same probability of developing carcinoma as the white lesion that Dabelsteen examined. Dr. Dabelsteen replied that this might indeed be worthwhile, but that he did not have access to that type of patient. Professor Kramer commented that out of the group of 63 patients with what he termed sublingual keratosis, marginally over 50% were, or became, malignant. Even if the epithelium histologically looked quiet, he still regarded such lesions as very high risk indeed. He also suggested that if sublingual epithelium is of endodermal origin, as opposed to most of the oral epithelium which is of ectodermal origin, this might account in part for the apparently different behavior of the sublingual mucosa. Dr. Mashberg proposed that this particular area deserved special attention in high risk patients, even to the extent of random biopsy in the absence of a clinically detectable lesion.

REFERENCES

Gohari, K. 1977. A quantitative morphological and cytochemical study of the synthetic and metabolic apparatus in hamster cheek pouch epithelium during chemical carcinogenesis. Ph.D. dissertation. University of Sheffield.

Marchetta, F. C., Sako, K., Camp, F. 1965. Multiple malignancies in patients with head and neck cancer. *Am. J. Surg.* **110**, 537–541.

Moertel, C. G. 1964. Incidence and significance of multiple primary malignant neoplasms. *Ann. N.Y. Acad. Sci.* **114**, 886–895.

Wynder, E. L., Dodo, H., Bloch, D. A., Gantt, R. C., Moore, O. S. 1969. Epidemiologic investigation of multiple primary cancer of the upper alimentary and respiratory tracts. I. A retrospective study. *Cancer* **24**, 730–739.